NEONATOLOGY AND BLOOD TRANSFUSION

DEVELOPMENTS IN HEMATOLOGY AND IMMUNOLOGY

Volume 39

The titles published in this series are listed at the end of this volume.

Neonatology and Blood Transfusion

Proceedings of the Twenty-Eighth International Symposium on Blood Transfusion, Groningen, NL
Organized by the Sanquin Division Blood Bank Noord Nederland

edited by

C.TH. SMIT SIBINGA

Sanquin Consulting Services and
Academic Institute for International Development of Transfusion Medicine,
Groningen, The Netherlands

and

N. LUBAN

Center for Cancer and Blood Disorders,
Children's National Medical Center,
Washington DC, U.S.A.

Springer

A C.I.P. Catalogue record for this book is available from the Library of Congress

ISBN-10 0-387-23599-X (HB)
ISBN-10 0-387-23600-7 (e-book)
ISBN-13 978-0-387-23599-8 (HB)
ISBN-13 978-0-387-23600-1 (e-book)

Published by Springer,
P.O. Box 17, 3300 AA Dordrecht, The Netherlands.

www.springeronline.com

Printed on acid-free paper

Printed in the Netherlands.

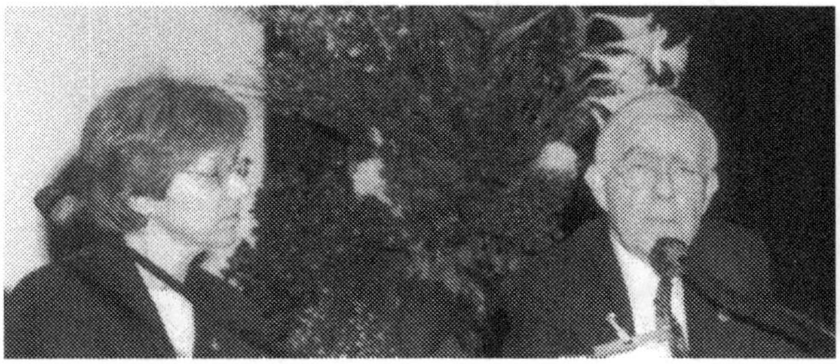

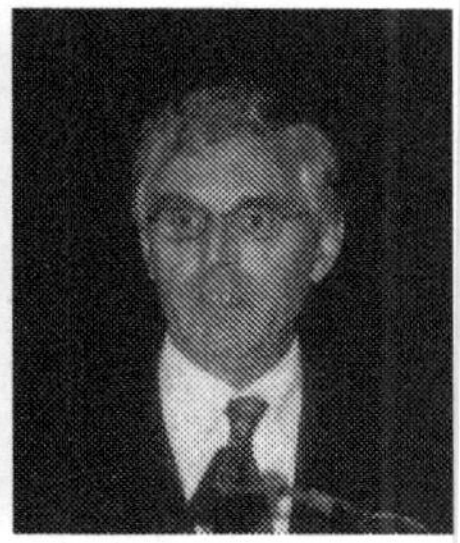

Naomi Luban — Cees Th. Smit Sibinga — Pieter J.J. Sauer

This 28th Sanquin International Symposium on Blood Transfusion was supported by WHO and International Society of Blood Transfusion and conducted under the auspices of the Sanquin Blood Supply Foundation.

ISBT SITS

Fresenius HemoCare

Acknowledgement

This publication has been made possible through the support of Fresenius HemoCare which is gratefully acknowledged.

INTRODUCTION

The 28 years tradition of annual international scientific symposia on blood transfusion in Groningen started in 1976 has come to an end.

Over the years the symposia have covered a wide range of themes in relation to blood transfusion, painting transfusion medicine in all its fascinating and colorful aspects on the canvas of daily practice, academic research and international development.

The strength of the symposia has not only been the format and the informality, but more explicitly the science, exploring the horizons of transfusion medicine as a vein to vein bridging science in a brain to brain fashion. These horizons always have provided the opportunities for bringing the various players in the field of transfusion medicine together for advanced discussion and cross-fertilisation.

The organisers thank the scientific contributors, the professional audience, the supporting industry, and the staff of the Sanquin Blood Bank Northeast for their loyalty and enthusiasm. Without them the tradition would never have occurred, the reputation never have been established and recognised, and the knowledge transfer never been managed and documented the way it happened.

Groningen, 10 October 2003
Prof. Dr. Cees Th. Smit Sibinga
Initiator

CONTENTS

III. Blood Transfusion in the Neonate

IV. Cellular Therapies in Neonatology

MODERATORS AND SPEAKERS

Moderators

N. Luban (chairman) – Center for Cancer and Blood Disorders, Chair, Laboratory Medicine & Pathology, Director, Transfusion Medicine/Donor Center, Children's National Medical Center, Washington, DC, USA

A. Brand – Sanquin Division Blood Bank Southwest, Leiden, NL

Chr. Dame – Department of Neonatology, Charité – Medical School University Berlin, Campus Virchow, Berlin, D

E.L. van Leeuwen – Concern Staff, Sanquin Blood Supply Foundation, Amsterdam, NL

C.Th. Smit Sibinga – Academic Institute for International Development of Transfusion Medicine, Faculty of Medical Sciences, University of Groningen WHO Collaborating Centre Groningen, Sanquin and AABB Consulting Services, Groningen, NL

R.G.Strauss – DeGowin Blood Center, University of Iowa College of Medicine, Iowa City, IA, USA

Speakers

J.B. Bussel – Weill Cornell Medical Center, New York, NY, USA

H.M. van den Berg – Pediatric Haematologist, University Hospital Utrecht, The Netherlands, Utrecht, NL

L. Lecchi – Milano Cord Blood Bank, Centro Trasfusionale e di Immunologia dei Trapianti, IRCCS Ospedale Maggiore,
Milan, I

C.S. Manno – The Children's Hospital of Philadelphia, Division of Hematology,
Philadelphia, PA, USA

P.T. Pisciotto – University of Connecticut Health Center, Farmington, Connecticut, USA

G.T. Rijkers – Department of Pediatric Immunology, Wilhelmina Children's Hospital, University Medical Center,
Utrecht, NL

B.L. Short – Chief, Division of Neonatology, Children's National Medical Center,
Washington, DC, USA

OPENING ADDRESS

I feel extremely privileged and honoured to give the opening address of the 28th Sanquin International Symposium on Blood Transfusion, especially because this will be the last in a long series of excellent symposia. Prof. Cees Th. Smit Sibinga started these symposia in 1976. Since then the symposium has been an annual event, every year with excellent topics and speakers. All different aspects of blood transfusion have been discussed.

Why would Cees Smit Sibinga have selected neonatology to be the topic of this last symposium? Paediatrics only was the topic of the symposium in 1980 neonatology never was a topic all these years. Would it have been that newborn infants like small adults are given only small amounts of blood? However, at the same time they are the most interesting creatures of human life. Everything that can go wrong in humans goes even more wrong in newborn infants. As a former neonatologist of course I am extremely glad that the topic now is the newborn, better late than never.

Neonatology for sure has a much shorter history than blood transfusions. Recently I read an interesting historical novel in which they claimed that the first blood transfusion was done in 1663 in Cambridge. Compare that to neonatology, the first clear description of the intensive care treatment of a tiny newborn is from 1945 in New York. Unfortunately, however, both the first patient after a blood transfusion and the newborn infant after neonatal intensive care treatment died, although of different complications. The historical novel does not explain the medical reasons why the old lady in 1663 receiving a transfusion died. It might have been of course blood group incompatibility. The newborn infant died, after discharge, at the age of 3 months as it was bitten by rats in a New York apartment!

When looking over the last years there have been many changes in the practice of transfusion in the newborn infant. 25 years ago we were used to give whole blood to newborn infants. This was understandable as the reason for a transfusion usually was blood taken for laboratory analysis. That we used whole blood was not only because there were no other products. We honestly believed that whole blood was to the benefit of the newborn child. We argued that when we took whole blood, we should replace it with whole blood. Secondly, we were highly convinced of the very healthy properties of whole blood including white cells, immunoglobulins and clotting factors.

We were also used to transfuse to relatively high levels. We believed that an infant needed a haematocrit of at least 0.40, the minimum of a haematocrit for a newborn infant. Later on we realized that a child at least without complications will do extremely well with haematocrit values as low as 0.25. This reduced the need of blood transfusions.

A second reason for needing help of the Blood Bank were the exchange transfusions. When I started my residency in paediatrics, there was almost one exchange transfusion per day in our unit. Exchange transfusions were performed with heparinised whole blood. This practice clearly has changed dramatically. Today exchange transfusions are extremely rare. Some of the residents leave our unit after 6 months without ever having done an exchange transfusion. Secondly, we are not using heparinised whole blood anymore. The Blood Bank is making specially tailored products for us. Tailored products such as reconstituted blood made of packed cells, plasma and perhaps other compounds. Also we are not using heparin anymore, but citrate or other anticoagulants.

Another reason for performing exchange transfusions 25 years ago were studies showing that patients with severe sepsis had a higher likelihood to survive when they were given an exchange transfusion with extremely fresh blood whereby we reasoned that the active white cells, immunoglobulines and other compounds in blood could help the newborn infant. Actually, the first abstract I ever wrote in my medical career was describing the outcome of infants with severe sepsis after an exchange transfusion. Of course the abstract indicated that the outcome was better after an exchange transfusion. However, we did not realize at that moment, that there were negative aspects of an exchange transfusion with very fresh whole blood as well. I do remember still today a 10 days old, very low birth weight infant where I performed an exchange transfusion. Two days later the child had all signs of Graft versus Host Disease, although we hardly recognized these signs at that time as being a Graft versus Host reaction.

The Blood Bank now recommends not to use whole blood and not to use fresh blood for blood transfusions. Instead, blood products or component us has been introduced in the unit. It is not, as will be discussed at this meeting, however, a simple answer which blood products should be used. Packed cells of course are extremely well known. However, at first we only used red cells at least 2 days old to reduce the risk of CMV infections. Because of fear for haemolysis, the cells should not be older than 2-3 weeks. Due to the risk of transfusion associated Graft versus Host the packed cells were first irradiated and then filtered. During this meeting you will hear the latest news about how to use red cells.

Another type of cells that has been used for some time in neonatology are white cell transfusions. White cells were separated and given to infants with severe infections. Very mixed results are published and probably infants developed Graft versus Host reactions, as indicated before. After some years and many studies the administration of white cells was abandoned. Another issue that also will be discussed extensively during this meeting is the transfusion of thrombocytes. Many newborn infants do have a low number of thrombocytes. However, does this mean that we have to transfuse thrombocytes? Only during the last years there is more knowledge regarding the cause of thrombocytopenia and we have obtained a better insight into the question whether or not to transfuse these infants. Over the last 10 years another topic in neonatology has been the use of growth factors - Erythropoietin, G-CSF and thrombopoietin are used with varying results. During this meeting you will hear the latest news about the use of these products. The hype some 10 years ago was that blood transfusions would not be needed anymore due to the use of these growth factors, in my opinion has at least partly faded away.

Prof. Cees Smit Sibinga, you put together an excellent programme covering all the important issues of transfusion in the newborn infant. Over the last 50 years many practices in transfusing the newborn infant were introduced and forgotten. I am extremely pleased that we will hear the "state of the art" during this meeting. On behalf of all paediatricians and neonatologists I thank you for composing this excellent programme. Finally, I do hope that, although this is the last symposium in a long series, there will be other meetings organised by you in the future. I wish you an excellent meeting.

Prof. Dr. Pieter J.J. Sauer,
Department of Paediatrics and Neonatology,
University Hospital Groningen, NL

I. FOETAL AND NEONATAL HAEMATOLOGY

REGULATION OF DEVELOPMENTAL HAEMATOPOIESIS BY GATA TRANSCRIPTION FACTORS[1]

Chr. Dame[2]

Introduction

The aim of this contribution is to summarize current data on the role of GATA transcription factors in the regulation of developmental haematopoiesis.

GATA transcription factors are a family of six zinc finger proteins, which bind to the (T/A)GATA(A/G) consensus sequence and play prominent roles in the regulation of cell differentiation and proliferation during development [1]. Each GATA transcription factor contains two highly conserved C4-type (Cys-X_2-Cys-X_{17}-Cys-X_2-Cys) zinc finger domains [2]. The carboxy-terminal zinc finger is necessary for the DNA-binding of the protein, the amino-terminal zinc finger is required for the interaction with other transcription factors or co-factors [3].

Based on their predominant expression in haematopoietic cells, GATA-1, -2, and -3 were designated as 'haematopoietic' GATA transcription factors, whereas GATA-4, -5, and -6 were categorized as 'endodermal' GATA factors due to their predominant expression in the heart, lung, liver, and gastrointestinal tract [4,5]. The functional role of GATA transcription factors in developmental processes has been most extensively studied in mice. Mice with targeted deletions of the genes encoding GATA-1, -2, or -3 die at embryonic stages of development and exhibit severe haematopoietic defects [6-9]. In contrast, mice with homozygous GATA-4 mutation die soon after implantation, and essential functions of GATA-4 in yolk sac vasculogenesis, heart morphogenesis, and the development of the visceral endoderm have been reported [10]. Transgenic mice with homozygous GATA-6 deletion also die also soon after implantation and display major deficits in the extra-embryonic tissue of the early mouse embryo [11,12].

However, the expression of the 'haematopoietic' GATA transcription factors is not restricted to haematopoietic cells. In mice, GATA-1 is also expressed in Sertoli cells of the testis [13]. GATA-2 is expressed in various tissues, including the liver, kidney, and nervous system [14-17]. GATA-3 is also expressed in a variety of non-haematopoietic organs, most abundantly in the developing central and peripheral nervous system, liver, kidney, adrenal gland, placenta, and thymus [16-22]. The functional implication of GATA-2 and -3 in the normal

---

1. Supported by the Deutsche Forschungsgemeinschaft (DA 484/2-1).

2. Assistant Professor, Charité – Universitätsmedizin Berlin, Department of Neonatology, Campus Virchow-Klinikum, Berlin, Germany.

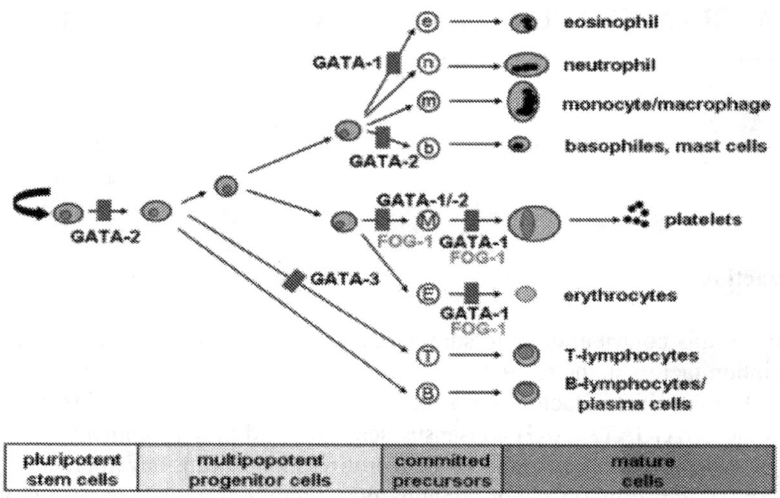

Figure 1. Illustration of the developmental steps in haematopoiesis that require the functional activity of GATA transcription factors. Red boxes depict the arrest in the development of haematopoietic cell lineages, if the respective factor is absent. In addition, the requirement of FOG-1 (*friend of GATA*) is indicated, since FOG-1 is an important co-factor to archive full biological activity of GATA-1. Abbreviations: e – eosinophil precursor, n – neutrophil precursor, m – myelocyte precusor, b – basophil precursor, M – megakaryocyte precursor, E – erythroid precursor, T – T cell precursor, B – B cell precursor. (M*odified from* Cantor and Orkin [124]).

development of various (non-haematopoietic) organs has been analyzed in different transgenic mice models [8,14-16,20, 23-25].

Mutations in human GATA genes have been identified to cause various congenital diseases. Haematopoietic abnormalities associated with GATA-1 mutations or mutations in a relevant GATA binding site of a target gene are summarized and discussed in detail later in this article. While human GATA-2 mutations have yet not been reported, GATA-3 haplo-insufficiency due to various forms of mutations causes HDR syndrome, a rare and complex disorder of hypoparathyreoidism, sensorineural deafness, and renal insufficiency (OMIM #131320 and #146255, respectively) [26-28]. Furthermore, somatic GATA-3 mutations have been recently identified in human breast tumours [29]. GATA-4 haplo-insufficiency causes human congenital heart malformation, in particular cardiac septal defects (OMIM #600576) [30,31].

Biology of 'haematopoietic' GATA transcription factors

Various developmental steps in haematopoiesis require the functional activity of 'haematopoietic' GATA transcription factors. A summary on these data is illustrated in Figure 1. In haematopoiesis, GATA transcription factors are embedded in a complex regulatory network. Therefore their exact biochemical function and molecular regulation is of high interest. The genes encoding haematopoietic GATA transcription factors usually contain two first exons, that are utilized tissue-specifically to restrict or activate gene expression in various haematopoietic or non-haematopoietic cell types, and five translated exons. Among the 'haematopoietic' GATA transcription factors, GATA-1 has the highest homology with GATA-2. Although these two GATA transcription factors recognize a similar DNA binding motif and share partially overlapping expression profiles in certain haematopoietic cell lineages, significant functional differences and unique biochemical characteristics have been identified. These differences are mediated by specific interactions with different co-activators or co-repressors and by the acquirement of distinct regulatory enhancers within the GATA genes [32,33].

GATA-1

GATA-1 is the founding member of the GATA family of transcription factors.[34] With the exception of Sertoli cells of the testis, in which the biological function is uncertain, GATA-1 expression is restricted to haematopoietic cells [13]. In haematopoietic cells, GATA-1 is most abundantly expressed in erythroid precursors, megakaryocyte progenitor cells, eosinophils, and mast cells [9,35-37]. Early, pluripotent haematopoietic progenitors express relatively low GATA-1 levels, and in haematopoietic stem cells, GATA-1 seems to be absent [6]. GATA-1 deficient mice die by day e12.5 due to inefficient haematopoiesis in the yolk sac, indicating that GATA-1 is necessary for differentiation of 'primitive' haematopoietic cells [9].

GATA-1 expression underlies a complex regulation. Regulatory mechanisms include the use of alternative promoter elements in Sertoli cells (distal first exon; IT exon) *vs.* haematopoietic cells (proximal first exon; IE exon) [13]. Furthermore, a GATA-1 haematopoietic regulatory domain (GATA-1 HRD) fragment, which contains at least three control regions (including a double GATA and a CACCC motif), and the enhancer are important for differential GATA-1 expression in various haematopoietic cell types [38-40]. While the haematopoietic GATA-1 promoter and the upstream region of the GATA-1 HRD fragment are sufficient for GATA-1 expression in 'primitive' erythroid cells, an additional sequence (intron S-P element) containing GATA repeats in the first intron is required for efficient GATA-1 expression in 'definitive' erythroid cells [39]. As in the globin gene locus, position effects may be required for some types of age-related epigenetic silencing in the GATA-1 locus [38]. More recent studies show that GATA-1 is able to form homodimers. In zebrafish homodimeric GATA-1 binds to the double GATA motif in the upstream region and activates GATA-1 gene transcription itself in an autoregulatory loop mechanism [41,42].

Full GATA-1 activity requires the presence of its essential co-factor *friend of GATA-1* (FOG-1), a zinc finger protein that interacts with the N-terminal zinc finger of GATA-1 and cooperates with GATA-1 to promote cellular differentiation of erythroid precursors and megakaryocytes [43]. The interaction with FOG-1 is cell type specific, since mast cells and eosinophils do not express FOG-1. Gene ablation of FOG-1 results in embryonic lethality between day e10.5 and e11.5 of murine gestation. These embryos exhibit a defect in the development of both 'primitive' and 'definitive' erythroid and in megakaryocyte progenitor cells. In contrast to GATA-1 -/- embryos, FOG-1 deficiency results in a complete failure of megakaryopoiesis, indicating that FOG-1 also has a GATA-1 independent role in early haematopoiesis [44]. In erythroblasts, the biological activity of GATA-1 is cleavaged by caspases, but this protein degradation is usually prevented by an Epo signal [45].

GATA-1 also displays its biological function in various haematopoietic cell types also with other specific co-factors. For example, in myelo-myeloid cells enforced GATA-1 expression perturbs cell differentiation due to direct interaction with PU.1, a member of the *ets* family of transcription factors. This interaction occurs through the DNA-binding domains of each of the respective proteins [46]. However, antagonistic effects of GATA-1 and PU.1 are mediated by different mechanisms: GATA-1 inhibits PU.1 by preventing it from interacting with the essential co-factor c-Jun, while PU.1 represses GATA-1 function by disrupting its ability to bind DNA [47].

GATA-2

GATA-2, which is highly expressed in haematopoietic stem cells and immature progenitors, is primary required for the proliferation and survival/self-renew of both 'primitive' and 'definitive' progenitors (Figure 1) [6,7]. In addition, GATA-2 mRNA is found in early, but not late erythroid precursors, mast cells, and megakaryocytes [7,48]. GATA-2 expression in progenitor cells is down regulated as they switch from proliferation to differentiation and lineage-specific maturation [6]. Loss of GATA-2 expression in transgenic mice leads to embryonic lethality at day e10.5 of gestation due to a severe reduction of 'primitive' erythroid cells [7].

Expression of GATA-2 is regulated by tissue-specific regulatory elements. The distal first exon (IS exon) of the GATA-2 gene drives transcription specifically in haematopoietic and neuronal cells, while the proximal GS exon directs expression in the other non-haematopoietic tissues [49,50]. In mice, this fragment, that extends 7 kb upstream of the haematopoietic first exon, allows to rise 'definitive' haematopoietic cells in the P-Sp and AGM (regions of the **p**ara-aortic **sp**lanchno-pleura and of the ventral aspect of the **a**orta, **g**enital ridge, and **m**esenephros) as well as the liver [51]. The haematopoietic GATA-2 enhancer contains a GATA binding site that functions as a dual gatekeeper for the stimulation or repression of GATA-2 activity in response to the differentiation of haematopoietic progenitor cells. In undifferentiated and non-induced early haematopoietic cells, GATA-2 binds to its enhancer element, in a positive regulatory loop, which correlates with a widespread histone H3 and H4 acetylation, reflecting transcriptional activity. However, as cells differentiate in response to GATA-1, GATA-1 binds to the same GATA site in the haematopoietic GATA-2 enhancer and suppresses GATA-2 activity [52]. In addition to GATA-1, FOG-1 is required to display GATA-2 from that regulatory element [53].

GATA-3

In the haematopoietic system GATA-3 is expressed in human fetal, neonatal and adult T cells [18]. GATA-3 is also expressed in early haematopoietic progenitor cells and homozygous GATA-3 deletion is accompanied with a severe failure of hepatic haematopoiesis [8,54]. The fact that GATA-3 over-expression in primary haematopoietic stem cells selectively induces a differentiation program towards erythropoiesis and megakaryopoiesis, but fail to expand bone marrow and to sustain multilineage haematopoiesis [55], suggests that a specific, most likely relatively constant GATA-3 expression level is required for normal haematopoiesis.

The tissue-specific expression of GATA-3 is regulated by distinct promoter elements, located in the complex GATA-3 gene locus [19,56-58]. However, the promoter element for GATA-3 expression in the thymus and in naïve T helper cells, in which GATA-3 is either down- or up-regulated in response to different cytokines, has not been identified yet, but lies presumably more than 450 kb upstream or more than 175 kb downstream of the GATA-3 gene [59].

Developmental changes in haematopoiesis

The development of the haematopoietic system is characterized by some fundamental changes, which are significantly influenced by the activity of GATA transcription factors. Major changes during the development of the haematopoietic system are (i) the switch from 'primitive' to 'definitive' haematopoiesis, (ii) the switch of the primary site of haematopoiesis from the mesoderm of the visceral yolk sac and the embryonic P-Sp and AGM to the foetal liver and later to the bone marrow, (iii) a developmental decrease in the proliferative activity of haematopoietic progenitor cells, (iv) the switch from embryonic and foetal to adult haemoglobins, and (v) the switch of the primary site of erythropoietin (Epo) production from the foetal liver to the mature kidney in infants [60, for review]. The pivotal role of GATA transcription factors in these developmental processes is reviewed herein.

GATA transcription factors in the switch from 'primitive' to 'definitive' haematopoiesis

The switch from 'primitive' to 'definitive' haematopoiesis is characterized by developmental changes in the morphology, maturation, and kinetics of the cell cycle of erythropoietic cells. 'Primitive' erythropoiesis is characterized by large $CD34^-$ erythroblasts (>20 μm), which differentiate with the blood vessels, remain nucleated, contain predominantly embryonic haemoglobin, and are not dependent on Epo [61,62]. In contrast, 'definitive' erythropoiesis is characterized by smaller (<20 μm) $CD34^+$ erythroblasts, which produce fetal or adult haemoglobins, exclude their nuclei, and are highly dependent on Epo [62,63]. While 'primitive' erythropoietic cells cycle continuously and do not pause for long periods to differentiate, 'definitive' erythropoietic cells remain in G_0 for extensive periods [64]. 'Primitive' erythroblasts normally undergo programmed cell death, whereas 'definitive' erythroblasts are able to self-renew [65].

Increasing evidence is given that GATA-1 and GATA-2 have an implication for developmental differences between 'primitive' and 'definitive' erythroblasts. In murine embryonic haematopoiesis, GATA-2 reduction severely reduces the production and expansion of haematopoietic stem cells in the AGM, while GATA-2 reduction in the foetal liver or adult bone marrow does not or only minimal affect the number haematopoietic stem cells [66]. As described above, the different activity of GATA-1 in 'primitive' *vs.* 'definitive' erythroblasts is mediated by a selective recruitment of gene regulatory elements. While the haematopoietic GATA-1 promoter and the upstream region of the GATA-1 HRD fragment are sufficient for GATA-1 expression in 'primitive' erythroid cells, sequences in the first intron are required for efficient GATA-1 expression in 'definitive' erythroid cells [39].

GATA transcription factors in the switch of the primary site of haematopoiesis

Medullary haematopoiesis starts around 10 weeks post conception (pc) with the development of blood forming units in the bone. As in the yolk sac, embryonic AGM, and foetal liver, medullary haematopoiesis begins also with 'primitive' erythropoiesis and switches to 'definitive' erythropoiesis. This switch is completed by 14 weeks pc. Beyond 16 weeks pc areas of dense haematopoietic activity are established in the bone, and the bone marrow becomes the primary site of haematopoiesis after 30 weeks pc [67,68].

Since gene ablation studies in mice have shown that GATA-1, -2, and -3 are critical for 'definitive' haematopoiesis, we analyzed their expression pattern during the development of human medullary haematopoiesis using immunohistochemistry and semi-quantitative RT-PCR [69]. Immunohisto-chemistry showed that the expression of GATA-1, -2, and -3 in bone marrow specimens from foetuses und neonates is restricted to haematopoietic cells without evidence for their expression in structural or stromal elements of the marrow. In human foetal and neonatal bone marrow specimens, the absence of pre-adipocytes and adipocytes, which express GATA-2 and GATA-3 [70], allowed a semi-quantitative analysis of GATA-1, -2, and -3 expression during that period of development. Among these transcription factors, only GATA-2 is expressed in the developmental stage II of medullary haematopoiesis (8.5 – 9 weeks pc, characterized by active chrondrolysis and detection of $CD34^+$ and $CD68^+$ cells in the bone cavity [68]). GATA-2 expression peaks at the onset of medullary haematopoiesis, declines from 16 to 30 weeks pc, and remains at a constant level from that time point onwards. In contrast, GATA-1 expression significantly increases with increasing haematopoietic activity in the bone marrow. After 30 weeks pc, when the bone marrow becomes the primary site of haematopoiesis, the ratio between GATA-2 and GATA-1 mRNA levels remains on a relatively constant level (Figure 2) [69].

These findings are concordant with *in vitro* and animal studies, indicating that GATA-2 is required for the self-renewal and proliferation of undifferentiated haematopoietic stem or progenitor cells, while GATA-1 is required for the terminal differentiation of erythroid and megakaryocyte precursor cells [4,48].

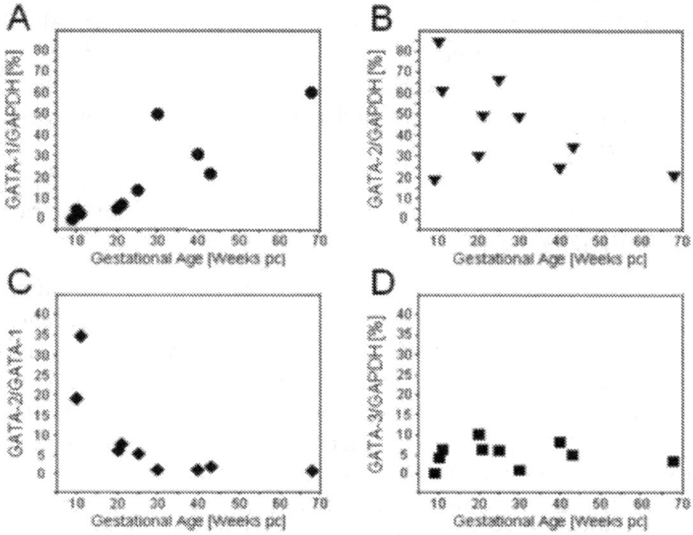

Figure 2. Expression of GATA-1, -2, and -3 in the human bone marrow during the ontogeny of medullary haematopoiesis as determined by semi-quantitative RT-PCR analysis; mRNA levels are given in relation to GAPDH. Panel C shows the ratio between GATA2 and GATA-1 during development (*with permission*) [69].

Importantly, GATA-2 is developmentally down regulated during the differentiation of early haematopoietic colony-forming cells derived from human embryonic stem cells [71]. Recent data highly suggest that GATA-1 is involved in this process by binding to regulatory elements in the GATA-2 gene locus [52]. In the absence of GATA-1, arrested erythroid precursor contain more than 50-fold higher GATA-2 levels than control cells [72]. GATA-2 over-expression inhibits the differentiation of haematopoietic progenitors to erythroid and megakaryocyte precursors [73]. These findings confirm that a complex network, which includes feedback mechanisms, modulates the activity of GATA transcription factors in the ontogeny of haematopoiesis. Furthermore, other regulators such as acetylases, polymerases, co-factors (e.g. FOG-1), and cytokines are required in this network. For example, Epo, which is expressed in the developing bone marrow, may exhibit paracrine effects [74]. *In vitro*, erythroleukaemic cells induced to differentiate into erythroid cells only by treatment with recombinant Epo exhibit increased GATA-1 expression levels, whereas GATA-2 expression declines as erythroid differentiation proceeds [6]. However, GATA-2 and GATA-3 have been implicated as negative regulators of Epo gene expression [75].

In contrast to GATA-1 and -2, GATA-3 expression levels are low and do not underlie developmental changes during the onset of medullary haematopoiesis [69]. GATA-3 is expressed in early haematopoietic cells derived from the AGM, and homozygous deletion of GATA-3 is accompanied with a severe failure of hepatic haematopoiesis [8,54]. GATA-3 over-expression in primary haematopoietic stem cells selectively induces a differentiation program towards erythropoiesis and megakaryopoiesis, but GATA-3 over-expressing cells fail to expand bone marrow and to sustain multilineage haematopoiesis [55]. This led us speculate that GATA-3 needs to be expressed on a specific and relatively constant level for proper development and maintenance of human medullary haematopoiesis [69].

GATA transcription factors in developmental changes of the proliferative activity of haematopoietic progenitor cells

The growth characteristics of haematopoietic progenitors and erythroid precursor cells are site-specific and change with age. The *in vitro* analysis of the long-term growth capacity of $CD34^{+}CD45^{RAlow}CD71^{low}$ cells, which were isolated from the human foetal liver (13-15 weeks pc), cord blood, and adult bone marrow and grown in serum-free media supplemented with interleukin (IL) -6, IL-3, stem cell factor (SCF), mast cell growth factor, and Epo, provided evidence for a significantly higher proliferation of haematopoietic stem cells derived from the foetal liver [76]. Own preliminary data indicate that GATA-2 expression in human liver specimens peaks with the highest haematopoietic activity in the liver (15-20 weeks pc). At this developmental stage, GATA-2 expression in hepatocytes is very low. GATA-2 expression in human hepatocytes does not increase before the neonatal period [Dame *et al.*, unpublished data].

Furthermore, modifications in the responsiveness of haematopoietic progenitors to growth factors, such as Epo, are also relevant for developmental changes in the proliferative activity of haematopoietic progenitor cells. In fact, erythroid burst-forming units (BFU-E) from human foetuses can be stimulated with Epo alone, whereas BFU-E from adults require additional factors, such as IL-3 or granulocyte-macrophage colony-stimulating factors (GM-CSF) [77]. Age-specific growth characteristics may result from different Epo receptor (Epo-R) isoforms being expressed during fetal gestation [78] or the level of Epo-R expression in haematopoietic progenitors and erythroid precursors.

Regulation of the Epo receptor by GATA-1 in haematopoietic progenitor cells

The expression of the Epo-R gene can be regulated at the transcriptional and post-transcriptional level as well as by post-translational modification [79-81]. At the transcriptional level Epo-R mRNA expression is controlled by *cis*-acting elements located upstream of the Epo-R gene. Reporter gene assays showed that various positive or negative regulatory domains exist within the 5'untranslated region (position *nt*-1050 to *nt*+135 of the transcription start site; GeneBank Accession No. S45332) [82]. The minimal promoter (*nt*-76 to *nt*+33) and a sequence located downstream of the transcription start site (*nt*+1 to *nt*+135) have both a specific implication for the transcriptional activation of Epo-R gene expression in erythroid progenitor cells. The minimal Epo-R promoter contains binding sites for the ubiquitous transcription factor Sp1 (CCGCCC) at *nt*-20 to *nt*-25 and GATA transcription factors at *nt*-44 to *nt*-47. The murine minimal

Epo-R promoter can be activated by co-transfection with GATA-1 [83,84]. Importantly, mice with targeted homozygous deletion of the Epo-R gene, which were transgenic for two different GATA-1 minigene cassettes with haematopoietic regulatory domains (GATA-1 HDR), can be rescued by each of these cassettes from the lethal defect of Epo-R deficiency [85].

GATA-1 also regulates the cell-cycle dependent regulation of Epo-R. As shown in cell-cycle of logarithmically growing Epo-dependent leukaemia cells (UT-7 cell line), both Epo-R and GATA-1 mRNA, but not GATA-2 mRNA levels, concomitantly decrease at the G_0/G_1 phase and later increase at the S and G_2/M phase. These dynamic changes in Epo-R mRNA expression parallel with the binding activity of GATA-1 in the Epo-R promoter element [86]. However, the increase of Epo-R mRNA expression seems to be dependent on other transcription factors than GATA-1 at the resting phases induced by growth factor starvation [86].

Cumulative data provide thereby evidence that GATA transcription factors are involved in the developmental regulation of the proliferative activity of multipotent haematopoietic progenitors and erythroid precursor cells.

Role of GATA transcription factors in the switch of globin genes during development

The genes of the α- and β-globin families (ζ, α_1/α_2 globins and ε, γ, δ, β globins, respectively) are expressed according to a strict ontogenetic schedule, and the quantitative expression of the genes from each of these families is strictly balanced and coordinated. The distinct intrachromosomal and interchromosomal control of globin gene expression implies complex regulatory mechanisms [87]. In the human β-globin locus, the most prominent distal regulatory element is the locus control region (LCR), located from about 6 to 22 kb upstream of the ε-globin gene [87]. The LCR is composed of five domains that exhibit extremely high sensitivity to DNase I (hysersensitive sites, HS) in erythroid cells and are required for high-level globin gene expression at all developmental stages [88]. More detailed information on the function of the LCR can be obtained from previous reviews [87,89].

The specific implication of GATA transcription factors in regulating the activity of the LCR is in focus of this chapter: Within the HS sites of the LCR various DNA sequence motifs have been identified, which are highly conserved among different species and bind specific proteins or protein complexes regulating the activity of the LCR. These elements include MARE (maf recognition element) and GATA bindings sites in the HS2, HS3, and HS4 as well as Krüppel-like factor (KLF) binding sites in HS2 and HS3, and an E-box motif (CANNTG) in HS2 [90]. The GATA sites in HS2, HS, and HS4 are bound by GATA-1 or GATA-2 [91].

GATA transcription factors are not only directly bound to the HS, they are also involved in protein-protein interactions. These interactions occur between GATA factors themselves and between GATA transcription factors and other transcription factors, such as the erythroid Krüppel-like factor (EKLF), LMO2/Tal1 (a complex of a LIM domain containing protein and a basic helix-loop-helix-protein), and the ubiquitously expressed transcription factor Sp1 [92-94].

Within the current multistep model for the human β-globin gene regulation, GATA transcription factors, in particular GATA-1, are involved in the initial generation of a highly accessible LCR holocomplex. This step is initiated by the partial unfolding of the chromatin structure containing the globin locus into a DNase I-sensitive domain. The initial unfolding of the chromatin structure is mediated by the diffusion of erythroid-specific proteins, such as GATA-1, into chromosomal domains that are not permissive for transcription. These proteins bind to sequences throughout the globin locus, leading to the partial unfolding and perhaps to hyperacetylation of the chromatin [89]. In this context, GATA-1 may rather act as a 'architectural' than as a 'traditional' transcriptional activator [95]. GATA transcription factors bound to the HS may also be required for the recruitment of chromatin-remodelling and transcription complexes to the LCR as second step in human β-globin gene regulation. Data on specific implications of GATA transcription factors on the following steps, namely the establishment of chromatin domains permissive for transcription and the transfer of transcription complexes to individual globin genes, are not given yet.

GATA transcription factors in the regulation of the switch of primary site of erythropoietin production

Another aspect of the developmental changes in haematopoiesis is the switch of the primary production site of circulating Epo from the liver in the foetus to the kidney in infants and adults. Such a switch of the primary site of hormone production from one to another organ is an unique phenomenon, which occurs in various mammalian species with a specific time of onset [74,78]. In humans the switch of Epo production may contribute to inadequately low Epo production in the anaemia of prematurity. Initially, it was thought that a different capacity in oxygen (pO_2) sensing in the foetal liver *vs.* kidney or that differences in the hypoxia-induced responsiveness of Epo production would be the physiological cause to switch the primary site of Epo production, but both could be excluded by animal experiments and the analysis of gene expression patterns in human foetal tissue specimens [78,96]. Moreover, data from organ ablation studies in sheep strongly suggested that the switch of Epo production site is transcriptionally regulated [97]. Analysis of transgenic animals indicated that conserved *cis*-acting elements both 5' and 3' of the Epo gene are important for its tissues-specific regulation in the liver and kidney [98, for review]. In a recent study, we identified GATA-4 as activator of Epo gene expression in the foetal liver by binding to its minimal 5' promoter. This mechanism is tissue–specific, since GATA-4 is not expressed in the foetal or adult kidney, and also developmental- stage specific, since GATA-4 is expressed in foetal, but not in adult hepatocytes [99]. In contrast, GATA-2 and/or GATA-3 bind to the same GATA site in the adult liver and inhibit thereby Epo gene expression [75,100]. The combined data result in a novel model for the developmental-

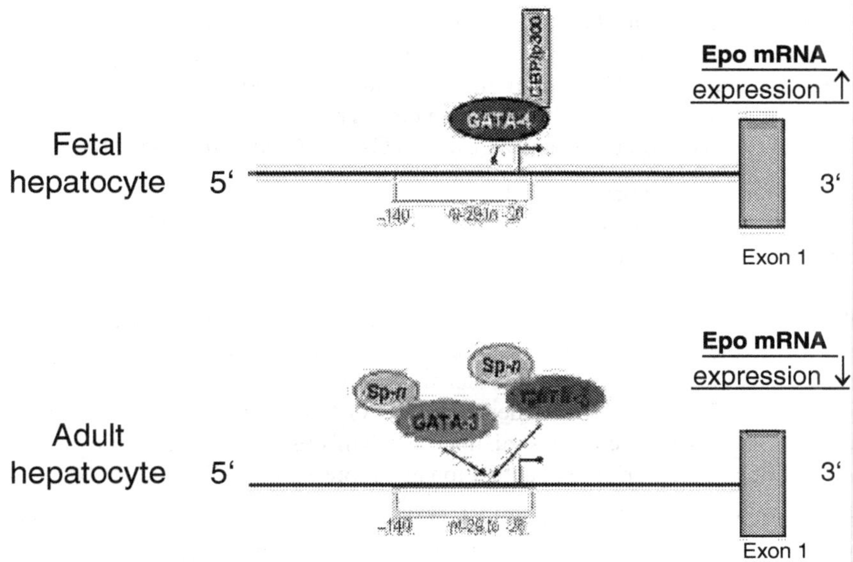

Figure 3. Current model of the role of GATA transcription factors in the regulation of the erythropoietin (Epo) gene expression in the foetal *vs.* adult liver. Recent data provide evidence that GATA-4 binds in foetal hepatocytes to the minimal promoter of the human Epo gene and activates its expression [99]. However, in the adult liver Epo gene expression may be inhibited by the binding of GATA-2 and/or GATA-3 to the Epo promoter [75].

stage specific regulation of Epo production in the foetal and adult liver (Figure 3). Thereby, evidence is given that a primarily 'non-haematopoietic' GATA transcription factor is also involved in developmental changes in haematopoiesis.

GATA transcription factors in congenital or acquired disorders of haematopoiesis

Increasing evidence exists that disturbances in the functional activity of GATA-1 cause various congenital or acquired disorders of haematopoiesis.

X-linked thrombocytopenia with or without anaemia

Mutations in the GATA-1 coding sequence (the GATA-1 gene is located on the X chromosome) have been found in X-linked thrombocytopenia and dyserythropoietic anaemia (poikilocytosis and anisocytosis) [101]. The G→A missense mutation at nucleotide 613 results in a substitution of valine by methionine at amino acid 205 (V205M) in the N-terminal zinc finger of the GATA-1 protein, leading to a reduced interaction of GATA-1 with its co-factor FOG-1. This study showed for the first time that a physical GATA-1-FOG-1 interaction is required *in vivo* for normal megakaryopoiesis and erythropoiesis in humans.

Two additional mutations have been found in X-linked thrombocytopenia without marked anaemia: Both single amino acids substitutions from aspartate to glycine in codon 218 (D218G) or glycine to serine in codon 208 (G208S) in the N-terminal zinc finger also affect, but to a lower degree, the interaction between GATA-1 and FOG-1 and not the binding of GATA-1 to DNA [102-

105]. In the D218G mutation platelets appear markedly immature and lack the membrane glycoproteins GPIbα, GPIbβ, GPIIIα, GPIX, and GPV.

In contrast to the D218G mutation, the substitution of aspartate by tyrosine in codon 218 (D218Y) of GATA-1 protein has found to be associated with a severe anaemia and profound macrothrombocytopenia. This mutations results in reduced affinity of GATA-1 to FOG-1 and a disturbed GATA-1 self-association [104].

X-linked thrombocytopenia with β-thalassaemia

An arginine to glutamine substitution in codon 216 (R216G) of the N-terminal zinc finger of GATA-1 causes X-linked thrombocytopenia with β-thalassaemia. This mutation affects rather the DNA binding of the protein to palindromic GATA-sites than the interaction with FOG-1 [106]. In the β-globin gene locus, the interaction between GATA-1 and FOG-1 has shown to be required for GATA-1 occupancy at select sites, such as HS2, but is dispensable at others, including the FOG-1-independent GATA-1 target gene EKLF. This indicates that FOG-1 employs distinct mechanisms when cooperating with GATA-1 during transcriptional activation and repression [107].

Acquired GATA-1 mutations in transient myeloproliferative disorder and acute myeloid leukaemia associated with trisomy 21 (Down syndrome)

Recently, acquired GATA-1 mutations have been identified as an early event in leukaemogenesis in individuals with Down syndrome (DS) [108]. At least 10% of infants with trisomy 21 develop - often already during foetal gestation – a transient myeloproliferative disorder (TMD), which is characterized by the accumulation of immature megakaryoblasts in liver, bone marrow, and peripheral blood. Although TMD undergoes spontaneous remission in most cases, approximately 30% of infants with TMD develop acute megakaryoblastic leukaemia (DS-AMKL) within 3 years [109]. TMD blasts are morphologically indistinguishable from AMKL blasts, classified as FAB M7 subtype. This led to the hypothesis that DS-AMKL is derived from TMD.

Given the fact that numerous mutations in the GATA-1 gene cause defective haematopoiesis, individuals with DS associated TMD and AMKL have been screened for GATA-1 mutations. Several groups described a very high incidence (about 85%) of various forms of GATA-1 mutations in DS-AMKL [108,110-113]. Importantly, GATA-1 mutations have not been detected in other types of leukaemia associated with DS or in individuals, who did not have DS, but suffered from AMKL or other subtypes of acute myeloid leukaemia (AML). Since the GATA-1 gene is not mutated in remission samples of patients who underwent chemotherapy due to DS-AMKL, it has been concluded that GATA-1 mutations are somatically acquired. Moreover, GATA-1 mutations have been found in nearly every neonate and infant (97%) with TMD associated to Down syndrome, again suggesting that GATA-1 mutagenesis is an early event in DS myeloid leukaemogenesis [110-114]. However, the exact time when individuals with DS acquire GATA-1 mutations is unclear. Since TMD occurs already in the neonatal period, it has been postulated that GATA-1 mutations arise *in utero* [115]. This assumption is further supported by the report of GATA-1 mutations in neonatal blood spots from 3 of 4 patients, who had clinically no TMD, but developed DS-AMKL 12 to 26 months later [108].

The majority of reported GATA-1 mutations in DS involves small deletions or insertions in the sequence encoding exon 2 and result in the expression of a short GATA-1 isoform (GATA-1s) due to a disruption of the normal reading frame [108,116]. GATA-1s is likely to arise from Met84 as alternative translation initiation site, downstream of each of the known mutations [116]. GATA-1s binds to DNA and interacts with FOG-1, but has a reduced transactivation potential due to the absence of the N-terminal activation domain [108,117]. However, GATA-1s is also a normal isoform of GATA-1, which is expressed – most likely by alternative splicing – in various human haematopoietic cell lines and in the murine foetal liver [116,118]. It has been speculated that GATA-1s may act as a negative-regulating protein, which down-modulates GATA-1 during normal haematopoiesis. If so, GATA-1s could fail to repress other factors, perhaps GATA-2. We and others are currently speculating that the implication of abnormal GATA-1s expression on TMD may depend on the time point of mutagenesis and haematopoietic microenvironment (liver *vs.* bone marrow). In this content, the spontaneous regression of TMD during infancy could be explained by the loss of the foetal haematopoietic environment. However, in about 30% of individuals with DS associated TMD/GATA-1 mutation, an additional, second event may be responsible for the development of DS-AML. This needs to be elucidated in the near future – both for understanding the leukaemogenesis in DS and for other forms of leukaemia.

Human disorders linked to *cis*-acting GATA sequences

An increasing number of mutations in a GATA binding site of critical *cis*-acting elements of various genetic disorders has been reported to be associated with hereditary diseases. These mutations result in an abolished or increased binding of GATA-1 to the following target genes: δ-globin (>> δ-thalassaemia), platelet membrane glycoproteins GPI-IX-V (>> Bernard-Soulier syndrome), PKLR (pyruvate kinase liver and red cell type) gene (>> pyruvate kinase deficient anaemia), and in the uroporphyrinogen III synthase (>> congenital erythropoietic porphyria) [119-123]. These data indicate that GATA-1 activity is required for a variety of genes expressed in erythroid cells and megakaryocytes, and that its binding to a particular *cis*-acting element is essential for the correct driving of the entire transcriptional machinery of these genes.

Summary

In summary, current data on the biology of GATA transcription factors show their major contribution on the development of the haematopoietic system. The GATA transcription factors orchestrate in a complex network of multiple factors and exhibit specific biochemical functions. The understanding of the pivotal role of GATA transcription factors in normal and disturbed development of haematopoiesis may be helpful to understand their implication in acquired haematologic diseases.

Acknowledgement

The author thanks the members of his laboratory, especially Iwona Palaszeweski and Malte Cremer, for the stimulating discussion on the biology of GATA transcription factors in developmental haematopoiesis and the critical reading of this manuscript.

References

1. Orkin SH. GATA-binding transcription factors in hematopoietic cells. Blood 1992;80:575-81.
2. Lowry JA, Atchley WR. Molecular evolution of the GATA family of transcription factors: conservation within the DNA-binding domain. J Mol Evol 2000;50:103-15.
3. Yang Z, Gu L, Romeo PH, et al. Human GATA-3 trans-activation, DNA-binding, and nuclear localization activities are organized into distinct structural domains. Mol Cell Biol 1994;14:2201-12.
4. Weiss MJ, Orkin SH. GATA transcription factors: key regulators of hematopoiesis. Exp Hematol 1995;23:99-107.
5. Molkentin JD. The zinc finger-containing transcription factors GATA-4, -5, and -6. Ubiquitously expressed regulators of tissue-specific gene expression. J Biol Chem 2000;275:38949-52.
6. Leonard M, Brice M, Engel JD, Papayannopoulou T. Dynamics of GATA transcription factor expression during erythroid differentiation. Blood 1993; 82:1071-79.
7. Tsai FY, Keller G, Kuo FC, et al. An early haematopoietic defect in mice lacking the transcription factor GATA-2. Nature 1994;371:221-6.
8. Pandolfi PP, Roth ME, Karis A, et al. Targeted disruption of the GATA3 gene causes severe abnormalities in the nervous system and in fetal liver haematopoiesis. Nat Genet 1995;11:40-44.
9. Pevny L, Simon MC, Robertson E, et al. Erythroid differentiation in chimaeric mice blocked by a targeted mutation in the gene for transcription factor GATA-1. Nature 1991;349:257-60.
10. Molkentin JD, Lin Q, Duncan SA, Olson EN. Requirement of the transcription factor GATA4 for heart tube formation and ventral morphogenesis. Genes Dev 1997;11:1061-72.
11. Morrisey EE, Tang Z, Sigrist K, et al. GATA6 regulates HNF4 and is required for differentiation of visceral endoderm in the mouse embryo. Genes Dev 1998;12:3579-90.
12. Koutsourakis M, Langeveld A, Patient R, Beddington R, Grosveld F. The transcription factor GATA6 is essential for early extraembryonic development. Development 1999;126:723-32.
13. Ito E, Toki T, Ishihara H, et al. Erythroid transcription factor GATA-1 is abundantly transcribed in mouse testis. Nature 1993;362:466-68.
14. Zhou Y, Lim KC, Onodera K, et al. Rescue of the embryonic lethal hematopoietic defect reveals a critical role for GATA-2 in urogenital development. Embo J 1998;17:6689-700.

15. Zhou Y, Yamamoto M, Engel JD. GATA2 is required for the generation of V2 interneurons. Development 2000;127:3829-38.
16. Nardelli J, Thiesson D, Fujiwara Y, Tsai FY, Orkin SH. Expression and genetic interaction of transcription factors GATA-2 and GATA-3 during development of the mouse central nervous system. Dev Biol 1999;210:305-21.
17. Ma GT, Roth ME, Groskopf JC, et al. GATA-2 and GATA-3 regulate trophoblast-specific gene expression in vivo. Development 1997;124:907-14.
18. George KM, Leonard MW, Roth ME, et al. Embryonic expression and cloning of the murine GATA-3 gene. Development 1994;120:2673-86.
19. Lakshmanan G, Lieuw KH, Lim KC, et al. Localization of distant urogenital system-, central nervous system-, and endocardium-specific transcriptional regulatory elements in the GATA-3 locus. Mol Cell Biol 1999;19: 1558-68.
20. Van Doorninck JH, van Der Wees J, Karis A, et al. GATA-3 is involved in the development of serotonergic neurons in the caudal raphe nuclei. J Neurosci 1999;19:RC12.
21. Labastie MC, Catala M, Gregoire JM, Peault B. The GATA-3 gene is expressed during human kidney embryogenesis. Kidney Int 1995;47:1597-603.
22. Debacker C, Catala M, Labastie MC. Embryonic expression of the human GATA-3 gene. Mech Dev 1999;85:183-87.
23. Lim KC, Lakshmanan G, Crawford SE, Gu Y, Grosveld F, Engel JD. Gata3 loss leads to embryonic lethality due to noradrenaline deficiency of the sympathetic nervous system. Nat Genet 2000;25:209-12.
24. Pata I, Studer M, van Doorninck JH, et al. The transcription factor GATA3 is a downstream effector of Hoxb1 specification in rhombomere 4. Development 1999;126:5523-31.
25. Karis A, Pata I, van Doorninck JH, et al. Transcription factor GATA-3 alters pathway selection of olivocochlear neurons and affects morphogenesis of the ear. J Comp Neurol 2001;429:615-30.
26. Van Esch H, Groenen P, Nesbit MA, et al. GATA3 haplo-insufficiency causes human HDR syndrome. Nature 2000;406:419-22.
27. Muroya K, Hasegawa T, Ito Y, et al. GATA3 abnormalities and the phenotypic spectrum of HDR syndrome. J Med Genet 2001;38:374-80.
28. Nesbit MA, Bowl MR, Harding B, et al. Characterization of GATA3 mutations in the hypoparathyroidism, deafness, and renal dysplasia (HDR) syndrome. J Biol Chem 2004;279:22624-34.
29. Usary J, Llaca V, Karaca G, et al. Mutation of GATA3 in human breast tumors. Oncogene 2004;23:7669-78.
30. Garg V, Kathiriya IS, Barnes R, et al. GATA4 mutations cause human congenital heart defects and reveal an interaction with TBX5. Nature 2003; 424:443-47.
31. Pehlivan T, Pober BR, Brueckner M, et al. GATA4 haploinsufficiency in patients with interstitial deletion of chromosome region 8p23.1 and congenital heart disease. Am J Med Genet 1999;83:201-06.

32. Takahashi S, Shimizu R, Suwabe N, et al. GATA factor transgenes under GATA-1 locus control rescue germline GATA-1 mutant deficiencies. Blood 2000;96:910-16.
33. Ohneda K, Yamamoto M. Roles of hematopoietic transcription factors GATA-1 and GATA-2 in the development of red blood cell lineage. Acta Haematol 2002;108:237-45.
34. Zon LI, Tsai SF, Burgess S, Matsudaira P, Bruns GA, Orkin SH. The major human erythroid DNA-binding protein (GF-1): primary sequence and localization of the gene to the X chromosome. Proc Natl Acad Sci USA 1990; 87:668-72.
35. Hirasawa R, Shimizu R, Takahashi S, et al. Essential and instructive roles of GATA factors in eosinophil development. J Exp Med 2002;195:1379-86.
36. Harigae H, Takahashi S, Suwabe N, et al. Differential roles of GATA-1 and GATA-2 in growth and differentiation of mast cells. Genes Cells 1998;3: 39-50.
37. Shivdasani RA, Fujiwara Y, McDevitt MA, Orkin SH. A lineage-selective knockout establishes the critical role of transcription factor GATA-1 in megakaryocyte growth and platelet development. Embo J 1997;16:3965-73.
38. McDevitt MA, Fujiwara Y, Shivdasani RA, Orkin SH. An upstream, DNase I hypersensitive region of the hematopoietic-expressed transcription factor GATA-1 gene confers developmental specificity in transgenic mice. Proc Natl Acad Sci USA 1997;94:7976-81.
39. Onodera K, Takahashi S, Nishimura S, et al. GATA-1 transcription is controlled by distinct regulatory mechanisms during primitive and definitive erythropoiesis. Proc Natl Acad Sci USA 1997;94:4487-92.
40. Yu C, Cantor AB, Yang H, et al. Targeted deletion of a high-affinity GATA-binding site in the GATA-1 promoter leads to selective loss of the eosinophil lineage in vivo. J Exp Med 2002;195:1387-95.
41. Kobayashi M, Nishikawa K, Yamamoto M. Hematopoietic regulatory domain of gata1 gene is positively regulated by GATA1 protein in zebrafish embryos. Development 2001;128:2341-50.
42. Nishikawa K, Kobayashi M, Masumi A, et al. Self-association of Gata1 enhances transcriptional activity in vivo in zebra fish embryos. Mol Cell Biol 2003;23:8295-305.
43. Tsang AP, Visvader JE, Turner CA, et al. FOG, a multitype zinc finger protein, acts as a cofactor for transcription factor GATA-1 in erythroid and megakaryocytic differentiation. Cell 1997;90:109-19.
44. Tsang AP, Fujiwara Y, Hom DB, Orkin SH. Failure of megakaryopoiesis and arrested erythropoiesis in mice lacking the GATA-1 transcriptional cofactor FOG. Genes Dev 1998;12:1176-88.
45. De Maria R, Zeuner A, Eramo A, et al. Negative regulation of erythropoiesis by caspase-mediated cleavage of GATA-1. Nature 1999;401:489-93.
46. Rekhtman N, Radparvar F, Evans T, Skoultchi AI. Direct interaction of hematopoietic transcription factors PU.1 and GATA-1: functional antagonism in erythroid cells. Genes Dev 1999;13:1398-411.

47. Zhang P, Behre G, Pan J, et al. Negative cross-talk between hematopoietic regulators: GATA proteins repress PU.1. Proc Natl Acad Sci USA 1999;96: 8705-10.
48. Minegishi N, Suzuki N, Yokomizo T, et al. Expression and domain-specific function of GATA-2 during differentiation of the hematopoietic precursor cells in midgestation mouse embryos. Blood 2003;102:896-905.
49. Minegishi N, Ohta J, Suwabe N, et al. Alternative promoters regulate transcription of the mouse GATA-2 gene. J Biol Chem 1998;273:3625-34.
50. Pan X, Minegishi N, Harigae H, et al. Identification of human GATA-2 gene distal IS exon and its expression in hematopoietic stem cell fractions. J Biochem (Tokyo) 2000;127:105-12.
51. Minegishi N, Ohta J, Yamagiwa H, et al. The mouse GATA-2 gene is expressed in the para-aortic splanchnopleura and aorta-gonads and mesonephros region. Blood 1999;93:4196-207.
52. Grass JA, Boyer ME, Pal S, Wu J, Weiss MJ, Bresnick EH. GATA-1-dependent transcriptional repression of GATA-2 via disruption of positive autoregulation and domain-wide chromatin remodeling. Proc Natl Acad Sci USA 2003;100:8811-16.
53. Pal S, Cantor AB, Johnson KD, et al. Coregulator-dependent facilitation of chromatin occupancy by GATA-1. Proc Natl Acad Sci USA 2004;101:980-85.
54. Labastie MC, Cortes F, Romeo PH, Dulac C, Peault B. Molecular identity of hematopoietic precursor cells emerging in the human embryo. Blood 1998;92:3624-35.
55. Chen D, Zhang G. Enforced expression of the GATA-3 transcription factor affects cell fate decisions in hematopoiesis. Exp Hematol 2001;29:971-80.
56. Lieuw KH, Li G, Zhou Y, Grosveld F, Engel JD. Temporal and spatial control of murine GATA-3 transcription by promoter- proximal regulatory elements. Dev Biol 1997;188:1-16.
57. Lakshmanan G, Lieuw KH, Grosveld F, Engel JD. Partial rescue of GATA-3 by yeast artificial chromosome transgenes. Dev Biol 1998;204: 451-63.
58. Asnagli H, Afkarian M, Murphy KM. Cutting edge: Identification of an alternative GATA-3 promoter directing tissue-specific gene expression in mouse and human. J Immunol 2002;168:4268-71.
59. Burch JB. Regulation of GATA gene expression during vertebrate development. Semin Cell Dev Biol 2005;16:71-81.
60. Dame C, Juul SE. The switch from fetal to adult erythropoiesis. Clin Perinatol 2000;27:507-26.
61. Luo HY, Liang XL, Frye C, et al. Embryonic hemoglobins are expressed in definitive cells. Blood 1999;94:359-61.
62. Wu H, Liu X, Jaenisch R, Lodish HF. Generation of committed erythroid BFU-E and CFU-E progenitors does not require erythropoietin or the erythropoietin receptor. Cell 1995;83:59-67.
63. Neubauer H, Cumano A, Muller M, Wu H, Huffstadt U, Pfeffer K. Jak2 deficiency defines an essential developmental checkpoint in definitive hematopoiesis. Cell 1998;93:397-409.
64. Zon LI. Developmental biology of hematopoiesis. Blood 1995;86:2876-91.

65. Dieterlen-Lievre F. Intraembryonic hematopoietic stem cells. Hematol Oncol Clin North Am 1997;11:1149-71.
66. Ling KW, Ottersbach K, van Hamburg JP, et al. GATA-2 plays two functionally distinct roles during the ontogeny of hematopoietic stem cells. J Exp Med 2004;200:871-82.
67. Kelemen E, Calvo W, Fliedner TM. Atlas of human haematopoietic development. New York: Springer; 1979.
68. Charbord P, Tavian M, Humeau L, Peault B. Early ontogeny of the human marrow from long bones: an immunohistochemical study of hematopoiesis and its microenvironment. Blood 1996;87:4109-19.
69. Dame C, Sola MC, Fandrey J, et al. Developmental changes in the expression of transcription factors GATA-1, -2 and -3 during the onset of human medullary haematopoiesis. Br J Haematol 2002;119:510-15.
70. Tong Q, Dalgin G, Xu H, Ting CN, Leiden JM, Hotamisligil GS. Function of GATA transcription factors in preadipocyte-adipocyte transition. Science 2000;290:134-38.
71. Kaufman DS, Hanson ET, Lewis RL, Auerbach R, Thomson JA. Hematopoietic colony-forming cells derived from human embryonic stem cells. Proc Natl Acad Sci USA 2001;98:10716-21.
72. Weiss MJ, Keller G, Orkin SH. Novel insights into erythroid development revealed through in vitro differentiation of GATA-1 embryonic stem cells. Genes Dev 1994;8:1184-97.
73. Ikonomi P, Rivera CE, Riordan M, Washington G, Schechter AN, Noguchi CT. Overexpression of GATA-2 inhibits erythroid and promotes megakaryocyte differentiation. Exp Hematol 2000;28:1423-31.
74. Dame C, Fahnenstich H, Freitag P, et al. Erythropoietin mRNA expression in human fetal and neonatal tissue. Blood 1998;92:3218-25.
75. Imagawa S, Yamamoto M, Miura Y. Negative regulation of the erythropoietin gene expression by the GATA transcription factors. Blood 1997;89: 1430-39.
76. Lansdorp PM, Dragowska W, Mayani H. Ontogeny-related changes in proliferative potential of human hematopoietic cells. J Exp Med 1993;178: 787-91.
77. Emmerson AJ, Westwood NB, Rackham RA, Stern CM, Pearson TC. Erythropoietin responsive progenitors in anaemia of prematurity. Arch Dis Child 1991;66:810-11.
78. Moritz KM, Lim GB, Wintour EM. Developmental regulation of erythropoietin and erythropoiesis. Am J Physiol 1997;273:R1829-44.
79. Komatsu N, Fujita H. Induced megakaryocytic maturation of the human leukemia cell line UT-7 results in down-modulation of erythropoietin receptor gene expression. Cancer Res 1993;53:1156-61.
80. Migliaccio AR, Jiang Y, Migliaccio G, et al. Transcriptional and posttranscriptional regulation of the expression of the erythropoietin receptor gene in human erythropoietin-responsive cell lines. Blood 1993;82:3760-69.
81. Migliaccio AR, Migliaccio G, D'Andrea A, et al. Response to erythropoietin in erythroid subclones of the factor-dependent cell line 32D is determined

by translocation of the erythropoietin receptor to the cell surface. Proc Natl Acad Sci USA 1991;88:11086-90.
82. Maouche L, Cartron JP, Chretien S. Different domains regulate the human erythropoietin receptor gene transcription. Nucleic Acids Res 1994;22:338-46.
83. Zon LI, Youssoufian H, Mather C, Lodish HF, Orkin SH. Activation of the erythropoietin receptor promoter by transcription factor GATA-1. Proc Natl Acad Sci USA 1991;88:10638-41.
84. Chiba T, Ikawa Y, Todokoro K. GATA-1 transactivates erythropoietin receptor gene, and erythropoietin receptor-mediated signals enhance GATA-1 gene expression. Nucleic Acids Res. 1991;19:3843-48.
85. Suzuki N, Ohneda O, Takahashi S, et al. Erythroid-specific expression of the erythropoietin receptor rescued its null mutant mice from lethality. Blood 2002;100:2279-88.
86. Komatsu N, Kirito K, Kashii Y, et al. Cell-cycle-dependent regulation of erythropoietin receptor gene. Blood 1997;89:1182-188.
87. Stamatoyannopoulos G, Grosveld F. Hemoglobin switching. In: Stamatoyannopoulos G, Nienhuis AW, Majerus PW, Varmus H, eds. The molecular basis of blood diseases. Philadelphia: W.B. Saunders Comp.; 2001:135-82.
88. Higgs DR. Do LCRs open chromatin domains? Cell 1998;95:299-302.
89. Levings PP, Bungert J. The human beta-globin locus control region. Eur J Biochem 2002;269:1589-99.
90. Hardison R, Slightom JL, Gumucio DL, Goodman M, Stojanovic N, Miller W. Locus control regions of mammalian beta-globin gene clusters: combining phylogenetic analyses and experimental results to gain functional insights. Gene 1997;205:73-94.
91. Horak CE, Mahajan MC, Luscombe NM, Gerstein M, Weissman SM, Snyder M. GATA-1 binding sites mapped in the beta-globin locus by using mammalian chIp-chip analysis. Proc Natl Acad Sci USA 2002;99:2924-29.
92. Wadman IA, Osada H, Grutz GG, Agulnick AD, Westphal H, Forster A, Rabbitts TH. The LIM-only protein Lmo2 is a bridging molecule assembling an erythroid, DNA-binding complex which includes the TAL1, E47, GATA-1 and Ldb1/NLI proteins. Embo J 1997;16:3145-57.
93. Crossley M, Merika M, Orkin SH. Self-association of the erythroid transcription factor GATA-1 mediated by its zinc finger domains. Mol Cell Biol 1995;15:2448-56.
94. Merika M, Orkin SH. Functional synergy and physical interactions of the erythroid transcription factor GATA-1 with the Kruppel family proteins Sp1 and EKLF. Mol Cell Biol 1995;15:2437-47.
95. Orkin S. Transcription factors that regulate lineage decisions. In: Stamatoyannopoulos G, Majerus PW, Perlmutter R, Varmus H, eds. The molecular basis of blood diseases. Philadelphia: W.B. Saunders Comp.; 2001:80-102.
96. Madan A, Varma S, Cohen HJ. Developmental stage-specific expression of the erythropoietin gene and the α- and β-subunits of the HIF-1 protein. Pediatr Res 1997;41:217A (abstract).
97. Flake AW, Harrison MR, Adzick NS, Zanjani ED. Erythropoietin production by the fetal liver in an adult environment. Blood 1987;70:542-45.

98. Ratcliffe P. Sites of erythropoietin production. In: Jelkmann W. ed. Erythropoietin: Molecular biology and clinical use. Mountain Home, TN; FP Graham Publishing Co.; 2003.
99. Dame C, Sola MC, Lim KC, et al. Hepatic erythropoietin gene regulation by GATA-4. J Biol Chem. 2004;279:2955-61.
100. Imagawa S, Suzuki N, Ohmine K, et al. GATA suppresses erythropoietin gene expression through GATA site in mouse erythropoietin gene promoter. Int J Hematol 2002;75:376-81.
101. Nichols KE, Crispino JD, Poncz M, et al. Familial dyserythropoietic anaemia and thrombocytopenia due to an inherited mutation in GATA1. Nat Genet 2000;24:266-70.
102. Freson K, Devriendt K, Matthijs G, et al. Platelet characteristics in patients with X-linked macrothrombocytopenia because of a novel GATA1 mutation. Blood 2001;98:85-92.
103. Freson K, Thys C, Wittewrongel C, Vermylen J, Hoylaerts MF, Van Geet C. Molecular cloning and characterization of the GATA1 cofactor human FOG1 and assessment of its binding to GATA1 proteins carrying D218 substitutions. Hum Genet 2003;112:42-49.
104. Freson K, Matthijs G, Thys C, et al. Different substitutions at residue D218 of the X-linked transcription factor GATA1 lead to altered clinical severity of macrothrombocytopenia and anemia and are associated with variable skewed X inactivation. Hum Mol Genet 2002;11:147-52.
105. Mehaffey MG, Newton AL, Gandhi MJ, Crossley M, Drachman JG. X-linked thrombocytopenia caused by a novel mutation of GATA-1. Blood 2001;98:2681-88.
106. Yu C, Niakan KK, Matsushita M, Stamatoyannopoulos G, Orkin SH, Raskind WH. X-linked thrombocytopenia with thalassemia from a mutation in the amino finger of GATA-1 affecting DNA binding rather than FOG-1 interaction. Blood 2002;100:2040-45.
107. Letting DL, Chen YY, Rakowski C, Reedy S, Blobel GA. Context-dependent regulation of GATA-1 by friend of GATA-1. Proc Natl Acad Sci USA 2004;101:476-81.
108. Wechsler J, Greene M, McDevitt MA, et al. Acquired mutations in GATA1 in the megakaryoblastic leukemia of Down syndrome. Nat Genet 2002;32: 148-52.
109. Zipursky A. Transient leukaemia--a benign form of leukaemia in newborn infants with trisomy 21. Br J Haematol 2003;120:930-38.
110. Hitzler JK, Cheung J, Li Y, Scherer SW, Zipursky A. GATA1 mutations in transient leukemia and acute megakaryoblastic leukemia of Down syndrome. Blood 2003;101:4301-04.
111. Groet J, McElwaine S, Spinelli M, et al. Acquired mutations in GATA1 in neonates with Down's syndrome with transient myeloid disorder. Lancet 2003;361:1617-20.
112. Rainis L, Bercovich D, Strehl S, et al. Mutations in exon 2 of GATA1 are early events in megakaryocytic malignancies associated with trisomy 21. Blood 2003;102:981-86.

113. Xu G, Nagano M, Kanezaki R, et al. Frequent mutations in the GATA-1 gene in the transient myeloproliferative disorder of Down syndrome. Blood 2003;102:2960-68.
114. Mundschau G, Gurbuxani S, Gamis AS, Greene ME, Arceci RJ, Crispino JD. Mutagenesis of GATA1 is an initiating event in Down syndrome leukemogenesis. Blood 2003;101:4298-300.
115. Taub JW, Mundschau G, Ge Y, et al. Prenatal origin of GATA1 mutations may be an initiating step in the development of megakaryocytic leukemia in Down syndrome. Blood 2004;104:1588-89.
116. Gurbuxani S, Vyas P, Crispino JD. Recent insights into the mechanisms of myeloid leukemogenesis in Down syndrome. Blood 2004;103:399-406.
117. Shimizu R, Takahashi S, Ohneda K, Engel JD, Yamamoto M. In vivo requirements for GATA-1 functional domains during primitive and definitive erythropoiesis. Embo J 2001;20:5250-60.
118. Calligaris R, Bottardi S, Cogoi S, Apezteguia I, Santoro C. Alternative translation initiation site usage results in two functionally distinct forms of the GATA-1 transcription factor. Proc Natl Acad Sci USA 1995;92:11598-602.
119. Moi P, Loudianos G, Lavinha J, et al. Delta-thalassemia due to a mutation in an erythroid-specific binding protein sequence 3' to the delta-globin gene. Blood 1992;79:512-16.
120. Matsuda M, Sakamoto N, Fukumaki Y. Delta-thalassemia caused by disruption of the site for an erythroid-specific transcription factor, GATA-1, in the delta-globin gene promoter. Blood 1992;80:1347-51.
121. Ludlow LB, Schick BP, Budarf ML, et al. Identification of a mutation in a GATA binding site of the platelet glycoprotein Ibbeta promoter resulting in the Bernard-Soulier syndrome. J Biol Chem 1996;271:22076-80.
122. Manco L, Ribeiro ML, Maximo V, et al. A new PKLR gene mutation in the R-type promoter region affects the gene transcription causing pyruvate kinase deficiency. Br J Haematol 2000;110:993-97.
123. Solis C, Aizencang GI, Astrin KH, Bishop DF, Desnick RJ. Uroporphyrinogen III synthase erythroid promoter mutations in adjacent GATA1 and CP2 elements cause congenital erythropoietic porphyria. J Clin Invest 2001; 107:753-62.
124. Cantor AB, Orkin SH. Transcriptional regulation of erythropoiesis: an affair involving multiple partners. Oncogene 2002;21:3368-76.

DEVELOPMENT OF THE IMMUNE SYSTEM IN THE FOETAL AND PERINATAL PERIOD

G.T. Rijkers[1], T. Niers[2], W. de Jager[1], P. Janssens[1], K. Gaiser[1], S. Wiertsema[1], S. Hoeks[3], L. van de Corput[1], E.A.M. Sanders[1].

During embryogenesis, the first haematopoietic cells develop outside the embryo, in the yolk sac. Then, in the 6th week of pregnancy, committed haematopoietic stem cells develop in the mesoderm of the fetus, the so-called aorta-gonad-mesonephros (AGM) region. Whether these haematopoietic stem cells are generated from endothelial cells within the aortic floor or originate from mesodermal cells (either within or below the aortic floor) remains a matter of debate [1]. Subsequently, haematopoietic stem cells migrate to the fetal liver and there initiate the erythropoiesis [2] In week 7 cells seed the developing thymus. Seeding into the bone marrow occurs much later (by week 20) [3, 4]. In the thymus, T lymphocytes develop that express either the $\alpha\beta$ T cell receptor or the $\gamma\delta$ receptor. The processes involved are rearrangement of the T cell receptors, positive selection on MHC followed by negative selection for self-antigens. Note that the development of the T cell repertoire is antigen independent. Development of Natural Killer (NK) cells as well as various dendritic cells (DC) also takes place in the thymus. In bone marrow, B lymphocytes, granulocytes, monocytes and DC develop. The development of lymphoid cells and organs is a complex process that requires timely expression of growth factors (cytokines, chemokines), receptors as well as adhesion molecules. As already stated above, development of the immune system is, apart from maternal-fetal transfer, independent of antigen (either bacterial, viral or allergenic).

Also for the immune system, birth marks a fundamental change in the demand put upon the system. When children are born, they emerge from the relatively sterile environment of the uterus into a world teeming with bacteria. Within the first days of life, mucosal surfaces of the gastrointestinal as well as respiratory tract become colonized with bacterial communities [5]. The neonate has passive acquired immunity as well as active immunity to combat these potential pathogenic micro-organisms.

Passive acquired immunity is provided by maternal immunoglobulins.During the last semester of pregnancy there is active transport of maternal IgG across the placenta so that after full term pregnancy the IgG levels in the neonate equal that of the mother (Figure 1). IgM and IgA antibodies are not able to be trans-

1. Wilhelmina Children's Hospital, Dept Pediatric Immunology, University Medical Center, Utrecht, NL.
2. item, Dept General Pediatrics, University Medical Center, Utrecht, NL.
3. item, Dept Neonatology, University Medical Center, Utrecht, NL.

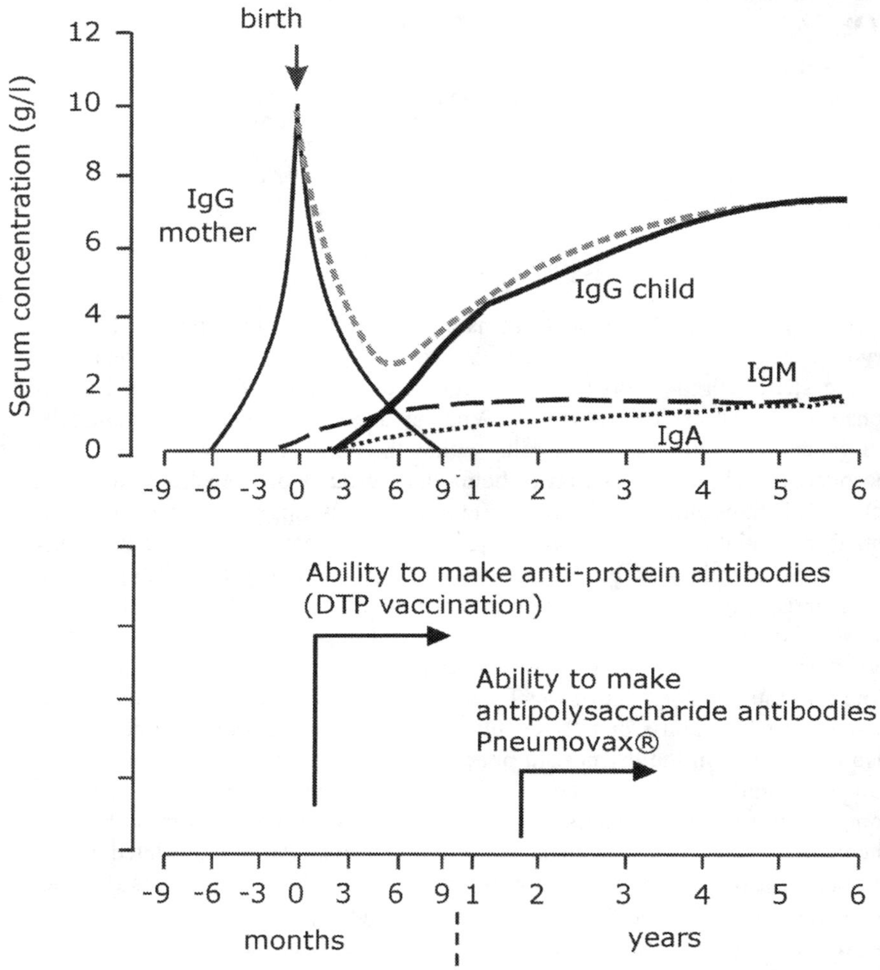

Figure 1. Development of immunoglobulin and antibody synthesis.

ported transplacentally and develop gradually. However, breast fed babies do receive IgA antibodies from their mother.

At birth, the lymphoid system although being developed, is not mature yet. All lymphocytes are naïve, i.e. have not yet encountered antigen. Naïve and memory T lymphocytes can be discerned by their respective expression of the CD45RA and CD45RO molecule. Figure 2 shows that all CD4 T lymphocytes of the human neonate are of the naïve phenotype (all CD8 T lymphocytes also are naïve; not shown). Activation of T lymphocytes results in a response that is biased towards a Th2 cytokine production pattern with relative little production of γ-interferon and more IL-4 and IL-5 [7]. The reasons for this skewing are unclear; it may be that the differentiation pathway in the absence of antigenic

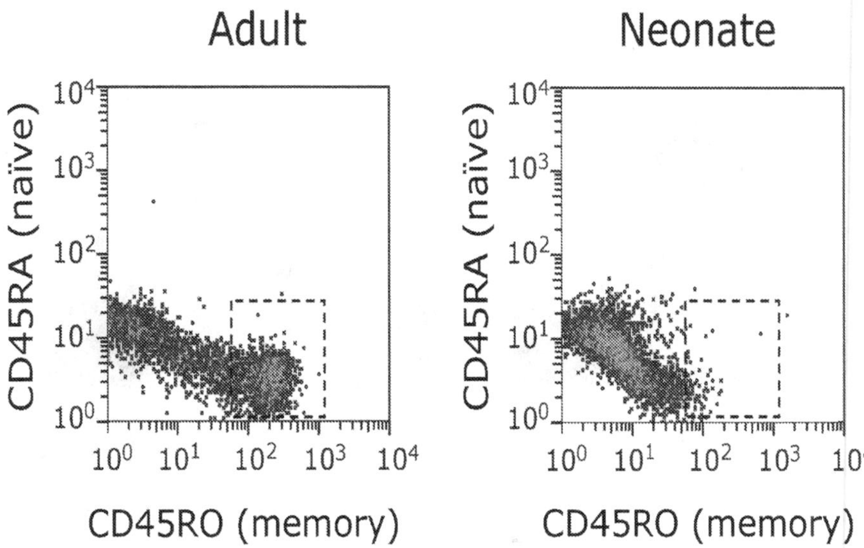

Figure 2. Phenotype of neonatal T lymphocytes. Cord blood and adult blood lymphocytes were stained with CD4-PerCP, CD45RO-PE, and FITC conjugated CD45RA. Depicted are CD45RA (naïve) and CD45RO (memory) expression on CD4 gated T lymphocytes. Boxed area encompasses $CD45RO^{+}CD45RA^{-}$ memory CD4 T cells.

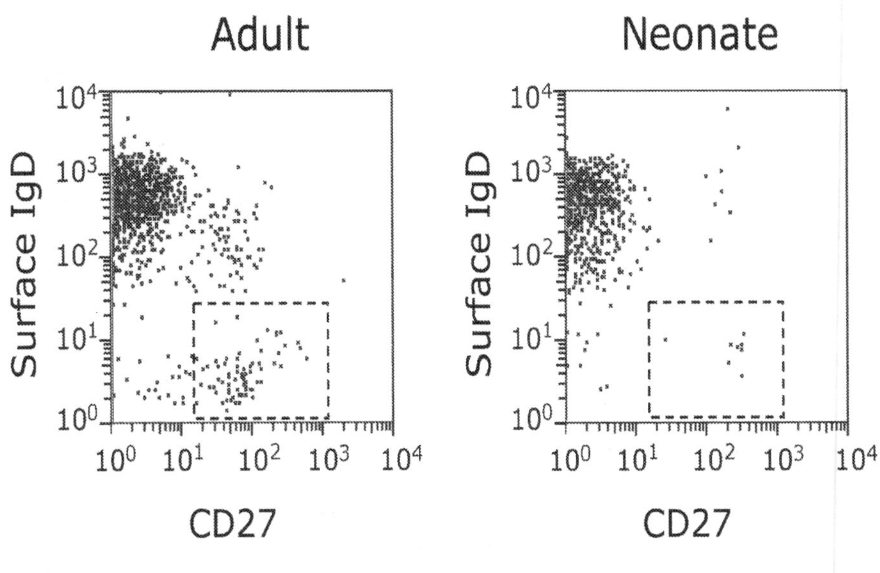

Figure 3. Phenotype of neonatal B lymphocytes. Cord blood and adult blood lymphocytes were stained with CD19-PerCP, CD27-PE, and FITC conjugated anti-IgD. Depicted are surface IgD and CD27 expression on CD19 gated B lymphocytes. Boxed area encompasses switched (surface IgD^{-}) memory ($CD27^{+}$) B cells.

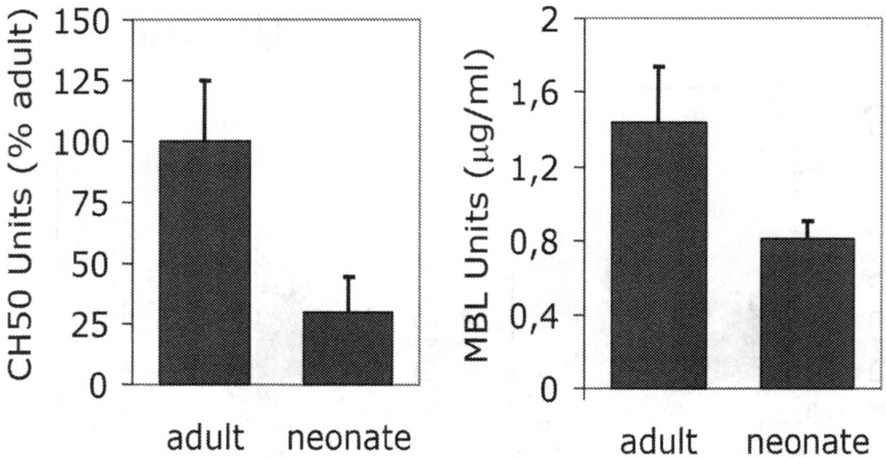

Figure 4. Complement activity in the newborn. Serum samples from 14 healthy adults and 32 (aterm and premature) neonates were tested for complement activity. Complement activity was initiated either through the classical pathway (CH50) on sheep red blood cells sensitized with rabbit antibodies (Amboceptor, RIVM, Bilthoven, The Netherlands) or through the mannose binding lectin (MBL) pathway. Latter pathway was activated by mannose on the surface of Saccharomyces cerevisae and measured as bystander lysis of chicken erythrocytes (Kuipers et al. JIM 2002). CH50 activity was expressed relative to pooled normal human serum; MBL activity was calibrated on a standard serum containing 1.670 µg/ml functional MBL.

stimuli is biased to Th2 [7]. Alternatively, the immature phenotypes of antigen presenting cells, or differential expression of signalling molecules (STAT4, STAT6) or transcription factors (T-bet, GATA3) may also contribute to this bias.

At birth, like the T lymphocytes, the B lymphocytes also are naïve and immature. Within the neonatal B cell population there is a high fraction of cells expressing the CD5 molecule, a population referred to as B1 B cells [8]. Furthermore, because memory B lymphocytes have not developed yet, the population of B lymphocytes which have lost expression of surface IgD and acquired expression of CD27 is absent in the neonate [9] (see also Figure 3). Yet, the neonate is able to mount an antibody response upon primary infection or upon primary vaccination with protein based vaccines. Neonates however are unable to respond to polysaccharide antigens, making them extra vulnerable to infections with polysaccharide encapsulated bacteria such as group B Streptococci and pneumococci. Limiting dilution analysis of neonatal B cells, which were polyclonally activated by a combination of phorbol esters and calcium ionophore, showed that polysaccharide B cells are present in cord blood, in a frequency comparable to that in adults [10]. Apparently, the necessary co-stimulatory molecules are not expressed on polysaccharide specific neonatal B lymphocytes. We have demonstrated that bacterial polysaccharides are able to activate complement through the alternative pathway and that C3d fragments which are generated during this process are bound on the polysaccharide molecule [11]. The complex of polysaccharide and C3d that is thus formed has the ability to co-crosslink the antigen receptors (on polysaccharide specific B lymphocytes) with the C3d receptor (CD21). CD21 is expressed on B lymphocytes in a molecular complex that also contains CD19 and CD81; the cytoplasmic domain of CD19 provides additional synergistic signals for B lymphocyte activation. B lymphocytes of neonates and young children show little or no expression of CD21 which precludes proper co-stimulation and therefore probably explains their inability to respond to polysaccharide antigens [12,13].

As indicated above, the neonatal immune system needs further maturation to reach full immunocompetence. This also holds true for the innate immune system. The most important form of humoral innate immunity is the complement system. The major routes of complement activation are the classical pathway, initiated by binding of C1q to antigen-antibody complexes and the MBL route, initiated by binding of mannose binding lectin to mannose residues on bacterial surfaces (as well as other bacterial compounds, for that matter) [15]. Both forms of complement are detectable in neonates, although the level of functional activity is reduced as compared to adults (see also Figure 4) .

Post-natally, the gastro-intestinal tract as well as the upper respiratory tract (nasopharynx) become colonized with micro-organisms [5]. The spectrum of commensal and pathogenic micro-organisms (and the corresponding pathogen-associated molecular patterns, PAMPs) to which the immune system is exposed is immense. The broad repertoire of the specific immune system allows to respond to virtually every trigger. It is now realized, however, that the immune system does not respond to every stimulus, but rather responds to "danger signals" from the environment. The emerging mechanism is that PAMPs are recognized by a polymorphic repertoire of receptors of the innate and adaptive immune system [15,16] and this will shape the direction of development of the immune system of child- and adulthood.

References

1. Le Douarin NM. The Claude Bernard lecture,.1987 Embryonic chimeras: a tool for studying the development of the nervous and immune systems. Proc R Soc Lond B Biol Sci, 1988;235:1-17.
2. Marshall CJ, Thrasher AJ. The embryonic origins of human haematopoiesis. Br J Haematol, 2001;112:838-50.
3. Bodey B, Bodey B Jr, Siegel SE, Kaiser HE. Intrathymic non-lymphatic hematopoiesis during mammalian ontogenesis. In Vivo, 1998;12:599-618.
4. Plum J, De Smedt M, Verhasselt B, et al. Human T lymphopoiesis. In vitro and in vivo study models. Ann N Y Acad Sci, 2000;917:724-31.
5. Favier CF, Vaughan EE, de Vos WM, Akkermans ADL. Molecular monitoring of succession of bacterial communities in human neonates. Appl Environm Microbiol, 2002; 68:219-16.
6. Liew FY. T(H)1 and T(H)2 cells: a historical perspective. Nature Rev Immunol, 2002;2:55-60.

7. Wills-Karp M, Santeliz J, Karp CL. The germless theory of allergic disease: revisiting the hygiene hypothesis. Nature Rev Immunol, 2001;1:69-75
8. Berland R, Wortis HH. Origins and functions of B-1 cells with notes on the role of CD5. Annu Rev Immunol, 2002;20:253-300.
9. Agematsu K, Nagumo H, Yang FC, et al. B cell subpopulations separated by CD27 and crucial collaboration of CD27+ B cells and helper T cells in immunoglobulin production. Eur J Immunol, 1997;27:2073-79.
10. Rijkers GT, Dollekamp I, Zegers BJ. 8-Mercaptoguanosine overcomes unresponsiveness of human neonatal B cells to polysaccharide antigens. J Immunol, 1988;141:2313-16.
11. Griffioen AW, Rijkers GT, Janssens-Korpela P, Zegers BJM. Pneumococcal polysaccharides complexed with C3d bind to human B lymphocytes via complement receptor type 2. Infect Immun, 1991; 59:1839-45.
12. Griffioen AW, Toebes EAH, Zegers BJM, Rijkers GT. Role of the CR2 in the human adult and neonatal in vitro antibody response to type 4 pneumococcal polysaccharide. Cell Immunol, 1992;143:11-22.
13. Peset LM, Harms G, Hardonk MJ, Timens W.. Human immune response to pneumococcal polysaccharides: complement- mediated localization preferentially on CD21-positive splenic marginal zone B cells and follicular dendritic cells. J Allergy Clin Immunol, 1996;97:1015-24.
14. Fujita T. Evolution of the lectin–complement pathway and its role in innate immunity. Nature Rev Immunol 2002;2:346-53.
15. Medzhitov R. Toll-like receptors and innate immunity. Nature Rev Immunol, 2001;1:135-45.
16. Kopp E, Medzhitov R. Recognition of microbial infection by Toll-like receptors. Curr Opin Immunol, 2003;15:396-401.

FOETAL AND NEONATAL IMMUNOHAEMATOLOGICAL RESPONSES: CONSEQUENCES FOR PRACTICAL MANAGEMENT?

A. Brand[1,2], F. Walther[3], S. Scherjon[4], J. v Beckhoven[1], H. Vietor[2], C. Meyer[5], M. Jansen[5], H.H.H. Kanhai[4]

Introduction

In physiological circumstances the foetal immune system matures in an environment which is – except the foeto-maternal exchange – sterile and devoid from alloantigens. The immune system of the new born is thought to be qualitatively normal, but naïve and memory cells have not yet been established. Indeed, clinical reports show at one hand that the foetus is capable to reject allogeneic haematopoietic stem cells from the 14-16th gestational week onwards [1]. At the other hand the quantitative response is impaired and cord blood transplantation in adults (albeit based on limited numbers) suggest that the capacity to respond in the Graft versus Host (GvHD) direction is reduced. At the level of the B cell, the neonate does not produce immunoglobulins, The neonatal B cells fail to up-regulate co-stimulatory factors, while also a lack of specific T cell helper factors may exist. With respect to the innate immune system, the foetal macrophages are capable of ADC (antigen dependent cytotoxicity) as reflected by alloimmune haemolytic disease, but resistance to microbial infections is impaired. This is attributed to impaired opsonizing capacity of granulocytes and macrophages due to the low levels of immunoglobulins and complement [2].

There are controversial in-vitro observations on the immunological potentials of neonates, in particular with functional tests. Some of these discrepancies can be explained by differences in techniques used. For example, for functional assays cells are washed and processed in-vitro, removing to a variable extent soluble factors present in neonatal plasma which may play a role. There is agreement that at birth, the neonatal cord blood (CB) of healthy new borns comprises almost exclusively of naïve, non-primed CD45RA+ T cells and a minority co-express the memory CD45RO phenotype. This differs from adult T cells, expressing in approximately 50% a memory CD45RO phenotype. In case of intrauterine infections CD45RO cells are up-regulated [3] in association with cytokine production and the foetus can produce considerable amounts of immu-

1. Sanquin Division Blood Bank Southwest, Leiden, NL.
2. Immunohaematology & Blood Tranfusion Service LUMC, Leiden, NL.
3. Department of Neonatology LUMC, Leiden, NL.
4. Department of Obstetrics LUMC, Leiden, NL.
5. Undergraduate students, University of Leiden, Leiden, NL.

.ature increased CD45RO expression and presence of IgA .ood are indicative for an intra-uterine infection. With respect .mune system the complement and mannin-binding lectin levels .n in adults, these levels are even lower in preterm neonates. Al- .ood products, either administered to the foetus or to the mother, may .ne foetus to foreign allo-antigens and to the immunomodulatory effects .od transfusions. The effects of blood transfusions on the foetal immune .tem have hardly been studied, while studies in neonates mainly addressed the question of allo-antibody formation, which is severely impaired. We evaluated some immunological effects of transfusion therapy in pregnancy, with emphasis on the cellular immune response.

Foetal and Neonatal Transfusions

The highest risk for foetal blood transfusions is present in otherwise healthy children with haemolytic disease due to maternal antibodies against a red cell- or platelet-antigen, inherited from the father. After birth alloimmune diseases are transient, although some (exchange) transfusions may be needed. Among neonates, preterm new borns in particular with a very low birth weight (VLBW) below 1000 gram, are most heavily transfused.

Because of reported cases of transfusion-associated GvHD and transmission of Cytomegalovirus, blood products intended for foetal or VLBW prematures are currently leukocyte reduced by filtration and gamma-irradiated [4,5]. In the sixty's and seventy's, blood transfusions for severe Rh-D haemolytic disease, were given in the foetal peritoneal cavity. These transfusions were neither leukocyte reduced, nor irradiated.

Most fetal and neonatal transfusions are red cell products. A minority receive platelet transfusions. Intrauterine platelet transfusions (IUPT) are administered to a fetus with severe potentially life-threatening alloimmune thrombocytopenia, often with a sibling with an intra-cranial haemorrhage. The primary treatment for fetal/neonatal alloimmune thrombocytopenia (FNAIT) is weekly maternal administration of high dose intravenous immunoglobulin (IVIG); while IUPT is reserved for treatment-resistant cases.

We studied the immune response to allogeneic transfusions in several cohorts of patients. Long-term effects could be studied in young adult patients surviving more than 20 years after intraperitoneal transfusions because of HDN and in infants treated for FNAIT. Short term effects of intrauterine transfusions, both for HDN and FNAIT, were measured in cord blood at birth. Besides changes in the T cell repertoire short-term effects showed decrease of natural killer (NK) cells after erythrocyte transfusions. This effect was further explored in premature children (Table 1).

Long-Term Effects of Intraperitoneal Transfusions with Non-Leukocyte Reduced, Non-Irradiated Red Cells

In older literature it was reported that in almost half of the cases after intra-peritoneal or neonatal exchange transfusions, a large proportion (up to 50%) of

Table 1. Populations studied for the effects of intrauterine /neonatal transfusions T cells (CTLp)

Research questions	Patients studied
Long-term effects: – Clinical outcome – Tolerance – Immunisation – Chimerism	Patients with HDN who survived 25 years after non-irradiated, non-leukocyte reduced intraperitoneal blood transfusions Infants of 2-7 years after NAIT treatment
Short-term effects in-utero and at birth: – Premature T cell maturation	Patients with HDN treated with intrauterine leukocyte reduced and irradiated red cells Newborns with NAIT treated with maternally high dose immunoglobulins
Immediate effects: – Innate immune system – Susceptibility for infections	Pre and post intrauterine red cell transfusions Effects of red cell transfusions in preterm new borns

donor leukocytes persisted for many years [6]. In the period 1966-75, in our centre 75 foetuses were treated with intraperitoneal non-irradiated, non-leukocyte reduced transfusions because of Rh-D haemolytic disease. Twenty-four (34%) were born alive and survived the neonatal period. Of these 24 infants, 2 died as child after renal transplantation and 1 as adolescent in a car accident and 1 suffered from broncho-pneumonial dysplasia with many hospitalisations. The remaining 20 young adults, between 21-28 years, showed an excellent clinical well-being and neuro-developmental outcome, not at variance with a matched control cohort. Of 9 of the 21 cases at least one of the donor(s) of intraperitoneal transfusions could be traced and consented to give blood for the study. We determined the cytotoxic precursor Table 1: Populations studied for the effects of intrauterine/neonatal transfusions T cells (CTLp) and helper precursor T cells (HTLp) against these donor(s) and compared this with the responses against an unrelated mismatched (third party) donor.

The CTLp and HTLp values were not depressed. In 3/9 cases even a higher response ($226\text{-}417/10^6$ CTLp) against the transfusion donor than against a third party control ($<162/10^6$) was observed. Further analysis made it however unlikely that the higher responses in these 3 cases were the result of memory cells, because the CTLp could be easily blocked by anti-CD8, while memory cells are in-vitro rather resistant against treatment with anti-CD8. The natural killer cell (NK) functions of all individuals was normal. Using X and Y-chromosome fluorescence in-situ hybridisation (FISH, sensitivity 0.1%)) there were no donor cells detectable in the circulation after this interval of at least 20 years. The results show that no long-term immunisation, tolerance or donor chimerism was present [7]. It should be realised however that the results may be biased by the fact that only surviving cases could be tested. Two-third of the children had died before or early after birth, most likely from haemolytic disease, but it is not excluded that transfusion-induced mortality e.g. by TA-GvHD might have played a role as well.

Effects of Maternally Administered High Dose Immunoglobulin (IVIG) and Platelet Transfusions (IUPT) in Infant Hood

Placental transmission of maternal IgG occurs from about 12 weeks of gestation onwards, resulting in passive immunity for the first months of life. IgA and IgM antibodies are virtually absent at birth and gradually increase in childhood in response to environmental antigens. Antenatal treatment for fetal/neonatal alloimmune thrombocytopenia (FNAIT) exposes the maturing fetal immune system to foreign alloantigens in IVIG and platelet transfusions. Besides, IVIG has immunomodulatory effects on several axis of the immune response [8]. Among other effects, IVIG skews the immune response towards a T helper 2 type direction.

We determined the health status, emphasising on infections and atopic constitution, of 50 children treated for FNAIT over a period of 10 years in our centre. Nine infants had been treated with IUPT alone, 26 with IUPT in combination with IVIG and 11 with IVIG alone. In four children only foetal blood sampling (FBS) was performed, revealing a normal foetal platelet count. The median period of maternal IVIG administration (1 g/kg/weekly) was 5 weeks (2-12 weeks) and the median number of IUPT was 1 (1-9). In the neonatal period eleven children needed platelet transfusion(s), four received platelet transfusion(s) and high dose IVIG and one received IVIG treatment alone.

Except one neonatal death (2 %) and one child lost to follow-up (2 %), the total follow-up rate was 96 % (48/50). The median age of the children at follow-up was 5.1 years (1.3-11.6 years). For follow-up we distinguished infants treated with IVIG with or without IUPT (n = 37) and 'No IVIG' (n = 13). The occurrence of higher airway infections and asthma was investigated with a standardized WHO-questionnaire [9]. In 17 children older than 5 years, plasma IgM-, IgA-, IgG-(subclasses) and IgE levels were measured.

Productive coughing occurred more frequently in the study group than in a normal population of Dutch school children (14 % and 1.7 %, respectively) . An unexpected observation was the influence of IVIG on the occurrence of ENT(ear-nose-throat) problems in the infants. ENT- and hearing problems were seen in the group of children treated with IVIG in 19 % and 3 %, respectively, which is comparable to the occurrence in the normal Dutch population, 20 % and 3 %, respectively [10]. However, in the group of children treated without IVIG, 58 % ENT- and 42 % hearing problems were reported. These results suggest possible adverse effects of fetal IUPT but no adverse effect or even a favorable influence of IVIG on susceptibility for ENT- and hearing problems compared to antenatal treatment without IVIG. The total IgG, IgG1-4 subclasses, IgA and IgM-levels were within the normal range for age and similar in children exposed to IVIG or not exposed to IVIG. Remarkably, in 7/10 children (70%) after maternal treatment with high dose IVIG, the IgE levels were higher than in the normal population adjusted for age and compared to the 1/7 children that had been treated for FNAIT without IVIG (15%) (p = 0.05) and compared to a normal population. But, these higher levels were not associated with clinical expressions of increased allergic or atopic reactions.

Table 2. Associations between antenatal treatment with or without IVIG and outcome

	IVIG **N = 37**	**No IVIG** **N =13**	**p**
Perinatal features:			
– GA wks – median (range)	37 (32-30)	38 (34-40)	NS
– BW (kg) – median (range)	2,8 (1,3-4,1)	2,9 (2,1-3,8)	NS
Susceptibility to:			
– ENT-problems	7/36 (19 %)	75/12 (42%)	0.02
– Hearing problems	1/36 (3 %)	5/12 (58 %)	0.002
– Pulmonary problems	4/36 (11 %)	4/12 (33 %)	NS
– Allergies	3/35 (9 %)	1/12 (8 %)	NS
– Eczema	6/36 (17 %)	2/12 (17 %)	NS

IVIG = maternal IVIG treatment ; No IVIG = fetal blood sampling (FBS) and/ or intrauterine platelet transfusion (IUPT), without IVIG; n = number; NS = not significant; GA = age of gestation; Preterm delivery <37 weeks; Pulmonary problems: Wheezing, productive coughing and pulmonary medication

High IgE and allergic diseases (asthma, rhinitis and dermatitis) are associated with an imbalance of Th-function towards an increased Th2-reaction [11]. However, none of those associated clinical manifestations of a Th2 was observed in any of the children. Increased IgG4-levels that have been described in atopic individuals were not found. An explanation for this intriguing finding is not unequivocal, since the immunomodulating effects of IVIG are described to be reversible [8]. In addition, due to the small number of our study population, confounding can not be excluded.

In conclusion antenatal treatment with IVIG in FNAIT seems to have less adverse effects than IUPT without IVIG. Antenatal IVIG seems to offer relative protection against infections and hearing problems in childhood when compared to antenatal treatment with IUPT/ FBS without IVIG [12] .Whether IVIG stimulates IgE antibodies and the clinical consequences on the longer term needs follow-up of larger patient cohorts.

Short Term Effects of Intrauterine Erythrocyte Transfusions (despite leukocyte reduction and gamma irradiation)

T Cell Maturation and NK Cell Suppression

For this purpose we compared the phenotypes of cord blood mononuclear cells from 14 new borns, treated with a mean of 3 (1-6) IUET. The first transfusion was administered between the 19th and 34th week (average 27 weeks) of gestation. Delivery took place at 37 weeks (range 32-39 weeks). Cord blood from 18 neonates, born after a gestational age of 40 weeks (38-41), served as control.

Haematological values of IUET treated new borns showed no difference in absolute number of leukocytes and leukocyte differentiation compared to controls. As expected the haemoglobin level of HDN children was lower and the proportion erythroblast and reticulocytes higher. Five of 14 HDN new borns had thrombocytopenia (platelet count 16-150 x 10^9/L) and the CD34 % was 3.1 % compared to 1% in the controls (Table 3).

Table 3: Cord blood values after IUET versus controls

	IUT (N=14) Mean (range)	Control (N=18) Mean (range)	P
Hb mmol/L	6.3 (3.6-8.9)	9.8 (8.4-10.7)	<0.0001
WBC x 109/L	15.2 (5.6-24.7)	16.8 (8.8-34.3)	NS
Reticulocytes109/L	0.03 (0-0.18)	0.00 (0-0.06)	NS
Erythroblasts109/L	80 (2-574)	6 (0-28)	0.026
Platelets109/L	173 (16-383)	235 (180-322)	0.0375
Lymphocytes (%)*	31 (12-52)	29 (12-45)	NS
Monocytes (%)	9 (4-13)	9 (3-19)	NS
NK (CD57)	0.0 (0-6)	1.4 (0-6)	0.0001 #
T cells:			
– CD3	49 (30-80)	51 (33-70)	NS
– CD3/CD4	31 (7-57)	33 (13-40)	NS
– CD3/CD8	20 (6-33)	19 (13-35)	NS
– CD3/CD45RA	43 (0-73)	47 (14-86)	NS
– CD45/RO	8 (0-28)	2 (0-7)	<0.0091$
B-cells:			
– CD19	19 (8-29)	16 (9-23)	NS
– CD19/CD5	7 (3-13)	6 (2-12)	NS
Activation markers:			
– CD25	2.9 (0-30)	2.9 (1-15)	NS
– HLA-DR	36 (14-63)	36 (25-50)	NS

Mean % and range % within CD45 cells after substraction of Glycophorin A+ cells.# Corrected P-value after multiparameter analysis 0.0016;$ p corrected for multivariate analysis 0.1493 (NS).

The proportion of CD4 and CD8 cells was similar in both groups, but the T cells expressing the memory phenotype CD45RO$^+$ was with 8% (0-28%) higher than the 2% (0-7%) observed in controls. Compared to controls, who compared to adults, already show a very low level of cytotoxic NK cells (CD56$^+$) and non-cytotoxic NK cells (CD57$^+$), these values are lower (CD16$^+$CD56$^+$) or even absent (CD57) in CB of IUET treated new borns. These differences were significant at the univariate level but, except CD57, lost significance after correction for the number of variables tested [13].

It can be concluded from this small study that after several IUET's there seems to be premature maturation of T cells, reflected by a higher average % of CD45RO$^+$ .A cut-off level of 17% is used as indication for intrauterine infection [14], which was not present in our patients, while 2/14 new borns showed levels of 20 and 27%. Our study confirmed the finding of the group of Nicolaides, who also found that NK cells and associated markers are depressed after IUET [15].

T-Cell Receptor V Beta Usage After IUET

In order to evaluate the nature of premature T cell maturation we compared the development of the 24 identified different T cell receptor V-beta (TCRBV) families of 5 foetuses before and 7-8 weeks after intrauterine transfusions with 5 newborns who underwent foetal blood sampling (FBS) but no transfusions. This approach was chosen because of a previous report in dialysis patients showing that pretransplantation blood transfusions could profoundly change the composition of the TCRVB repertoire [16] and that prolonged survival of donor leukocytes was associated with complete deletions of some TCRBV families [17]. We first investigated all identified 24 TCRVB family members by semi-quantitative PCR using TCRVB family-specific oligonucleotide primers [18]. Subsequently we performed spectratyping of a selection of families that showed changes by semi-quantitative PCR. All except 1 foetus expressed all (24) TCRVB families at the moment of the first foetal blood sampling, while 1 HDN patient lacked TCRVB 17 and 19-24 gene expression in the CD 4^+ population at 32 weeks. At birth these genes were detectable at low levels. In IUET treated patients and FBS controls the TCRBV repertoire within the $CD8^+$ T subset underwent considerable alterations in usage frequencies during gestation. This rather reflects ongoing maturation within this T cell compartment and this prohibited to conclude on transfusion induced alterations. In contrast the TCRVB repertoire of the $CD4^+$ T cell subset seems to be completed at the gestational time of first FBS and did not show alterations in the control group. But in 4 out of 5 patients with HDN significant changes in the TCRVB usage within the $CD4^+$ T cell subset had occurred. Although this was probably induced by transfusions we cannot rule out a role for HDN itself. Transfusions did not cause alterations in specific TCRVB families but resulted in apparently random increase and decrease of usage of several families. We subsequently evaluated whether the semi-quantitative changes of some TCRVB usage observed by PCR could be confirmed by determination of the length of the complementary determining region 3 (CDR3) sizes by spectratyping. We found no indication of qualitative differences in CDR3 lengths before and after transfusions and must therefore conclude that all differences were quantitative. Even in 1 foetus of 23 weeks old, who had received a HLA-B,DR shared transfusion and responded with an enormous expansion of the TCRVB21 family within the $CD4^+$ population in the PCR, spectratyping showed no changes in the distribution of the CDR3 lengths.

Finally we tested the alloproliferative responses of IUET treated foetuses against their IUT donors and against third party cells and found a stronger responses against the IUT donors, indicative of establishment of memory cells.

In conclusion, IUET induce alloreactive T cell responses in the fetus and can establish memory cells upon transfusion as early as 23 weeks of gestational age. We found no specific changes or deletions in the TCRVB repertoire associated with these alloresponses [18]. The nature of these response and the kinetics after birth warrants further research.

In contrast to IUET the foetal administration of IUPT with or without concomitant IVIG do not affect NK cells in cord blood and only 1/15 FNAIT children showed an increased CD4/CD45RO percentage, of 22%, in cord blood.

Immediate Effects of IUET

For this purpose we investigated the pre and post IUET transfusion haematological values after 253 transfusions administered to 81 patients. The motivation to do this study was based on an observation of Fenwick et al. [19], who observed transient leukocytosis within 4 hours after transfusion in critically ill intensive care patients. After IUT a similar observation was done by Yankowitz and Weiner [20]. With IUET, a fairly large volume load in relation to the small fetoplacental volume, is administered with a high speed of 2-5 ml/min. and is completed after an average interval of 28 minutes. After transfusion of leukocyte-depleted RBC we observed an absolute small decrease of 4% leukocytes, in contrast with an expected reduction in WBC count. due to haemodilution. Indeed a large 49 % decrease of the platelet count was observed. When corrected for the transfused volume the relative increase in leukocytes was 41% on account of monocytes and basophils and a relative slight decrease in lymphocytes. The lymphocyte sub-population distribution (CD3, CD4, CD8, CD20 and CD56 cells) did not change. We postulate that the large volume induces vascular stress factors that cause leukocytosis by demargination, although a role of cytokines present in blood products cannot be excluded. At the moment of the next IUET, 2-4 weeks later, all values were restored to base-line levels, in accordance with the transient effect lasting 24 hours in intensive care patients [21].

Premature Infants

In 2002, our neonatal centre received 288 infants born after a gestational age <36 weeks. Sixteen were excluded because of an a priori indication for transfusions, such as HDN or NAIT. Of 272 new borns 35.3% (n=96)were transfused the first month of life.. In total 242 paediatric units were administered (median=0.00, min=0,max=9). Most transfusions were required the first week of life (n=106), in the second week 58 units and in the third week 78 units were administered respectively (Table 4).

From this investigation it is clear that there is a strong correlation between gestational age and the receipt of blood transfusions and with mortality. The association between transfusions and mortality may not at all be causal. We assumed that if blood transfusions have an immunosuppressive effect with clinical implications that this would be most likely a transient effect by suppression of NK cell and macrophage functions, during 3 months we evaluated all (n=18) neonates born after a gestational age <32 weeks and who developed an infection (defined as a positive blood and/or liquor culture) We compared this group with a matched control cohort of 36 new borns who did not develop an infection. The groups were matched for gestational age, birth weight, gender, intubation, intravascular access and way of delivery (Table 5). Positive cultures in the case group were present in 22% within 3 days, after the first week 56% of the infections had occurred and this increased to 89% at the end of the second week. A minority (11%) developed an infection between the 15 and 30 days. We compared the infected group and the non-infected control group for

Tabel 4. Preterm infants in 2002

Variables			**N =272**
Gestational age (weeks)	24-27^{+6}		34
	28-29^{+6}		46
	30-31^{+6}		60
	32-33^{+6}		40
	34-35^{+6}		92
Gender	Male/female		152/120
Birth weight (g)	<1000		38
	1000-1499		78
	1500-1999		78
	2000-2499		53
	≥2500		25
Way of delivery	Vaginal/CS		165/107
Hospitalisation (days)	<7		144
	8-14		61
	15-30		46
	>30		21
Hospitalisation Unit	Intensive Care		203
	High/medium Care		50/19
Transfusions	Transfused/No BT		96/176
<32 weeks	N=140	Transfused	82/59%
>32-36 weeks	N=132	Transfused	14/11%
Deceased	Total N=272		30/10.6%
	<32 weeks		29/20.7%
	>32-36 weeks		1/0.75%

Table 5. Erythrocyte transfusions administered in the first week of life and neonatal infections

Cases	N=18 Infected	Controls N=36 No infections	P
Gest age (days)	204 (181-219)	204 (181-221)	NS
Birth w (grams)	1137 (720-1690)	1197 (707-2163)	NS
Intubated	13 (72%)	24 (67%)	NS
Ivlines	18 (100%)	32 (89%)	NS
>24hr ruptured membrane	3 (17%)	9 (25%)	NS
Maternal antibiotics	7 (39%)	11 (31%)	NS
Vaginal delivery	9 (50%)	22 (61%)	NS
Primary Caesarian section	6 (33%)	8 (22%)	NS
Sec Caesarian section	2 (11%)	6 (17%)	NS
Number of BT (mean)	2.3 units	1.6 units	0.04
Number of pat transfused <7 days			
	N=9 (50%)	N=17 (47%)	NS

being transfused the first week of life. A similar % of new borns were transfused in both groups (Table 5). Although the infected group received more BT (0.7 unit/patient), most transfusions were administered after a positive blood/ cerebrospinal flood culture was established. In the infected group in 7/18 (39%) of the new borns a positive culture anytime during the first month was preceded by at least one erythrocyte transfusion in the 5 days preceding the positive culture. Of the total 34 positive cultures in the 18 patients 13 (38%) were preceded by a transfusion the 5 days before and 21 of the positive cultures were not preceded by a transfusion within this interval.

Although the numbers are small we found no indication that transfusions enhanced the susceptibility for severe infections.

Conclusion

Intrauterine erythrocyte transfusions are possible from the 17th gestational week onwards and contribute significantly to the survival of these otherwise healthy children, which are threatened *in utero* by maternal antibodies. It is reassuring that no long term immunomodulatory effects could be identified more than 20 years after intraperitoneal non-leukocyte reduced and non-irradiated transfusions, but serious effects such as TA-GvHD may have been missed because 60% of the children died before or soon after birth.

Modern treatment uses ultrasound guided intravascular transfusions and blood products with optimal precautionary safety measurements .The greatest advantage is that transfusion treatment can be started earlier in gestational life. Survival increased to > 85%. Nevertheless, despite precautionary safety measurements, on the short term these IUET's induce premature T cell maturation towards the CD45RO phenotype in association with quantitative alterations in the TCRVB family usage within the CD4^{+} T cell sub-populations. We observed increased (memory) proliferative responses against the transfusion donor after transfusion to a foetus as young as 23th weeks of age. In contrast to reports with pretransplantation immunomodulatory transfusions we observed no deletions within the TCR family repertoire.

A point of concern is the depression of the innate immune system reflected by reduced NK cells observed by other groups as well. It remains to be investigated how long this effect lasts and if this compromises resistance to infections in early life. Despite we found in a preliminary study in preterm neonates that neonatal erythrocyte transfusions do not enhance susceptibility for infections this must be further evaluated in a larger group. The usage of autologous cord blood may offer a product with less immunosuppressive effects [22].

The observations in FNAIT pregnancies are intriguing as prenatal administration of IVIG seems to protect against post natal ear-nose and throat infections in this group. Longer follow-up and larger patient cohorts however are needed to exclude that this treatment enhances allergy in later life. In contrast to IUET transfused foetuses this neonates show no NK suppression in cord blood and hardly a shift from naïve to memory T cells. It may well be that the fact that often maternal platelet transfusions were used and the concomitant maternal IVIG treatment suppresses alloreactive T cell activation.

Summarising, there are no obvious deleterious clinical effects of foetal and neonatal transfusions, despite premature T cell activation. The probably transient, effect on the innate immune response deserves further investigations. Prenatal IVIG exposure on the other hand may skew the immune response towards a Th2-type, although clinical sequellae have not been observed. Further studies to evaluate negative effects or to exploit a beneficial effect of maternal IVIG are warranted.

References

1. Westgren M, Ringden O, Eik-Ness S et al. Lack of evidence of permanent engraftment after in-utero fetal stem cell transplantation in congenital hemoglobinopathies. Transplantation 1996;61:1176-79.
2. Fujiwara T, Taniuchi S, Hattori K et al. Effect of immunoglobulin therapy on phagocytosis by polymorphonuclear leucocytes in whole blood of neonates. Clin Exp Immunol 1997;107:435-39.
3. Bruning T, Daiminger A, Enders G. Diagnostic value of CD45RO expression on circulating T lymphocytes of fetuses and newborn infants with pre-, peri- or early post-natal infections. Clin Exp Immunol 1997;107:306-11.
4. Bohm N, Kleine W, Enzel U. Graft-versus-host disease in two newborns after repeated blood transfusions because of rhesus incompatibility. Beitr Pathol 1977;160:381-400.
5. Parkman R, Mosier D, Umansky I et al. Graft-versus-host disease after intrauterine and exchange transfusions for hemolytic disease of the newborn. New Engl J Med 1974;290:359-63.
6. Turner JH, Hutchinson DL,HayashinTT et al. Fetal and maternal risks associated with intrauterine transfusion procedures. Am J Obstet Gynecol 1975; 123:251-56.
7. Vietor HE, Hallensleben E, van Bree SPMJ et al. Survival of donor cells 25 years after intrauterine transfusion Blood 2000;95:2709-14.
8. Kazathkine M, Kaveri SV Immunomodulation of autoimmune and inflammatory diseases with intravenous immune globulin. N. Engl. J. Med. 2001; 10:747-55.
9. Steenbekkers A, Boer de A, Brunekreef B, Groot B, Rijcken B. [Een vergelijking van twee vragenlijsten naar luchtwegsymptomen bij kinderen. I: Vergelijking van prevalenties]. Tijdschr Soc Gezondheidsz 1990;68:478-82.
10. Schaapveld K, Hirasing RA. (ed.) Een praktisch overzicht van preventieprogramma's voor huisartsen, verloskundigen en medewerkers van de jeugdgezondheidszorg. Preventiegids, 2d edition, Van Gorcum & Comp B.V., Assen, the Netherlands, 1997:60-63.
11. Van Bever HP. Early events in atopy. Eur J Pediatr 2002;161:542-46.
12. Radder CM, de Haan HJJ, Brand A et al. Follow-up of children after antenatal treatment for fetal or neonatal Alloimmune Thrombocytopenia. Vox Sang 2003;84:318-25.
13. Vietor HE, Bolk J, Vreugdenhil GR et al. Alterations in cord blood leukocyte subsets of patients with severe hemolytic disease after intrauterine transfusion therapy. J of Pediatrics 1994;130:718-24.

14. Michie C, Harvey D. Can expression of CD45R), a T cell surface molecule, be used to detect congenital infection ? Lancet 1994;343:1259-60.
15. Thilaganathan B, Makrydimas G, Plachouras N, Nicolaides KH. Fetal lymphocyte subpopulations in red blood cell iso-immunised pregnancies. Br J Obstet Gynaecol. 1994;101:315-18.
16. Hanto DW, Ruger JK, Rossi SJ. Alloresponses in-vitro and in-vivo show restricted T-cell receptor V gene usage, Transplant Proc 1995;27:491-93.
17. Munson JL, van Twuyer E, Mooijaart RJ et al. Missing T-cell receptor V families following blood transfusion. The role of HLA in development of immunization and tolerance. Hum Immunol 1995;42:43-53.
18. Vietor HE, Hawes GE, van den Oever C et al. Intrauterine transfusions affect fetal T-cell immunity. Blood 2000;95:2709-14.
19. Fenwick JC, Cameron M, Naiman SC et al. Blood transfusions as a cause of leucocytosis in critically ill patients. Lancet 1994;344:855-56.
20. Yankowitz J, Weiner CP. Blood transfusions for haemolytic disease as a cause of leukocytosis in the fetus. Prenatal Diagn 1996;16:719-22.
21. Vietor HE, Klumper F, Meerman R-J H et al. Intrauterine transfusions influence fetal leukocyte count and subsets. Prenatal Diagnosis 1998;18:325-31.

BIOLOGY OF THROMBOPOIETIN IN THE HUMAN FOETUS AND NEONATE[1]

Chr. Dame[2]

Introduction

The aim of this contribution is to summarize the current data on the biology of thrombopoietin (Tpo) in the human foetus and neonate.

Discovery and terminology of thrombopoietin and its receptor c-mpl

In 1994, several groups reported almost simultaneously on the identification and cloning of Tpo [1-6]. Based on the identification of Tpo as primary regulator of megakaryopoiesis and platelet production, the pathomechanisms of several inherited thrombocytopenias and familiar thrombocythaemia have been elucidated. The term thrombopoietin was introduced in 1958 by Kelemen et al., who postulated a specific humoral regulator of platelet production [7]. In 1992, Vigon et al. identified the human cellular homologue of the v-mpl, the oncogene of the murine myeloproliferative leukemia virus (MPLV), as a member of the haematopoietic growth factor receptor family. This gene was named c-mpl (cellular mpl) [8]. C-Mpl was found to be mainly expressed on $CD34^+$ cells, megakaryocytes, and platelets. The search for the c-Mpl ligand finally resulted in the discovery of Tpo, which was also named megakaryocyte growth and development factor (MGDF) [5].

Cellular biology of thrombopoietin

Tpo acts primary as a lineage-specific growth factor in megakaryopoiesis, but also in early haematopoiesis. It induces the commitment of early haematopoietic stem and progenitor cells into lineage-specific megakaryoblastic differentiation and stimulates the proliferation and differentiation of megakaryocyte progenitor cells [3,9]. The role of Tpo in megakaryopoiesis increases gradually with preceding proliferation and differentiation of the progenitor cells. However, Tpo seems not to be required for pro-platelet formation and platelet release as final stages of thrombopoiesis [10]. Analysis of transgenic animals with Tpo or c-mpl (Tpo receptor/Tpo-R) deficiency confirmed the essential role of Tpo in mega-

1. Authors' work is supported by the Deutsche Forschungsgemeinschaft (DA 484/2-1).

2. Assistant Professor, Charité – Universitätsmedizin Berlin, Department of Neonatology, Campus Virchow-Klinikum, Berlin, D.

karyopoiesis. Mice with targeted homozygous gene deletion of Tpo or c-mpl have platelet counts of about 5–15% of normal; heterozygous mice have platelet numbers of 50% of normal, indicating the lack of a compensatory increase from the remaining allele [9,11].

Besides Tpo, other cytokines or haematopoietic growth factors are relevant for megakaryopoiesis, including stem cell factor (SCF), interleukin-1 (IL-1), IL-3, IL-6, IL-11, leukaemia inhibitory factor (LIF), granulocyte-macrophage colony-stimulating factor (GM-CSF), and erythropoietin (Epo) [12-14]. However, the remaining platelet production in c-mpl -/- mice results neither from the effects of GM-CSF, IL-3, IL-6, IL-11, nor LIF [15-17].

The cellular effects of Tpo are mediated by its binding to c-Mpl on megakaryocyte and non-megakaryocyte/early haematopoietic progenitor cells, respectively. Importantly, the responsiveness of bone marrow-derived megakaryopoietic progenitor cells to recombinant Tpo (rTpo) is age-dependent. A higher sensitivity of neonatal megakaryocyte progenitor cells has been demonstrated in comparison to adult megakaryocyte progenitor cells. It is still unclear, why the in vitro responsiveness of megakaryocyte progenitor cells of thrombocytopenic neonates to rTpo is lower than in neonates with normal platelet counts [18].

Besides its lineage-specific effects on the proliferation of megakaryocyte progenitor cells, Tpo stimulates the expression of platelet specific membrane proteins, such as the fibrinogen receptor glycoproteins (GP) IIb/IIIa, von Willebrand receptor GP Ib/V/IX and GP VI [3,19-21]. Tpo also enhances megakaryocyte adhesion through the activation of glycoprotein IIb/IIIa and very late antigens (VLA)-4 and VLA-5 [22,23].

Molecular biology of thrombopoietin

The human Tpo is encoded by a single copy gene with six exons, which is located on chromosome 3q26-27 [6]. The primary translation product of human Tpo is composed of 332 amino acids and characterized by two distinct domains plus an additional 21 amino acids secretory leader sequence. The N-terminal receptor binding domain (residues 1-152) shares 20 % sequence identity plus 25 % sequence homology with Epo ("Epo-like" domain) and is predicted to fold into a four helix bundle protein [2,24]. This domain is essential for the signalling and the proliferative activity of the molecule [5]. Several essential receptor binding residues have been identified (D_8, K_{14}, K_{52}, K_{59}, K_{136},K_{138}, and R_{140}) [1,2,25,26]. The C-terminal domain (residues 153-332) specifically characterizes the Tpo molecule and is termed the Tpo glycan domain. This domain contains six potential N-linked glycosylation sites and many sites (≥ 5) of O-linked glycosylation [25,27]. The human full-length Tpo protein has an apparent molecular weight of approximately 70 kDa (68-85 kDa as analyzed in SDS page electrophoresis), again indicating considerable glycolysation, as the predicted molecular weight for the non-glycolysated molecule is 38 kDa [28].

Besides the full-length Tpo mRNA, five alternative splice variants of Tpo mRNA and heterogenous circulating Tpo proteins have been identified in humans and mice [28-30]. In comparison to the full-length Tpo mRNA (Tpo-1), the isoforms are characterized by various deletions in exon 6 (affecting the N- or

C-terminal domain, or both) or by a 60-bp insert (part of exon 5, containing a stop codon) between exons 5 and 6 in combination with a 116-bp deletion in exon 6 (Tpo-6). These Tpo protein variants show a reduced extracellular secretion, poor protein synthesis, or diminished biological half-life time, resulting in a loss of biological activity [28,30-32].

Data on the expression of Tpo isoforms in normal foetal, neonatal, or adult tissues are very limited, but organ-specific expression patterns are strongly suggested. For example, the ratio of Tpo-2/Tpo-1 mRNA expression in normal human adult kidney is 0.4, but 0.75 in brain tissue [33]. Furthermore, certain isoforms (e.g. Tpo-3, Tpo-5, and Tpo-6) are not detectable in the foetal kidney [34].

Both in human neonates and adults, the liver is the primary site of Tpo gene expression, followed by the kidneys. Tpo is also expressed to a less amount in other organs, such as the bone marrow, skeletal muscle, intestine, spleen, placenta, and central nervous system [5,33-36]. In situ hybridization and immunohistochemistry showed that Tpo production is localized in hepatocytes, in interstitial cells of the proximal and distal tubules of the kidneys, in endothelial cells, and in bone marrow stroma cells [37].

Regarding human development, the earliest Tpo gene expression has been described in organs from an eight-week old foetus, where the most intense signals for Tpo transcripts were found in the liver [35]. By competitive RT-PCR, we described the highest Tpo mRNA expression in the liver, contributing to more than 90 % of the combined Tpo mRNA expression in liver, kidney, and spleen at a gestational age between 17 and 36 weeks post conception. These findings indicate that, in contrast to Epo, Tpo production does not undergo a developmental switch of the primary production site [36,38]. In contrast to adults, Tpo mRNA is strongly expressed in the foetal bone marrow. In some foetal bone marrow specimens, Tpo mRNA levels are as high as in the corresponding liver or kidneys [36]. This raises the question about an essential role of Tpo in the ontogeny of medullary megakaryopoiesis by modifying the specific microenvironment of the stroma.

Molecular biology of c-mpl, the thrombopoietin receptor

The human Tpo-R is encoded by a single copy gene with 12 exons, which is located on chromosome 1p34. The Tpo-R belongs to the cytokine receptor family. The translation product consists of 610 amino acids and is composed of a 466-amino acid extracellular ligand-binding domain, which includes two cytokine receptor motifs (encoded by exons 2-5 and exons 6-8, respectively), a 22-residue transmembrane domain (encoded by exon 9), and a 122-amino acid cytoplasmic domain (encoded by exons 10 and 11) [39]. The distal cytokine receptor motif of the extracellular domain seems to be responsible for ligand-binding. In the absence of Tpo, it puts a break on the constitutive signalling activity of the membrane proximal cytokine receptor motif [40]. The juxtamembrane WSXWS motif (tryptophan-serine-X (any amino acid)-tryptophan-serine), which is a common motif in each member of the cytokine receptor family, is thought to be responsible for maintaining the proper structural conformation of the extracellular domain as well as for the internalization and signal transduction. The intracellular domain is characterized by a box 1 motif, located 17-20 residues from the transmembrane domain, and a box 2 motif located 30 residues downstream of the box 1 motif. Box 1 and box 2 are highly conserved and vital for full biological activity of the Tpo-R [41]. In the cytoplasmic domain five tyrosine residues have been identified, two of which become phosphorylated upon ligand-binding [42]. Binding analysis with radiolabeled rTpo revealed a single class of receptors with a binding affinity of approximately 560 pmol. Although precise data are not available, it is assumed that megakaryocyte progenitor cells display a significant higher number of Tpo-R on their surface than platelets, which display approximately 220 receptors per cell [43].

In humans, two co-linear forms of c-Mpl (Mpl P and Mpl K) have been found. Mpl K derives from an alternative reading frame that eliminates the box1 and box2 motifs as well as all other signalling motifs of the intracellular domain by introducing a stop codon [39]. Furthermore, a soluble human Tpo-R originates from alternative splicing of the primary transcript between exon 8 and exon 10, resulting in the deletion of the transmembrane region and signalling motifs of the intracellular domain [44]. It is unlikely that any of the alternative forms of Tpo-R bind Tpo or initiate signal transduction. However, it remains unclear whether the activity of Tpo-R is regulated by such mechanisms during development.

Previous studies on the cellular implication of the Tpo-R focused primarily on its expression on CD34+ cells, pluripotent early haematopoietic progenitor cells, megakaryocytes, and platelets [45]. However, c-Mpl is also expressed on endothelial cells, Purkinje cells in the cerebellum, and neuronal cells in the human cerebral cortex, as most recently reported [46,47].

Regulation of Tpo

The current model of Tpo regulation is based on the relationship between Tpo gene expression levels, circulating Tpo concentrations, and the mass of Tpo-R bearing megakaryocyte progenitor cells and platelets. Hepatic Tpo mRNA expression does not change in thrombocytopenia, implicating that Tpo production is mainly constitutive [43,48]. Therefore, Tpo-R bearing cells play a major role in regulating Tpo protein concentrations. Functional Tpo receptors remove Tpo by absorption and internalization of the cell surface complex. Several studies on circulating Tpo concentrations, megakaryopoietic activity, and platelet counts led to the concept of an 'end-cell-mediated regulation' of Tpo. Circulating Tpo concentrations are high, if a low number of Tpo-R bearing cells are available, such as in thromboctyopenia resulting from primary reduced megakaryopoiesis [49]. In contrast, Tpo concentrations are normal or in the upper normal range if thrombocytopenia results from platelet destruction, since Tpo has been already bound to the mass of Tpo-R bearing cells [50,51].

However, more recent data demonstrate that the regulation of Tpo is more complex and shows organ-specific differences:

a) In reactive thrombocytosis, Tpo concentrations do not inversely correlate with the mass of platelets [52,53]. Longitudinal Tpo measurements in infants and children with acute infection show indeed that an elevation of Tpo concentrations precedes thrombocytosis [54]. In vitro and in vivo experiments provide evidence that inflammatory cytokines increase Tpo gene expression in hepatocytes and in (murine) liver endothelial cells [55-58]. Increased Tpo mRNA levels and/or protein concentrations have been also described after stimulation with hepatic growth factor (HGF) and in a model of liver regeneration [59].

b) In the bone marrow, Tpo gene expression underlies other regulatory mechanisms. In contrast to the liver, Tpo gene expression in the stroma increases in response to thrombocytopenia [37,60]. Although the exact type of stroma cell expressing Tpo in the bone marrow has still not been identified, studies in primary bone marrow cultures indicate that various platelet α-granular proteins are involved in the regulation of Tpo mRNA expression. The amount, to which the bone marrow contributes to total Tpo production, is still unclear and of interest.

Clinical biology of Tpo

Measurements of Tpo concentrations in health and disease contributed significantly to the understanding of pathomechanisms leading to neonatal thrombocytopenias and thrombocytosis. As previously reviewed, the interpretation of determined circulating Tpo concentrations need some general considerations [61]: In the present studies, various antibodies have been used for the immunoassays, but they are not standardized yet. Tpo concentrations are given either in arbitrary units, fmol/ml, or pg/ml – as in the majority of studies. Assays using polyclonal antibodies may be sensitive to truncated forms of Tpo, which have no or less biological activity. Although highly correlated, Tpo values are somewhat higher in serum than in plasma, most likely due to the detection of internalized Tpo/c-Mpl complexes, which are released from platelets during blood clotting [62-64].

The summary of published data on neonatal Tpo concentrations allow the conclusion that normal Tpo concentrations in cord blood are <300 pg/ml in plasma samples and <320 pg/ml in serum samples (2 SD above the mean). Tpo concentrations between 300-1000 pg/ml should be interpreted as moderately elevated; Tpo concentrations higher than 1000 pg/ml as severely increased [61]. Decreased Tpo concentrations may be under the detection limit (<15 pg/ml) of the one commercially available ELISA system.

In cord blood, circulating Tpo concentrations are similar in preterm and term neonates [61]. In some studies, higher Tpo concentrations have been reported in preterm than in term neonates [64-67], but this finding has not been confirmed in the majority of the studies [35,36,68-72]. Relevant developmental changes in circulating Tpo concentrations during foetal gestation have been finally excluded by the longitudinal analysis of fetal blood samples [73-75]. Our longitudinal analysis of foetal blood samples obtained by cordiocentesis in non-thrombocytopenic, non-hydropic foetuses with haemolytic disease of the neonate (HDN) showed no changes in circulating Tpo concentrations during gestation [76].

However, Tpo concentrations are significantly higher in non-thrombocytopenic neonates than in healthy adults [63,64,73-75,77]. In contrast to the prenatal period, Tpo concentrations underlie age-related changes during postnatal development. Neonatal Tpo concentrations increase after birth with a peak on the second day of life, before they return to levels found in cord blood by the end of the first month. Then, they gradually decrease until the end of the first year of life, where they are still somewhat higher than in adults [64]. An additional study on Tpo concentrations of low-birth-weight preterm neonates (<2.500g) shows the same phenomenon on postnatal changes in Tpo concentrations, but the absolute Tpo concentrations in cord blood and at day 2 are significantly higher than in term neonates studied at the same respective time-points [67]. The mechanisms that are responsible for these phenomena are still unclear.

Biology of thrombopoietin in inherited neonatal thrombocytopenias

Studies on the biology of Tpo have clarified the pathogenic mechanisms of some rare inherited thrombocytopenias, in particular of thrombocytopenia with absent radii (TAR) syndrome and congenital amegakaryocytic thrombocytopenia (cAMT).

In neonates and children with TAR syndrome, extremely increased circulating Tpo concentrations exclude a defect in Tpo-production (own unpublished data) [78-81]. Contrary data have been reported on the expression of Tpo-R/c-mpl. While Ballmaier et al. found normal c-mpl expression, Letestu et al. reported decreased c-mpl mRNA levels in platelets of TAR patients and a different ratio in the expression of the two main c-Mpl isoforms (lower Mpl-P to Mpl-K ratio) compared with controls [78,82]. Although no mutations in the c-mpl gene locus have been found [82,83], platelets from TAR patients show a defective reactivity to Tpo [78]. These data suggest that the disorder of megakaryopoiesis is caused by a defect in the signal transduction after binding of Tpo to its receptor [78]. This conclusion is further supported by the incomplete in vitro response of megakaryocyte colony forming units (CFU-Meg) to rTpo. Letestu et al. also found a differentiation blockage at the stage of megakaryocyte precursors in TAR syndrome [82]. Although suggested by findings of thrombocytopenia and radial/ulnar malformations in mutant mice with targeted disruption of certain genes of the homeobox family (HoxA10, HoxA11, and HoxD11), an implication of transcription factor of the homeobox gene family in the pathogenesis of TAR syndrome has not been found in humans [84]. It is also still unclear what causes the thrombocytopenic crisis following cow milk ingestion in infants with TAR syndrome, and why platelet counts often increase and stabilize in older children [85].

Congenital amegakaryocytic thrombocytopenia (cAMT) is defined by a severe isolated thrombocytopenia with absence of megakaryocytes in the bone marrow. As expected, Tpo plasma concentrations are exceptionally high in neonates and children with cAMT, indicating that Tpo production is intact [80, 86-88]. Bone marrow derived $CD34^+$ cells revealed a defective in vitro response

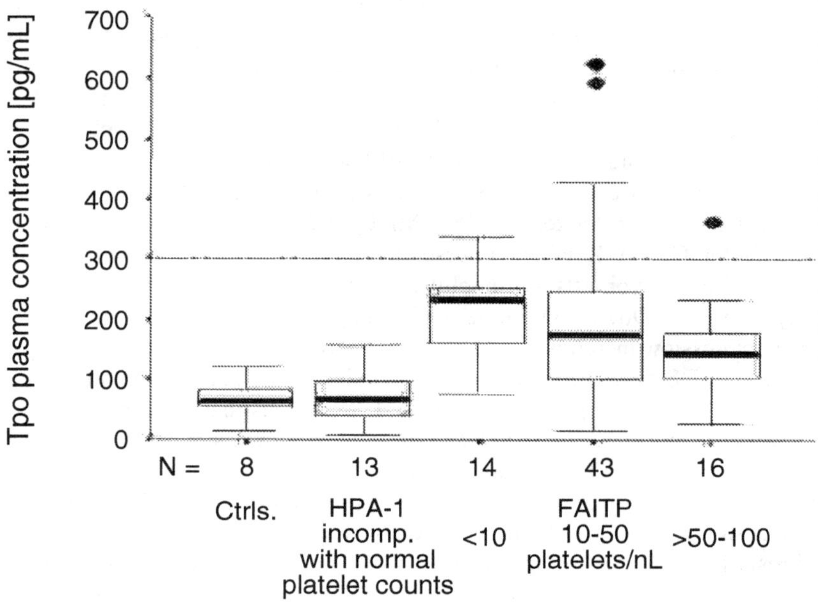

Figure 1. Plasma Tpo concentrations in foetuses with incompatible foeto-maternal human platelet antigen (HPA-1) constellation, who suffered from foetal alloimmune thrombocytopenia (FAITP) or were at risk for that. Blood samples from foetuses with HPA-1 incompatibility were longitudinally analyzed in the original publication [51]. Reference data have been obtained in plasma samples taken from foetuses with normal haematopoiesis, who underwent foetal blood sampling for diagnostic purposes. Data are analyzed in relation to the degree of foetal thrombocytopenia and presented as box plots with the median and the 25th and 75th percentile defining the box. Error bars indicate the 10th and 90th percentile, respectively. Single data points that lie outside the 10th and 90th percentile are also shown. Both outliers in the group of samples with a corresponding platelet count between 10-50/nL were found in the only foetus (out of 14), who suffered from intracranial haemorrhage already during gestation. Normal Tpo plasma concentrations are below the scattered line [61].

to rTpo [88]. Furthermore, platelet activation with rTpo did not result in an increased response to adenosine diphosphate (ADP) and thrombin receptor agonist peptide (TRAP). Different mutations in the c-mpl (frame-shifts, nonsense and point mutations) cause cAMT [86,88,89]. Importantly, specific c-mp1 mutations correlate with the clinical course and the progression of cAMT into pancytopenia [86]. These findings provide clinical evidence that Tpo has a non-redundant role in controlling the self-renew, proliferation, and differentiation of haematopoietic stem cells. Recently, it has been shown that Tpo induces the expression of HoxB4 mRNA in primitive haematopoietic cells, which may be one mechanism for the favorable effect of Tpo on these cells [90]. Tpo is also involved in regulation of the biological activity of other members of the homeobox family of transcription factors. Most recently, Tpo has been found to regulate HoxA9 at the posttranscriptional level by inducing its transport into the nucleus of immature haematopoietic cells [91].

Neonates and infants with trisomy 21 (Down syndrome) and associated transient myeloproliferative disorder (TMD) represent another group of patients with thrombocytopenia due to impaired megakaryopoiesis. At least 10% of infants with trisomy 21 develop – often already during foetal gestation – TMD, which is characterized by the accumulation of immature megakaryoblasts in liver, bone marrow, and peripheral blood. Although TMD undergoes spontaneous remission in most cases, approximately 30% of infants with TMD develop acute megakaryoblastic leukemia (DS-AMKL) [92]. Mutagenesis of the transcription factor GATA-1, which is essential for normal development of erythroid cells, megakaryoblasts, eosinophils, and mast cells, has been described as an early event in Down syndrome leukaemogenesis [93,94]. From normal GATA-1 expression in remission samples of patients who underwent chemotherapy due to DS-AMKL, it has been concluded that GATA-1 mutations are somatically acquired. Importantly, GATA-1 mutations have been found in nearly every infant (97%) with TMD associated to Down syndrome [94]. The majority of reported GATA-1 mutations in Down syndrome are located in the sequence encoding exon 2 and result in the expression of a short GATA-1 isoform (GATA-1s) [93,94]. TMD is often complicated by severe liver dysfunction and fibrosis [95,96]. Regarding the effects of Tpo on the megakaryoblasts as well as the production of Tpo in case of severe liver dysfunction, data on Tpo in neonates and infants with Down syndrome are of particular interest. In six neonates with Down syndrome and associated TMD Tpo concentrations were low or even undetectable. Tpo concentrations increased remarkably with the regression of blast cells in the surviving patients. C-Mpl is expressed on the blast cells, and changes in Tpo concentrations seem to be primarily regulated by binding to c-Mpl bearing cells. However, severe liver dysfunction was found in both patients who died and in one surviving patient who had relatively low Tpo concentrations. Autopsy showed diffuse liver fibrosis with massive destruction of the hepatic structure, suggesting that diminished hepatic Tpo production, in addition to increased Tpo protein binding uptake by blasts, contributed to low Tpo concentrations [97].

Biology of thrombopoietin in acquired neonatal thrombocytopenias

Data on Tpo in acquired neonatal thrombocytopenias have been reported in fetal alloimmune thrombocytopenia (FAITP), thrombocytopenia associated with HDN, infection/sepsis, and thrombocytopenias associated with maternal diabetes, pregnancy-induced hypertension, intrauterine growth retardation, or hypoxia.

Five studies reported on fetal and/or neonatal Tpo concentrations in FAITP [51,70,72,73,75]. The summary on the data gives evidence that in most foetuses and neonates with FAITP Tpo concentrations are in the normal range, as expected according to the model of the 'end-cell mediated regulation' of Tpo. A trend towards a higher (median) Tpo concentration in foetuses with HPA-1 incompatibility and severe thrombocytopenia (platelets < 50/nL) is obvious, although these concentrations are still in the upper normal range or only moderately elevated (Figure 1) [51,73]. As shown in our study on the longitudinal analysis of foetal Tpo plasma concentrations, single foetuses with severe FAITP may have significantly increased Tpo concentrations, indicating insufficient megakaryopoiesis [51]. Further data are required to confirm whether exhausted megakaryopoiesis is indeed associated with a higher risk of prenatal bleeding complications, such as intracranial haemorrhage, as suggested by our data. If so, measurement of foetal Tpo concentrations as a parameter to estimate on foetal megakaryopoietic activity may be useful for further decisions on the indication and frequency of intrauterine platelet transfusion therapy.

Foetal blood samples taken prior to intrauterine red blood cell transfusions in HDN without associated thrombocytopenia have been analyzed to generate reference values for Tpo concentrations during gestation [74,75]. However, severe HDN is well-known to be associated with thrombocytopenia [98,99]. While Kell antigens are expressed on megakaryocyte progenitor cells and Kell-related antibodies inhibit the proliferation of CFU-Meg, Rhesus antigens are not expressed on the surface of megakaryocytes [100,101]. In a preliminary analysis, we found significantly increased Tpo concentrations in more than 50% of blood samples from thrombocytopenic foetuses with severe HDN due to Rhesus incompatibility [76]. This may reflect suppressed megakaryopoiesis, probably as result of the extreme stimulation of erythropoiesis. However, some foetuses, who suffered from thrombocytopenia and hydrops, had Tpo concentrations in the normal range. Since Rhesus hydrops is often associated with liver dysfunction, these Tpo concentrations may be inadequately low, contributing to thrombocytopenia, as known in other conditions of liver dysfunction [76,102].

If one summarizes current data on Tpo concentrations in neonates with infection/sepsis, the heterogeneity in the design of these studies needs to be considered. In sepsis with thrombocytopenia (platelet count < 150/nl), Tpo concentrations are normal or only moderately elevated [66,71,103]. However, if sepsis with thrombocytopenia is complicated by disseminated intravascular coagulation, Tpo concentrations vary widely from undetectable up to 2500 pg/ml [71]. The wide range of Tpo concentrations suggests that various pathomechanisms may contribute to thrombocytopenia, including a reduced or inadequate Tpo production in the liver. More studies, which also analyze the megakaryopoietic activity, are required to determine whether these neonates, who have often prolonged thrombocytopenia, would benefit from a treatment with megakaryopoietic growth factors [104].

Neonatal thrombocytopenia associated with maternal diabetes, pregnancy-induced hypertension, intrauterine growth retardation, or hypoxia occurs frequently, particularly in sick preterm babies. Watts et al. measured serially Tpo concentrations over the first 12 d after birth and determined the number of circulating megakaryocyte progenitor cells in preterm neonates with early-onset thrombocytopenia (< 48h after birth). Although the numbers of megakaryocyte progenitor cells were significantly lower than in controls, circulating Tpo concentrations were only slightly increased. Importantly, at the nadir of thrombocytopenia Tpo concentrations were significantly lower than in older thrombocytopenic children. By day 12, platelet counts, megakaryocyte progenitors, and Tpo concentrations returned to normal levels [69]. Two other studies also suggested impaired or inadequate low Tpo production as factor contributing to early-onset thrombocytopenia in preterm babies and in neonates, who are small for gestational age [68,70].

Towards a rational to treat neonatal thrombocytopenia in sick preterm and term neonates

Based on the current understanding of the biology of Tpo in inherited and acquired neonatal thrombocytopenias, it became clear that only a certain group of neonates may benefit from future treatment strategies using rTpo, Tpo mimetic peptides, or other megakaryopoietic growth factors/cytokines, such as IL-11, to prevent bleeding and requirement for platelet transfusions [61,104,105]. Although rTpo stimulates in vitro megakaryocyte precursor and progenitor cells of preterm and term neonates [68,69,106], it needs to be considered that the platelet count will start to rise about 6 days after the beginning of rTpo treatment and peaks after 10-12 days, as shown in newborn rhesus monkeys [107]. Therefore, rTpo is unlikely to prevent bleeding complications in critically sick neonates with rapid progression of thrombocytopenia and risk of disseminated intravascular coagulation. Coupled with the increase of endogenous Tpo in the acute phase response to infection and due to the higher sensitivity of megakaryocyte progenitor cells of (preterm) neonates to rTpo [67,68], rTpo could additionally contribute to reactive thrombocytosis [108]. In conclusion, only babies with severe, persistent thrombocytopenia and inadequate Tpo production may be candidates for a treatment with rTpo. However, the examination of liver function and megakaryopoietic activity combined with the measurement of endogenous Tpo concentrations may be required to identify these babies. Enthusiasm for using certain forms of rTpo, in particular pegylated recombinant megakaryocyte growth and development factor (PEG-rHu-MGDF), has been destroyed due to the development of pancytopenia by antibodies, which cross-reacted with endogenous Tpo and neutralized its biological activity in PEG-rHu-MGDF treated adults [109,110]. Current studies using recombinant full-length human Tpo in adults may contribute to outline future studies on using rTpo in thrombocytopenic neonates.

Novel therapeutic approaches are provided by Tpo mimetic peptides or minibody agonists of the Tpo-R. Very recently, minibody agonists, which base on IgG antibodies against Tpo-R and include diabody or sc(Fv)2 as potent natural ligand, have been successfully developed. Such minibody agonists have been shown to bind and to activate two types of dysfunctional mutant c-mpl that cause cAMT [111].

New aspects of the developmental biology of thrombopoietin

Recent work on the developmental biology of Tpo focuses on its expression and function in the nervous system. Several haematopoietic cytokines, such as erythropoietin (Epo) or stem cell factors (SCF), are expressed in the central nervous system (CNS) and exert favourable biological function [112,113]. For example, Epo and Epo-R are expressed in the nervous system in a developmental-stage specific manner [114-118]. Epo mRNA expression can be also up-regulated by hypoxia, and Epo acts as a neuroprotective and neurotrophic agent [112,119,120]. To achieve these effects, Epo must be available in the tissue within a critical time frame of up to 4 h (in single animal models even longer) after the insult [112]. These effects have been shown in a variety of in vitro experiments and animal models representing different mechanisms of tissue damage such as oxidative stress, ischaemia/stroke, spinal cord and peripheral-nerve trauma, experimental autoimmune encephalomyelitis, neuronal damage related to human immunodeficiency virus infection, and retinal damage [121]. In adults with acute stroke, a phase I-II clinical trial showed that high-dose rEpo treatment is safe and ameliorates the neurological outcome [122]. Interestingly, Tpo shares within its functional N-terminal domain a significant homology with various neutrophins and a small homology with Epo [123]. In addition to Tpo, c-Mpl is also expressed in the human brain [124]. However, little is known about the biological function of Tpo and c-Mpl in the nervous system. Although no major neurological defects have been reported in mice with targeted homozygous deletion of Tpo or c-mpl, the association between cerebral and cerebellar hypoplasia and c-mpl mutations in the ligand-binding and transmembrane domains of the receptor, leading to cAMT, is striking [28,29].

In our recent study on the expression of Tpo in the developing human CNS, we found Tpo transcripts in tissue specimens of the myelencephalon, metencephalon, diencephalons, and telencephalon taken between 23 and 41 weeks post-conception [34]. Considerable differences were obvious in the intensity of Tpo expression in various areas of the CNS. Highest Tpo mRNA levels were found in the spinal cord, cerebellum, and cortex cerebri, where the amount of Tpo mRNA per µg total RNA was as high as in the liver and kidney, which are the primary organs producing circulating Tpo [34]. Differences in the degree of Tpo gene expression in the CNS may depend on the cellular composition of the tissues. In adult rats, neuronal cells, but neither oligodendrocytes nor astrocytes, of the hippocampus and the cerebellar cortex contain Tpo mRNA. In the cerebellum, Tpo is expressed in Purkinje cells [46]. Differences in the expression of Tpo isoforms in the developing vs. the adult brain suggest that Tpo activity in the nervous system may be down-regulated by alternative splicing [33,34]. Since Tpo protein may be required to archive biological effects of c-Mpl activation and endogenous Tpo may not cross the intact blood brain barrier due its high molecular weight, we analyzed also Tpo protein concentrations in the cerebrospinal fluid and detected low Tpo concentrations, which were relatively equal to the corresponding Tpo serum concentration [34]. Most recently, preliminary in vitro data on the biological function of Tpo in the nervous system have been reported. In this study, Tpo has been shown to stimulate the growth of c-mpl expressing murine neuronal cells and to exert an antiapoptotic effect [47].

Acknowledgement

The author thanks Malte Cremer, MD, and Iwona Palaszewski, Dipl.-Ing. Biotechnology, for the critical reading of the manuscript.

References

1. de Sauvage FJ, Hass PE, Spencer SD, et al. Stimulation of megakaryocytopoiesis and thrombopoiesis by the c-Mpl ligand. Nature 1994;369:533-38.
2. Lok S, Kaushansky K, Holly RD, et al. Cloning and expression of murine thrombopoietin cDNA and stimulation of platelet production in vivo. Nature 1994;369: 565-68.
3. Kaushansky K, Lok S, Holly RD, et al. Promotion of megakaryocyte progenitor expansion and differentiation by the c-Mpl ligand thrombopoietin. Nature 1994;369: 568-71.
4. Wendling F, Maraskovsky E, Debili N, et al. cMpl ligand is a humoral regulator of megakaryocytopoiesis. Nature 1994;369:571-74.
5. Bartley TD, Bogenberger J, Hunt P, et al. Identification and cloning of a megakaryocyte growth and development factor that is a ligand for the cytokine receptor Mpl. Cell 1994;77:1117-24.
6. Sohma Y, Akahori H, Seki N, et al. Molecular cloning and chromosomal localization of the human thrombopoietin gene. FEBS Lett 1994;353:57-61.
7. Kelemen E, Cserhati I, Tanos B. Demonstration and some properties of human thrombopoietin in thrombocythaemic sera. Acta Haematologica Basel 1958;20:350-55.
8. Vigon I, Mornon JP, Cocault L, et al. Molecular cloning and characterization of MPL, the human homolog of the v-mpl oncogene: identification of a member of the hematopoietic growth factor receptor superfamily. Proc Natl Acad Sci USA 1992; 89:5640-44.
9. de Sauvage FJ, Carver-Moore K, Luoh SM, et al. Physiological regulation of early and late stages of megakaryocytopoiesis by thrombopoietin. J Exp Med 1996;183 :651-56.
10. Choi ES, Hokom M, Bartley T, et al. Recombinant human megakaryocyte growth and development factor (rHuMGDF), a ligand for c-Mpl, produces functional human platelets in vitro. Stem Cells 1995;13:317-22.
11. Gurney AL, Carver-Moore K, de Sauvage FJ, Moore MW. Thrombocytopenia in c-mpl deficient mice. Science 1994;265:1445-47.
12. Kaushansky K. Thrombopoietin: the primary regulator of platelet production. Blood 1995;86:419-31.
13. Debili N, Masse JM, Katz A, Guichard J, Breton-Gorius J, Vainchenker W. Effects of the recombinant hematopoietic growth factors interleukin-3, interleukin-6, stem cell factor, and leukemia inhibitory factor on the megakaryocytic differentiation of CD34+ cells. Blood 1993;82:84-95.
14. Yang M, Li K, Chui CM, Yuen PM, et al. Expression of interleukin (IL) 1 type I and type II receptors in megakaryocytic cells and enhancing effects of IL-1beta on megakaryocytopoiesis and NF-E2 expression. Br J Haematol 2000;111:371-80.
15. Scott CL, Robb L, Mansfield R, Alexander WS, Begley CG. Granulocyte-macrophage colony-stimulating factor is not responsible for residual thrombopoiesis in mpl null mice. Exp Hematol 2000;28:1001-07.

16. Gainsford T, Roberts AW, Kimura S, et al. Cytokine production and function in c-mpl-deficient mice: no physiologic role for interleukin-3 in residual megakaryocyte and platelet production. Blood 1998;91:2745-52.
17. Gainsford T, Nandurkar H, Metcalf D, Robb L, Begley CG, Alexander WS. The residual megakaryocyte and platelet production in c-mpl-deficient mice is not dependent on the actions of interleukin-6, interleukin-11, or leukemia inhibitory factor. Blood 2000;95:528-34.
18. Sola MC, Du Y, Hutson AD, Christensen RD. Dose-response relationship of megakaryocyte progenitors from the bone marrow of thrombocytopenic and non-thrombocytopenic neonates to recombinant thrombopoietin. Br J Haematol 2000; 110:449-53.
19. Eisbacher M, Khachigian LM, Khin TH, Holmes ML, Chong BH. Inducible expression of the megakaryocyte-specific gene glycoprotein IX is mediated through an Ets binding site and involves upstream activation of extracellular signal-regulated kinase. Cell Growth Differ 2001;12:435-45.
20. Doubeikovski A, Uzan G, Doubeikovski Z, et al. Thrombopoietin-induced expression of the glycoprotein IIb gene involves the transcription factor PU.1/Spi-1 in UT7-Mpl cells. J Biol Chem 1997;272:24300-07.
21. Holmes ML, Bartle N, Eisbacher M, Chong BH. Cloning and analysis of the thrombopoietin-induced megakaryocyte-specific glycoprotein VI promoter and its regulation by GATA-1, Fli-1, and Sp1. J Biol Chem 2002; 277:48333-41.
22. Zauli G, Bassini A, Vitale M, et al. Thrombopoietin enhances the alpha IIb beta 3-dependent adhesion of megakaryocytic cells to fibrinogen or fibronectin through PI 3 kinase. Blood 1997;89:883-95.
23. Cui L, Ramsfjell V, Borge OJ, Veiby OP, Lok S, Jacobsen SE. Thrombopoietin promotes adhesion of primitive human hemopoietic cells to fibronectin and vascular cell adhesion molecule-1: role of activation of very late antigen (VLA)-4 and VLA-5. J Immunol 1997;159:1961-69.
24. Geddis AE, Linden HM, Kaushansky K. Thrombopoietin: a pan-hematopoietic cytokine. Cytokine Growth Factor Rev 2002;13:61-73.
25. Hoffman RC, Andersen H, Walker K, et al. Peptide, disulfide, and glycosylation mapping of recombinant human thrombopoietin from Ser1 to Arg246. Biochemistry 1996;35:14849-61.
26. Pearce KH, Jr., Potts BJ, Presta LG, Bald LN, Fendly BM, Wells JA. Mutational analysis of thrombopoietin for identification of receptor and neutralizing antibody sites. J Biol Chem 1997;272:20595-602.
27. Foster D, Hunt P. The biological significance of truncated and full-length forms of mpl ligand. In: Kuter DJ, Hunt P, Sheridan W, Zucker-Franklin D, eds. Thrombopoiesis and Thrombopoietins: Molecular, cellular, preclinical and clinical biology. Totowa, NJ: Humana Press Inc.; 1997:203-14.
28. Gurney AL, Kuang WJ, Xie MH, Malloy BE, Eaton DL, de Sauvage FJ. Genomic structure, chromosomal localization, and conserved alternative splice forms of thrombopoietin. Blood 1995;85:981-88.
29. Chang MS, McNinch J, Basu R, et al. Cloning and characterization of the human megakaryocyte growth and development factor (MGDF) gene. J Biol Chem 1995;270:511-14.

30. Sasaki Y, Takahashi T, Miyazaki H, et al. Production of thrombopoietin by human carcinomas and its novel isoforms. Blood 1999;94:1952-60.
31. Stoffel R, Wiestner A, Skoda RC. Thrombopoietin in thrombocytopenic mice: evidence against regulation at the mRNA level and for a direct regulatory role of platelets. Blood 1996;87:567-73.
32. Muto T, Feese MD, Shimada Y, et al. Functional analysis of the C-terminal region of recombinant human thrombopoietin. C-terminal region of thrombopoietin is a "shuttle" peptide to help secretion. J Biol Chem 2000;275: 12090-94.
33. Li B, Pan H, Winkelmann JC, Dai W. Thrombopoietin and its alternatively spliced form are expressed in human amygdala and hippocampus. Blood 1996;87:5382-84.
34. Dame C, Wolber EM, Freitag P, Hofmann D, Bartmann P, Fandrey J. Thrombopoietin gene expression in the developing human central nervous system. Brain Res Dev Brain Res 2003;143:217-23.
35. Sola MC, Juul SE, Meng YG, et al. Thrombopoietin (Tpo) in the fetus and neonate: Tpo concentrations in preterm and term neonates, and organ distribution of Tpo and its receptor (c-mpl) during human fetal development. Early Hum Dev 1999;53:239-50.
36. Wolber EM, Dame C, Fahnenstich H, Hofmann D, Bartmann P, Jelkmann W, Fandrey J. Expression of the thrombopoietin gene in human fetal and neonatal tissues. Blood 1999;94:97-105.
37. Sungaran R, Markovic B, Chong BH. Localization and regulation of thrombopoietin mRNa expression in human kidney, liver, bone marrow, and spleen using in situ hybridization. Blood 1997;89:101-07.
38. Dame C, Fahnenstich H, Freitag P, et al. Erythropoietin mRNA expression in human fetal and neonatal tissue. Blood 1998;92:3218-25.
39. Mignotte V, Vigon I, Boucher de Crevecoeur E, Romeo PH, Lemarchandel V, Chretien S. Structure and transcription of the human c-mpl gene (MPL). Genomics 1994;20:5-12.
40. Sabath DF, Kaushansky K, Broudy VC. Deletion of the extracellular membrane-distal cytokine receptor homology module of Mpl results in constitutive cell growth and loss of thrombopoietin binding. Blood 1999;94:365-67.
41. Drachman JG, Miyakawa Y, Luthi JN, et al. Studies with chimeric Mpl/ JAK2 receptors indicate that both JAK2 and the membrane-proximal domain of Mpl are required for cellular proliferation. J Biol Chem 2002; 277:23544-53.
42. Drachman JG, Kaushansky K. Dissecting the thrombopoietin receptor: functional elements of the Mpl cytoplasmic domain. Proc Natl Acad Sci USA 1997;94:2350-55.
43. Fielder PJ, Gurney AL, Stefanich E, et al. Regulation of thrombopoietin levels by c-mpl-mediated binding to platelets. Blood 1996;87:2154-61.
44. Skoda RC, Seldin DC, Chiang MK, Peichel CL, Vogt TF, Leder P. Murine c-mpl: a member of the hematopoietic growth factor receptor superfamily that transduces a proliferative signal. Embo J 1993;12:2645-53.

45. Debili N, Wendling F, Cosman D, et al. The Mpl receptor is expressed in the megakaryocytic lineage from late progenitors to platelets. Blood 1995; 85: 391-401.
46. Nakanishi K, Tajima F, Osada H, et al. Thrombopoietin expression in normal and hypobaric hypoxia-induced thrombocytopenic rats. Lab Invest 1999;79:679-88.
47. Yang M, Xia WJ, Li K, et al. Identification of TPO Receptors on Central Nervous System-A Preliminary Report. Zhongguo Shi Yan Xue Ye Xue Za Zhi 2004;12: 494-97.
48. Cohen-Solal K, Villeval JL, Titeux M, Lok S, Vainchenker W, Wendling F. Constitutive expression of Mpl ligand transcripts during thrombocytopenia or thrombocytosis. Blood 1996;88:2578-84.
49. Kuter DJ, Rosenberg RD. The reciprocal relationship of thrombopoietin (c-Mpl ligand) to changes in the platelet mass during busulfan-induced thrombocytopenia in the rabbit. Blood 1995;85:2720-30.
50. Ichikawa N, Ishida F, Shimodaira S, Tahara T, Kato T, Kitano K. Regulation of serum thrombopoietin levels by platelets and megakaryocytes in patients with aplastic anaemia and idiopathic thrombocytopenic purpura. Thromb Haemost 1996;76:156-60.
51. Cremer M, Dame C, Schaeffer HJ, Giers G, Bartmann P, Bald R. Longitudinal thrombopoietin plasma concentrations in fetuses with alloimmune thrombocytopenia treated with intrauterine PLT transfusions. Transfusion 2003; 43:1216-22.
52. Hsu HC, Tsai WH, Jiang ML, et al. Circulating levels of thrombopoietic and inflammatory cytokines in patients with clonal and reactive thrombocytosis. J Lab Clin Med 1999;134:392-97.
53. Cerutti A, Custodi P, Mduranti, Cazzola M, Balduini CL. Circulating thrombopoietin in reactive conditions behaves like an acute phase reactant. Clin Lab Haematol 1999;21: 271-75.
54. Ishiguro A, Suzuki Y, Mito M, et al. Elevation of serum thrombopoietin precedes thrombocytosis in acute infections. Br J Haematol 2002;116:612-18.
55. Wolber EM, Jelkmann W. Interleukin-6 increases thrombopoietin production in human hepatoma cells HepG2 and Hep3B. J Interferon Cytokine Res 2000;20:499-506.
56. Kaser A, Brandacher G, Steurer W, et al. Interleukin-6 stimulates thrombopoiesis through thrombopoietin: role in inflammatory thrombocytosis. Blood 2001;98: 2720-25.
57. Cardier JE, Dempsey J. Thrombopoietin and its receptor, c-mpl, are constitutively expressed by mouse liver endothelial cells: evidence of thrombopoietin as a growth factor for liver endothelial cells. Blood 1998;91:923-29.
58. Wolber EM, Fandrey J, Frackowski U, Jelkmann W. Hepatic thrombopoietin mRNA is increased in acute inflammation. Thromb Haemost 2001;86: 1421-24.

59. Yamashita K, Matsuoka H, Ochiai T, et al. Hepatocyte growth factor/scatter factor enhances the thrombopoietin mRNA expression in rat hepatocytes and cirrhotic rat livers. J Gastroenterol Hepatol 2000;15:83-90.
60. Nagata Y, Shozaki Y, Nagahisa H, Nagasawa T, Abe T, Todokoro K. Serum thrombopoietin level is not regulated by transcription but by the total counts of both megakaryocytes and platelets during thrombocytopenia and thrombocytosis. Thromb Haemost 1997;77:808-14.
61. Dame C. Developmental biology of thrombopoietin in the human fetus and neonate. Acta Paediatr Suppl 2002;91:54-65.
62. Folman CC, von dem Borne AE, Rensink IH, et al. Sensitive measurement of thrombopoietin by a monoclonal antibody based sandwich enzyme-linked immunosorbent assay. Thromb Haemost 1997;78:1262-67.
63. Ikeno K, Koike K, Takeshita A, et al. Stressful delivery influences circulating thrombopoietin (TPO) levels in newborns: possible role for cortisol in TPO-mpl binding. Early Hum Dev 2000;58:225-35.
64. Ishiguro A, Nakahata T, Matsubara K, et al. Age-related changes in thrombopoietin in children: reference interval for serum thrombopoietin levels. Br J Haematol 1999;106: 884-88.
65. Albert TS, Meng YG, Simms P, Cohen RL, Phibbs RH. Thrombopoietin in the thrombocytopenic term and preterm newborn. Pediatrics 2000;105: 1286-91.
66. Oygur N, Tunga M, Mumcu Y, et al. Thrombopoietin levels of thrombocytopenic term and preterm newborns with infection. Am J Perinatol 2001; 18:279-86.
67. Matsubara K, Baba K, Nigami H, et al. Early elevation of serum thrombopoietin levels and subsequent thrombocytosis in healthy preterm infants. Br J Haematol 2001;115: 963-68.
68. Murray NA, Watts TL, Roberts IA. Endogenous thrombopoietin levels and effect of recombinant human thrombopoietin on megakaryocyte precursors in term and preterm babies. Pediatr Res 1998;43:148-51.
69. Watts TL, Murray NA, Roberts IA. Thrombopoietin has a primary role in the regulation of platelet production in preterm babies. Pediatr Res 1999; 46:28-32.
70. Sola MC, Calhoun DA, Hutson AD, Christensen RD. Plasma thrombopoietin concentrations in thrombocytopenic and non-thrombocytopenic patients in a neonatal intensive care unit. Br J Haematol 1999;104:90-92.
71. Colarizi P, Fiorucci P, Caradonna A, Ficuccilli F, Mancuso M, Papoff P. Circulating thrombopoietin levels in neonates with infection. Acta Paediatr 1999;88:332-37.
72. Dame C, Cremer M, Ballmaier M, et al. Concentrations of thrombopoietin and interleukin-11 in the umbilical cord blood of patients with fetal alloimmune thrombocytopenia. Am J Perinatol 2001;18:335-44.
73. Sainio S, Javela K, Kekomaki R, Teramo K. Thrombopoietin levels in cord blood plasma and amniotic fluid in fetuses with alloimmune thrombocytopenia and healthy controls. Br J Haematol 2000;109:330-35.

74. Jilma-Stohlawetz P, Homoncik M, Jilma B, et al. High levels of reticulated platelets and thrombopoietin characterize fetal thrombopoiesis. Br J Haematol 2001;112: 466-68.
75. Porcelijn L, Folman CC, de Haas M, et al. Fetal and neonatal thrombopoietin levels in alloimmune thrombocytopenia. Pediatr Res 2002;52:105-08.
76. Dame C, Fahnenstich H, Schaaff F, Schild R, Bartmann P. Longitudinal determinations of fetal thrombopoietin concentrations in severe Rhesus hemolytic disease. Pediatric Research 2000;47:332A (abstract).
77. Walka MM, Sonntag J, Dudenhausen JW, Obladen M. Thrombopoietin concentration in umbilical cord blood of healthy term newborns is higher than in adult controls. Biol Neonate 1999;75:54-58.
78. Ballmaier M, Schulze H, Strauss G, et al. Thrombopoietin in patients with congenital thrombocytopenia and absent radii: elevated serum levels, normal receptor expression, but defective reactivity to thrombopoietin. Blood 1997; 90:612-19.
79. Sekine I, Hagiwara T, Miyazaki H, et al. Thrombocytopenia with absent radii syndrome: studies on serum thrombopoietin levels and megakaryopoiesis in vitro. J Pediatr Hematol Oncol 1998;20:74-78.
80. Cremer M, Schulze H, Linthorst G, et al. Serum levels of thrombopoietin, IL-11, and IL-6 in pediatric thrombocytopenias. Ann Hematol 1999;78: 401-07.
81. al-Jefri AH, Dror Y, Bussel JB, Freedman MH. Thrombocytopenia with absent radii: frequency of marrow megakaryocyte progenitors, proliferative characteristics, and megakaryocyte growth and development factor responsiveness. Pediatr Hematol Oncol 2000;17:299-306.
82. Letestu R, Vitrat N, Masse A, et al. Existence of a differentiation blockage at the stage of a megakaryocyte precursor in the thrombocytopenia and absent radii (TAR) syndrome. Blood 2000;95:1633-41.
83. Strippoli P, Savoia A, Iolascon A, et al. Mutational screening of thrombopoietin receptor gene (c-mpl) in patients with congenital thrombocytopenia and absent radii (TAR). Br J Haematol 1998;103:311-14.
84. Fleischman RA, Letestu R, Mi X, et al. Absence of mutations in the HoxA10, HoxA11 and HoxD11 nucleotide coding sequences in thrombocytopenia with absent radius syndrome. Br J Haematol 2002;116:367-75.
85. Hedberg VA, Lipton JM. Thrombocytopenia with absent radii. A review of 100 cases. Am J Pediatr Hematol Oncol 1988;10:51-64.
86. Ballmaier M, Germeshausen M, Schulze H, et al. c-mpl mutations are the cause of congenital amegakaryocytic thrombocytopenia. Blood 2001;97: 139-46.
87. Muraoka K, Ishii E, Tsuji K, et al. Defective response to thrombopoietin and impaired expression of c-mpl mRNA of bone marrow cells in congenital amegakaryocytic thrombocytopenia. Br J Haematol 1997;96:287-92.
88. Van Den Oudenrijn S, Bruin M, Folman CC, et al. Mutations in the thrombopoietin receptor, mpl, in children with congenital amegakaryocytic thrombocytopenia. Br J Haematol 2000;110:441-48.

89. Ihara K, Ishii E, Eguchi M, et al. Identification of mutations in the c-mpl gene in congenital amegakaryocytic thrombocytopenia. Proc Natl Acad Sci USA 1999;96: 3132-36.
90. Kirito K, Fox N, Kaushansky K. Thrombopoietin stimulates Hoxb4 expression: an explanation for the favorable effects of TPO on hematopoietic stem cells. Blood 2003; 102:3172-78.
91. Kirito K, Fox N, Kaushansky K. Thrombopoietin induces HOXA9 nuclear transport in immature hematopoietic cells: potential mechanism by which the hormone favorably affects hematopoietic stem cells. Mol Cell Biol 2004;24:6751-62.
92. Zipursky A. Transient leukaemia--a benign form of leukaemia in newborn infants with trisomy 21. Br J Haematol 2003;120:930-38.
93. Wechsler J, Greene M, McDevitt MA, et al. Acquired mutations in GATA1 in the megakaryoblastic leukemia of Down syndrome. Nat Genet 2002;32: 148-52.
94. Gurbuxani S, Vyas P, Crispino JD. Recent insights into the mechanisms of myeloid leukemogenesis in Down syndrome. Blood 2004;103:399-406.
95. Schwab M, Niemeyer C, Schwarzer U. Down syndrome, transient myeloproliferative disorder, and infantile liver fibrosis. Med Pediatr Oncol 1998; 31: 159-65.
96. Ruchelli ED, Uri A, Dimmick JE, et al. Severe perinatal liver disease and Down syndrome: an apparent relationship. Hum Pathol 1991;22:1274-80.
97. Bonno M, Azuma E, Kawasaki H, et al. Thrombopoietin level is inversely related to blast count, not platelet number, in Down syndrome neonates with transient myeloproliferative disorder. Am J Hematol 1998;58:267-72.
98. Koenig JM, Christensen RD. Neutropenia and thrombocytopenia in infants with Rh hemolytic disease. J Pediatr 1989;114:625-31.
99. Saade GR, Moise KJ, Jr., Copel JA, Belfort MA, Carpenter RJ, Jr. Fetal platelet counts correlate with the severity of the anemia in red-cell alloimmunization. Obstet Gynecol 1993;82:987-91.
100. Wagner T, Bernaschek G, Geissler K. Inhibition of megakaryopoiesis by Kell-related antibodies. N Engl J Med 2000;343:72.
101. Brown EJ, Zipursky A. Isoimmune hemolytic disease. In: Nathan DG, Oski FA, eds. Hematology of infancy and childhood. Philadelphia: WB Saunders; 1987:44-73.
102. Wolber EM, Ganschow R, Burdelski M, Jelkmann W. Hepatic thrombopoietin mRNA levels in acute and chronic liver failure of childhood. Hepatology 1999;29: 1739-42.
103. Paul DA, Leef KH, Taylor S, McKenzie S. Thrombopoietin in preterm infants: gestational age-dependent response. J Pediatr Hematol Oncol 2002; 24:304-09.
104. Sola MC, Dame C, Christensen RD. Toward a rational use of recombinant thrombopoietin in the neonatal intensive care unit. J Pediatr Hematol Oncol 2001;23:179-84.
105. Roberts IA, Murray NA. Thrombocytopenia in the newborn. Curr Opin Pediatr. 2003;15:17-23.

106. Sola MC, Du Y, Hutson AD, Christensen RD. Dose-response relationship of megakaryocyte progenitors from bone marrow and peripheral blood of thrombocytopenic neonates to recombinant thrombopoietin. Pediatr Res 1999;45:153A (abstract).
107. Sola MC, Christensen RD, Hutson AD, Tarantal AF. Pharmacokinetics, pharmacodynamics, and safety of administering pegylated recombinant megakaryocyte growth and development factor to newborn rhesus monkeys. Pediatr Res. 2000;47: 208-14.
108. Dame C, Sutor AH. Primary and secondary thrombocytosis in childhood. Br J Haematol. 2005;in press.
109. Li J, Yang C, Xia Y, Bertino A, Glaspy J, Roberts M, Kuter DJ. Thrombocytopenia caused by the development of antibodies to thrombopoietin. Blood 2001;98:3241-48.
110. Basser RL, O'Flaherty E, Green M, et al. Development of pancytopenia with neutralizing antibodies to thrombopoietin after multicycle chemotherapy supported by megakaryocyte growth and development factor. Blood 2002;99:2599-602.
111. Orita T, Tsunoda H, Yabuta N, et al. A novel therapeutic approach for thrombocytopenia by minibody agonist of the thrombopoietin receptor. Blood 2004; prepublished online, September 16.
112. Dame C, Juul SE, Christensen RD. The biology of erythropoietin in the central nervous system and its neurotrophic and neuroprotective potential. Biol Neonate 2001;79:228-35.
113. Zhang SC, Fedoroff S. Modulation of microglia by stem cell factor. J Neurosci Res 1998;53:29-37.
114. Dame C, Bartmann P, Wolber E, Fahnenstich H, Hofmann D, Fandrey J. Erythropoietin gene expression in different areas of the developing human central nervous system. Brain Res Dev Brain Res 2000;125:69-74.
115. Juul SE, Anderson DK, Li Y, Christensen RD. Erythropoietin and erythropoietin receptor in the developing human central nervous system. Pediatr Res 1998;43:40-49.
116. Marti HH, Wenger RH, Rivas LA, et al. Erythropoietin gene expression in human, monkey and murine brain. Eur J Neurosci 1996;8:666-76.
117. Chin K, Yu X, Beleslin-Cokic B, et al. Production and processing of erythropoietin receptor transcripts in brain. Brain Res Mol Brain Res 2000; 81:29-42.
118. Knabe W, Knerlich F, Washausen S, et al. Expression patterns of erythropoietin and its receptor in the developing midbrain. Anat Embryol (Berl) 2004;207:503-12.
119. Chikuma M, Masuda S, Kobayashi T, Nagao M, Sasaki R. Tissue-specific regulation of erythropoietin production in the murine kidney, brain, and uterus. Am J Physiol Endocrinol Metab 2000;279:E1242-48.
120. Stolze I, Berchner-Pfannschmidt U, Freitag P, et al. Hypoxia-inducible erythropoietin gene expression in human neuroblastoma cells. Blood 2002; 100:2623-28.
121. Lipton SA. Erythropoietin for neurologic protection and diabetic neuropathy. N Engl J Med 2004;350:2516-17.

122. Ehrenreich H, Hasselblatt M, Dembowski C, et al. Erythropoietin therapy for acute stroke is both safe and beneficial. Mol Med 2002;8:495-505.
123. Li B, Dai W. Thrombopoietin and neurotrophins share a common domain. Blood 1995; 86:1643-44.
124. Columbyova L, Loda M, Scadden DT. Thrombopoietin receptor expression in human cancer cell lines and primary tissues. Cancer Res 1995;55:3509-12.

DISCUSSION

Moderators: N. Luban and C.Th. Smit Sibinga

M.S. Harvey (Leiden, NL): Dr. Rijkers, you said that neonates and young children can't mount an immune response against polysaccharide. However, children do develop IgM, anti-A and anti-B in the first year of life. Why?

G.T. Rijkers (Utrecht, NL): Because that are polysaccharide antigens. The antibodies are probably induced by polysaccharide containing micro-organisms in the intestinal tract and cross-react with blood group antigens. The question is why can you develop these antibodies at an early age . We don't know for sure. The most proper explanation is that on the surface of those bacteria the polysaccharides are complexed with proteins. That creates what in the vaccine world is named a polysaccharide-protein conjugate. If you vaccinate a young baby with a polysaccharide-protein conjugate, you do get a response and polysaccharide-specific B cells that are present can be activated. This is probably the most proper explanation for the relatively early onset of anti blood group antibodies.

S. Moeslichan (Jakarta, Ind): A question to the panel about the recommendation of dosage and velocity (transfusion rate/minute) of blood transfusion in neonates, especially in very low birth weight babies.

A. Brand (Leiden, NL): I think doctor Strauss is presenting a meta-analyses, evidenced based. I can only give my own opinion on dosage. We use ten millilitres of red cells per kilogram bodyweight for the premature. But that doesn't solve your question I think.

N. Luban (Washington DC, USA): You will get your questions answered by doctor Strauss and others. They will present what is in the literature and what is wrong with what is in the literature. Some recommendations will surely come out from that. They maybe varied among different countries actually.

J.B. Bussel (New York, NY, USA): I want to make a comment and ask doctor Brand a question. We had done follow-up in foetuses, that we have treated with maternal IVIG primarily. We compared 75 sibling pairs where the elder sibling was the one where the diagnoses of alloimmune thrombocytopenia was made after birth and than the foetus subsequently treated. We did not do anything like the elegant immunology studies you did, but we tried to do more of a neuro-developmental follow-up. We didn't see in that pairing an increased number of hearing losses or other infections, but we did think that the babies did better develop mentally. We used a questionnaire and the babies who were treated did better on the adaptability scale. So the question I have for you is whether you did any neuro-developmental work in your follow-up of the transfusion effect.

A. Brand: In the neonatal alloimmune study we did follow-up, but in comparison with the Dutch population matched for birth age, gestational age, and we didn't find differences in neuro-development either. Only in those cases who had an intracranial haemorrhage, you find of course retardation. If I understand you well, you say you compare those children, the first born who wasn't treated with IVIG and platelet transfusions, with the second child who was treated with IVIG and platelet transfusions? Than you see no difference between the second child and the first child? But corrected I think for those who develop intracranial damage. So in fact we have the same results.

J.F. Harrison (London, UK): Dr. Dame, is there any incidence of naturally occurring antibodies to thrombopoietin? Because we know that in the United States, where volunteers were given the genetically engineered thrombopoietin, there was an incidence of development of thrombopoietin antibodies which resulted in a long term thrombocytopenia in these people.

C. Dame (Berlin, D): It is correct that in the trials you are referring to, in which PEGylated recombinant thrombopoietin [from Amgen] has been used, patients developed antibodies resulting in long-term thrombocytopenia. Natural anti-thrombopoietin antibodies have not been reported to my knowledge.

J.B. Bussel: Can I comment on that. There is an article that is in press[1] looking at 205 patients with ITP, who were studied for that and none of them were found to have an antibody to thrombopoietin. Using a different preparation specifically engineered to not have the biochemical structural problems of the PEG-ylated form, in 24 patients with ITP treated at different dose levels. This was presented at ASH this year[2]. There were no antibodies detected to the different form and none in 30 controls either.

R.G. Strauss (Iowa City, IA, USA): If I can make a comment on this question. In terms of recombinant growth factors, there are antibodies described – the G-CSF, GM-CSF, erythropoietin, the PEG-ylated form of thrombopoietin. Particularly, alterations in the carbohydrate structures seem to cause an immunologic response. Most are non-neutralising antibodies; they don't interfere with the

1. Aledort, LM, Hayward, C, Chen, MG, Nichol, J, Bussel, JB. Prospective Screening of 205 Patients with ITP including Diagnosis, Serological Markers, and the Relationship of Platelet Counts, Endogenous Thrombopoietin, and Circulating Anti-Thrombopoietin Antibodies. Am J Hematol, 2004 (in press).
2. Bussel, JB, George, JN, Kuter, et al. An Open-label, Dose-finding Study Evaluating the Safety and Platelet Response of a Novel Thrombopoietic Protein (AMG531) in Thrombocytopenic Adult Patients With Immune Thromboctyopenia Purpura (ITP). Blood, 2003;102: ASH Abstract.

natural hormones. But with erythropoietin there are a few that have interacted with the natural hormone, and with thrombopoietin there was the problem also. So the point is that there are a lot of things about recombinant growth factors that are not so innocent as we suspect. We are very careful about how they are being used, particularly in infants. Now, infants may not make antibodies against growth factors very well, and perhaps this will not be a problem, but I think we have to be very cautious about how growth factors are being used. Antibodies might cause a problem, also in normal blood donors. Stimulating normal donors with erythropoietin and thrombopoietin to get larger numbers of blood cells to harvest is different, in terms of risk-benefit, compared to a patient with whom you are willing to take a risk, in the autologous donation setting, because you are likely to help them.

But the question for Dr. Dame is: are we in danger of drawing incorrect conclusions by only looking at plasma levels of erythropoietin and thrombopoietin, rather than looking at paracrine effects in the bone marrow. For example, if you bleed somebody and look at the erythropoietin levels, they shoot up very high in plasma. Erythropoietin levels then fall, yet, the marrow effects go on for quite a while afterwards. In studying thrombopoietin levels, does looking at plasma levels alone really relate to what goes on in the bone marrow. My concern is that if we look at plasma only, are we sometimes going to miss something or draw the wrong conclusion about marrow activity? What are your thoughts about how cautious we ought to be?

C. Dame: I totally agree with you. It was one of my intentions to show you the potential pitfalls you can make if you measure thrombopoietin concentrations only. I think, particularly looking at megakaryopoietic activity, it is important to accept that we need a bone marrow examination. There are some attempts going on to optimise the detection of megakaryopoietic activity. For example, *Martha Sola* is looking at the level of reticulated platelets[1]. But I think this alone will not generate the answer. I agree that we must to do more then measuring thrombopoietin concentrations to understand the situation of the patient.

A. Brand: Dr. Dame, you showed that the TPO receptor is expressing brain like the EPO receptor, and that the EPO receptor of course is inducible by hypoxia. EPO is even proposed as a protection against cerebral brain damage. Have you any idea when the receptor is upregulated in the brain?

C. Dame: I showed you data on the thrombopoietin expression in the brain. We have no data yet on the thrombopoietin receptor expression in the brain. You may assume that the thrombopoietin receptor is there as well, but this needs to be investigated. Do we have different information on erythropoietin in the central nervous system? We know that erythropoietin is expressed in the brain in a hypoxia dependent manner. We also know the erythropoietin receptor is expressed. Furthermore we know that preconditioning increases the expression of

---

1. Sola MC. Evaluation and treatment of severe and prolonged thrombocytopenia in neonates. Clin Perinatol. 2004;31:1-14.

the erythropoietin receptor, which is important to get an optimal response or effect of erythropoietin, which induces anti-apoptotic pathways in neuronal cells. I think we have to wait a little bit before we know what thrombopoietin is really doing in the brain. But I would like to give an outlook that we have most likely a situation as for erythropoietin that a cytokine or haematopoietic growth factor has another implication in other organs.

R.G. Strauss: I just wanted to ask one question about these brain findings. Erythropoietin and erythropoietin receptor are expressed in brain. There is much literature suggesting that these are neuro-protective in some way and that it is very helpful.

But the two questions are, if I remember correctly, erythropoietin given systemically doesn't pass into the brain. The erythropoietin in spinal fluid is actually made within the brain. But I am not certain if that is true for thrombopoietin. Actually, almost all foetal and infant tissues have erythropoietin and erythropoietin receptor genetic machinery.

I assume these receptors and the proteins that are being made probably at physiologic concentration have a neuro-protective effect. If we give pharmacologic doses of these agents to infants for example, are we at more danger, potentially causing a problem because of the extraordinarily high doses with extra-systemic effects possible?

C. Dame: This is a very complex question. We know that erythropoietin (34 kDa) crosses the intact blood brain barrier most like in a concentration lower than one percent. So, going back to Christensen's and Juul's data[1] , it is very plausible that we see after asphyxia different erythropoietin levels in the cerebrospinal fluid versus in the circulation. But II think, this is one part of the whole picture. The other point is that erythropoietin may cross the blood brain barrier to a higher degree if the blood brain barriers is damaged. These are data coming from animal experiments[2], where erythropoietin concentrations in the central nervous system gradually increase with the degree of the damage of the blood brain barrier. These data are the rational for current studies, which are ongoing for example in Göttingen[3]. In adults suffering from stroke, Ehrenreich et al. gave erythropoietin in very high concentration within the first three hours. They have the concept that erythropoietin needs to be given systemically in very high concentrations so that a relevant amount crosses into the central nervous system and acts there. However, there are conflicting data. In mutant mice over-expressing erythropoietin in the brain, the size of an infarct is bigger as in the

1. Juul SE, Stallings SA, Christensen RD. Erythropoietin in the cerebrospinal fluid of neonates who sustained CNS injury. Pediatr Res. 1999;46:543-7.
2. Alafaci C, Salpietro F, Grasso G, et al. Effect of recombinant human erythropoietin on cerebral ischemia following experimental subarachnoid hemorrhage. Eur J Pharmacol. 2000;406:219-25.
3. Ehrenreich H, Hasselblatt M, Dembowski C, et al. Erythropoietin therapy for acute stroke is both safe and beneficial. Mol Med. 2002;8:495-505.

controls[1]. The authors conclude regard that this finding results perhaps from circulatory problems, but it may be that we seen a side effect.

C.Th. Smit Sibinga (Groningen, NL): Dr Rijkers, given the outcome of the long-term effects of blood transfusion in haemolytic disease of a newborn in intra-uterine transfusion as Dr. Brand showed, do you think that the absence of tolerance, but also the absence of any type of chimerism relates to the late development of the B-cell types and the absence of the Th1 responses, and specifically the late development of the memory cells?

G.T. Rijkers: That is a very good question, but I am not sure whether I can answer that correctly. I don't think it has anything to do with development of B-lymphocytes, because those cells will not be activated by the T-cells of the mother. From the data of Dr. Brand I don't know whether you can conclude very firmly whether there is absolutely no memory to those cells. It is of course a limited set of data. The intra-individual variation is rather large, so maybe there still is some memory. But on the other hand those transfusions are given relatively early during embryogenesis. There are certainly the dendritic cell populations that are most vital in antigen presentation, are not fully developed yet. I speculate that it is one of the factors why there is not such a long study impact on the immune system.

A. Brand: We used in the group the long term follow-up of whole blood. So the donor antigen presenting cells (APCs) are quite viable and capable to induce T-helper cell proliferations. We had effective antigen presenting cells, the more intriguing it is that we didn't find memory cells. Maybe you should repeat the experiment, but than you should select for the CD45 cells and then look whether you see an increase of persisting memory cells, but we didn't do that. If you take as a model that memory cells are easier, are not inhibited by monoclonal CD8, are less dependent on IL-2, so you don't need to add IL-2 if you have potent memory cells. If you use that definition we didn't find memory cells. So they were depending on IL-2 and they were inhabitable by CD8 monoclonals. So, I agree that there can be additional work done really to prove that they are virtually absent.

E.F. van Leeuwen (Amsterdam, NL): Dr. Rijkers and Dr. Brand, isn't it true that the induction of immune tolerance happens earlier in premature infants, that it is also depending on the dose of antigens you expose the child and the frequency you expose the child with the same antigens. Dr. Brand has given transfusions only from the donor once and not several times the same donor – I don't know, that is perhaps the reason why you haven't seen any immune tolerance. It is a good practice to use only one unit of blood for a premature infant during the first month to reduce the donor exposure, but perhaps than you induce immune

---

1. Wiessner C, Allegrini PR, Ekatodramis D, Jewell UR, Stallmach T, Gassmann M. Increased cerebral infarct volumes in polyglobulic mice overexpressing erythropoietin. J Cereb Blood Flow Metab. 2001;21:857-64.

tolerance. When grown up, the child may develop more autoimmune diseases or not?

G.T. Rijkers: It is not one question, but there are many questions. You are completely right that the induction of tolerance depends on dose, frequency, route of immunisation, that is constant in this. But also on whether you have additional co-stimulatory factors or not. Maybe, that last one is important. The other issue, that there are arguments to save one unit of blood for one infant to reduce the exposure. That of course are multiple doses and may give tolerance to that one particular donor. But that is only one donor, and tolerance is specific. So you may become tolerant to that single specificity. However, that doesn't mean that you will be tolerant to all other potential donors. I am not afraid that will cause a major problem.

N. Luban: It would be a good idea for the group to comment on the incidence of auto-immune diseases that have been reported in 20 to 40 year olds who were exposed to transfusion early on. I think there are now at least three articles in the literature on that[1,2,3]. Perhaps you would like to speak to that.

A. Brand: That is another large and different area!

N. Luban: Well, it could be our area in the future since we are exposing the children to blood transfusion and now these individuals have scleroderma, multiple sclerosis, etc.

A. Brand: To start to answer the question. For the intrauterine transfusions we didn't use the same donor. So we used different donors. But you should realise that the intrauterine transfusions are relatively massive transfusions. As I understand, you get immune tolerance with lower doses of antigens. Or not? Second, we evaluated tolerance only against the lymphocytes of the transfusion donor, so that was the model. We can't say that we didn't induce tolerance. We can only say that we didn't observe that certain clones have been deleted by the transfusion donor, as was one of the suggestions in, for instance transplantation-induced modulation – deletion of certain T-cell receptor families. That we didn't observe. We always observed a positive response. But you need a clinical model to show that you really have not induce tolerance.

---

1. Lee TH, Paglieroni T, Ohto H, et al. Survival of donor leukocyte subpopulations in immunocompetent transfusion recipients: Frequent long term microchimerism in severe trauma patients. Blood 1999;93:3127-39.
2. Evans PC, Lambert N, Maloney S, et al. Long-term fetal microchimerism in peripheral blood mononuclear cell subsets in health women and women with scleroderma. Blood 1999;93:2033-37.
3. Nardo B, Valdiral A, Catera F, et al. Evidence of microchimerism after pretransplant blood transfusion and FK504 in liver xenograft. Transplant Proc 2000;32:2710-12.

II. IMMUNOHAEMATOLOGY AND HAEMOSTASIS

MANAGEMENT OF RED CELL ALLOIMMUNIZATION IN PREGNANCY

I.L. van Kamp, H.H.H. Kanhai[1]

History of Red Cell Alloimmunization

Haemolytic disease of the foetus and newborn, also known as erythroblastosis foetalis, used to be one of the main causes of perinatal mortality for many centuries. Although the clinical picture of extremely hydropic and icteric stillborns was already described in the 17 century, the pathogenesis of the disease was not understood until the early 1940s. Darrow published in 1934 an extensive overview on the clinical picture and etiologic considerations of neonatal haemolytic disease [1]. From the observation that the disease frequently occurred in the offspring in one family, Darrow hypothesized that the placenta may be the means of transmission of a destructive influence from mother to foetus [1]. Subsequently, Levine and Stetson managed to identify an unknown red-cell antigen in the blood of a woman who was delivered from a stillborn hydropic baby [2]. The woman had massive uterine bleeding and appeared to suffer from a life-threatening transfusion reaction, after being transfused with her husbands blood. As husband and wife both had blood type 0, Levine and Stetson called this unknown phenomenon "intra-group agglutination" [2,3]. Simultaneously, Landsteiner and Weiner discovered an agglutinating factor in th serum of rodents, sensitised with blood from a Macacus Rhesus monkey [4]. As this factor caused agglutination of the blood of 85% of New York's population, it was initially assumed to be similar to the human antibody causing erythroblastosis foetalis. Eventually, the antibody appeared comparable, though not identical to the human antibody, but by that time it had been erroneously called "Rhesus". After the discovery of the alloimmune origin of haemolytic disease, more insight and knowledge was gained on this pathological process by several studies [5]. In these years a beneficial effect of maternal and paternal ABO incompatibility on the severity of haemolytic disease was observed [6].

Neonatal exchange transfusion as a method of treatment of hyperbilirubinaemia was described by Wallerstein in 1946 [7]. This was the first impor tant step in the prevention of kernicterus, the most serious and feared complication of neonatal hyperbilirubinaemia, followed in 1958 by the introduction of fototherapy. However, until the 1960s severe foetal haemolytic disease could

1. Department of Obstetrics, Leiden University Medical Center, Leiden, NL.

neither be diagnosed nor be treated. Elective preterm delivery of a foetus, assumed to be viable, was the policy in most pregnancies complicated by maternal Rhesus (D) alloimmunization, aiming to prevent foetal demise and to be able to start neonatal treatment.

To assess the severity of foetal haemolysis, Liley introduced in 1961 amniotic fluid bilirubin measurements by spectrophotometry at 450 nm (ΔOD450) [8]. With this technique, a first tool became available to acquire information on the severity of foetal disease. Despite the invasive nature of the procedure, Liley's method is still widely used. In 1963 both Clarke et al. and Freda et al. described a method to prevent Rhesus(D) sensitisation, by administering human anti-Rhesus(D) immunoglobulin (anti-D) to Rh(D) negative individuals having blood contact with the Rh(D) antigen [9-11]. This finding is considered to be a milestone in the management of Rhesus(D) alloimmunization, as by this an important reduction in the incidence of this potentially serious disease was attained. The first prevention programs were introduced in most developed countries from 1968 onwards, and consisted of the administration of Rhesus(D) immunoglobulin to Rhesus(D) negative women after the delivery of a Rhesus(D) positive baby [12-15]. To prevent sensitisation, resulting from foetomaternal haemorrhage during pregnancy, antenatal prophylaxis has appeared to be effective and is nowadays introduced in many countries [16-18].

Another milestone in the management of Rhesus(D) alloimmunization, was the introduction in 1963 of intrauterine intraperitoneal foetal transfusions by Liley [19]. This method of treatment of foetal anaemia was based on the fact that red cells can be absorbed from the foetal peritoneal cavity and enter the circulation. In 1966, Liley reported a survival rate of 38% after intraperitoneal transfusion in 52 pregnancies [20]. Intraperitoneal transfusions were performed for over 20 years, in centres all over the world. Initially X-ray was used at the transfusion procedure, but with increasing experience, ultrasonography appeared to be a reliable and safer method to guide intrauterine needling [21]. Due to improvements in both technique and in neonatal intensive care, the overall survival after intraperitoneal transfusions increased from 30% in the early years to about 70% (90% in the absence of hydrops) in the 1980s [22-24].

The intravascular intrauterine foetal transfusion was first introduced by Rodeck in 1981 [25]. Initially, intravascular intrauterine transfusions were performed by the use of foetoscopy [25]. However, soon after the first publication of foetal blood sampling by ultrasound guided percutaneous cordocentesis by Daffos in 1983, this method to assess the fetal haematological status also became the preferable technique to perform foetal intravascular transfusions [26-28]. Thus far, many series have shown that this method of direct intravascular foetal transfusion is superior to the intraperitoneal technique, with improved survival rates especially of foetuses with hydrops and of those having severe anaemia very early in gestation [22-24]. Nowadays, the overall perinatal survival rate of foetuses treated with intravascular transfusions in published series is approximately 90% [29].

From 1970 onwards, the development of advanced ultrasonography resulted in its application in pregnancies complicated by maternal red blood cell alloimmunization. In the first years, ultrasonography was not routinely applied as a tool to assess foetal anaemia, but merely used to diagnose foetal and placental hydrops [30,31]. By refinement of ultrasound equipment and progress in skills in the 1980s, it became possible to suspect foetal anaemia and foetal compromise more accurate and earlier in gestation [21,32]. Ultrasonographic liver and spleen measurements, based on the assumption that compensatory increased foetal erythropoiesis causes hepatosplenomegaly, appeared to be useful in the management of red-cell alloimmunization [33, 34]. To assess foetal condition, biophysical profile scoring (BPS) was introduced in 1980, combining ultrasound parameters with the results of cardiotocography [35]. However, given the fact that foetal heart rate tracings were not performed in the second trimester, the value of BPS appeared to be limited to the third trimester of pregnancy. Also in these years, ultrasonographic Doppler flow measurements were introduced, and these appeared to be promising in diagnosing foetal anaemia by assessing the hyperdynamic circulation, resulting from a decrease in blood viscosity in anaemic conditions [36-43].

Although cordocentesis is clearly the most accurate method to assess the severity of foetal anaemia, this technique never became widely used for pure diagnostic reasons in red-cell alloimmunization, due to the estimated procedural loss rate of about 2% and the additional risk of enhanced maternal sensitisation [44, 45]. Alternative measures, such as the administration of promethazine or corticosteroids to the mother and oral desensitisation to the Rh(D) antigen, appeared to have no clear beneficial effect on the onset or severity of foetal or neonatal haemolytic disease [46-49]. When Clarke stated in 1982 that: "In a lifetime there has been witnessed not only the discovery of a disease but a way of preventing it", he could not be aware of the availability and efficacy of a method to treat foetal anaemia with intrauterine transfusions in the next decade [50]. Reviewing the developments in the field of Rhesus(D) alloimmunization in the past century, it seems right to conclude nowadays, that in a lifetime not only insight in the pathogenesis and prevention of the disease was gained, but furthermore that a safe and effective treatment of foetal anaemia with intravascular intrauterine transfusions was developed and implemented in this timescale.

Prevention of Red Cell Immunisation

Immunoprophylaxis

Since the introduction of Rh(D) immunoprophylaxis in 1963, prevention programs were formulated and implemented in most developed countries [12-15,51]. In the early years it was established, that sensitisation after a transfusion volume of 10 ml Rh(D) positive blood, may be prevented by administering 100 mcg of Rh(D) immunoglobulin [52].

Despite its widespread use and efficacy, the mechanism of action of anti-D in preventing red-cell alloimmunization is unproven. As recently hypothesized by Kumpel, not only destruction of antigenic red blood cells is a contributing factor, but also down-regulation of antigen-specific B cells through co-ligation of B cell receptors and inhibitory IgG Fc receptors [53]. Anti-D immunoglobulin appeared not only to be effective in the prevention of red cell alloimmunization, but also in the treatment of autoimmune thrombocytopenic purpura in Rh(D) positive individuals [54-57].

In the Netherlands, post-delivery Rh(D) prophylaxis was introduced in 1969, and consisted of the routine administration of 200 micrograms (1000 IU) of anti Rh(D) immunoglobulin to Rh(D) negative women, delivering from a Rh(D) positive baby [15,58]. In addition, in later years it was advised to administer anti-D also in situations with a certain risk of foetomaternal haemorrhage, such as abortion, trauma, invasive procedures and external version of the fetus. Kleihauer-Betke test was frequently used in situations, likely to be associated with foetomaternal haemorrhage, in order to administer an adjusted dose of Rh(D) immunoglobulin. Similar recommendations are current in other countries [59]. In the Netherlands, the post-delivery prophylaxis program resulted in a reduction of new Rh(D) immunizations from 3.5% in 1969 to 0.6% in 1995 [60]. Comparable rates of reduction of new immunizations were found in the United Kingdom [17].

However, approximately 1% of Rh(D) negative women develop Rh(D) antibodies as a result of usually small and silent foetomaternal haemorrhages, especially occurring during the last trimester of pregnancy [61].To prevent sensitisation during pregnancy, different schemes of antenatal prophylaxis have been studied in several countries [62,63]. Studies focused not only on efficacy but also on cost-effectiveness of antenatal Rh(D) immunoprophylaxis [14,61-64]. Recently a meta-analysis showed that the antenatal administration of 100 mcg of anti-D at 28 and 34 weeks of gestation reduces the risk of immunization from about 1.5% to about 0.2% without any adverse effects [18]. Implementation of antenatal prophylaxis started in the 1990s and became part of red-cell alloimmunization prevention programs in most developed countries [65,66]. In the Netherlands, antenatal immunoprophylaxis was started in 1998 and consists of the administration of 200 mcg (1000 IU) anti-D at 30 weeks gestation to Rh(D) negative women with no living child. For this regimen was chosen as supplies of human anti-D were limited and as the highest cost-effectiveness was reported in primigravidae [64]. Although it is assumed, that monoclonal anti-D may replace the currently used human polyclonal anti-D in future, the safety and efficacy of these preparations in the prevention of anti-D sensitisation is still subject to further studies [67].

Matched Blood Transfusions

As was already observed by Levine in 1955, clinically significant haemolytic disease can also be caused by non-Rh(D) red-cell alloantibodies, of which Rhesus(c) and Kell are the most frequently observed [68-72]. However, Fy and Rhesus(E) and Rhesus(C) immunization may occasionally also result in significant foetal or neonatal disease [73-76]. Contrary to other sensitisations, inducing foetal anaemia by haemolysis of circulating red blood cells, Kell antibodies cause anaemia in the foetus by specifically inhibiting the growth of erythroid Kell positive progenitor cells [77-78].

Most of the non-Rh(D) immunizations occur following unmatched blood transfusions. Prevention of a potentially hazardous immunization after blood transfusion is only possible by routinely screening and matching of donor blood for those antigens, for which sensitisation may cause alloimmune haemolytic disease. In the Netherlands, the advice to transfuse Rhesus(c), Rhesus(E) and Kell compatible blood to all women till the age of 45 years, was formalized in 1994. However, not all blood banks adopted this advice. Moreover, as immunoprophylaxis is not available for non-Rh(D) disease, immunizations during pregnancy will continue to occur.

Maternal Serum Testing

Antibody Assessment

Until recently, only Rh(D) negative women were screened in pregnancy for the presence of red-cell alloantibodies. Nowadays, most caregivers in the western world assume it to be good clinical practice, to perform a red-cell antibody screen at least in the first trimester of every pregnancy, a regimen also implemented in the Netherlands in 1998 [79]. A positive screen test should only be followed by serial assessment of antibody titres, if one or more of the detected antibodies are known to cause foetal haemolysis and anaemia. Antibodies of the IgM type do not cross the placenta and therefore neither result in foetal nor neonatal haemolysis.

Ever since the discovery of alloimmune Rh(D) antibodies, a relation between antibody concentration and the severity of haemolytic disease has been assumed [80]. Antibody levels may be assessed as titres, respectively with saline, albumin or with the indirect antiglobulin (Coombs) test, or alternatively be quantified in IU/ml, the latter being general practice in the United Kingdom. Due to these different techniques, it is difficult to universally assess a critical anti-D titre or concentration for haemolytic disease. A risk for significant foetal or neonatal disease is frequently assumed to exist at a minimum anti-D titre of 1:16 in the albumin method, and therefore invasive testing is frequently initiated from this cut-off level [81]. Bowell et al. postulated a critical anti-D concentration of 4 IU/ml [80]. In contrast, Nicolaides et al. found severe foetal anaemia at cordocentesis only, if the maternal anti-D concentration exceeded 15 IU/ml, and consequently they considered this concentration as a threshold for invasive antenatal intervention [82]. From the study of Moise et al., it may be concluded that adjustment of all formerly assumed critical titres is necessary [83]. We recently found, that foetal disease is not to be expected with anti-D titres below 1:128 in the indirect globulin test [84].Our study and those of others indicate that the value of any critical titre in predicting haemolytic disease is highly debatable [83-86].

The poor correlation between antibody titre and severity of disease may be explained by the composition of IgG subclasses [87, 88]. Anti-D antibodies of the IgG3 subclass are known to induce more severe haemolysis than that of the

IgG1 subclass. This phenomenon is probably caused by a difference in binding capacity to the Fc receptor of monocytes [89]. IgG2 and IgG4 anti-D antibodies have even less clinical significance [87]. Another reason for the poor predictive value of serum antibody levels may be the protective effect of maternal FcR-blocking IgG alloantibodies, that are directed against HLA-DR antigens. This mechanism was described in 1993 by Dooren et al., and may explain the incidental occurrence of mild haemolytic disease after prior pregnancies with severe disease [90].

As there is a poor correlation of non-Rh(D) antibody titres and foetal or neonatal haemolytic disease, careful foetal monitoring is advisable in these cases, independent of the antibody level.

Functional Bioassays

Nowadays, several functional bioassays are available and may be superior to antibody testing in predicting the severity of haemolytic disease [91-94]. Many studies have been performed on the value of the following bioassays: the monocyte monolayer assay (MML), the chemiluminescence test (CL) and the antibody-dependent cell-mediated cytotoxicity assay (ADCC test), in the management of alloimmune haemolytic disease. Studies on the value of ADCC testing in red cell alloimmunization were performed in the early 1980s by Urbaniak et al., but also in the department of immunohaematology of the Central Laboratory of the Netherlands Red Cross Blood Transfusion Service in Amsterdam [89,91]. Mollison compared the predictive values of different functional bioassays and concluded that the antibody-dependent cell-mediated cytotoxicity assay (ADCC test) was the best predictor for the severity of Rh(D) haemolytic disease [95]. ADCC testing was routinely used in Leiden in the management of red-cell alloimmunization in pregnancy, during the past 20 years. The clinical usefulness of the ADCC test in predicting foetal alloimune haemolytic disease, was confirmed in our recent retrospective study [84].As foetal anaemia warranting transfusion in Rh(D) alloimmunization does not occur at ADCC values less than 30%, it was concluded that referral to specialized centres for non-invasive and if necessary invasive monitoring may be restricted to those women having ADCC values exceeding 30 to 50% [84].

Paternal Zygosity and Foetal Typing

Determination of the paternal Rh(D) status should always be the next step after the detection of maternal Rh(D) alloantibodies. Approximately 85% of the white population of Europe and North America is Rh(D) positive. In case of paternal Rh(D) positivity, heterozygosity is expected in 56%, with a subsequent chance of 50% for the fetus to be Rh(D) negative. Until recently paternal Rh(D) zygosity could only be assessed with a 95% certainty. As the molecular structure of the Rh gene cluster is nowadays defined, paternal zygosity can be determined with certainty using PCR techniques [96]. The assessment of paternal blood type and zygosity is equally important in clinically relevant non-Rh(D) maternal immunizations.

If the father is heterozygous for the antigen concerned, it is advantageous to determine the foetal antigen when possible. Different invasive methods, such as cordocentesis, chorionic villi sampling and amniocentesis have been used, starting in the 1970s, with the aim to assess the antigen status on thus acquired foetal material [97-99]. Being the lesser invasive and safest technique, amniocentesis is nowadays preferred and routinely offered in most centres for both foetal Rh(D) and Kell typing, by means of multiplex PCR analysis of amniocytes [100-102]. To avoid the risk on foetomaternal haemorrhage, transplacental needling at amniocentesis should be avoided in the presence of maternal red-cell alloimmunization [103,104]. Chorionic villus biopsy carries a higher risk on foetomaternal bleeding and subsequent enhanced sensitisation and should therefore preferably not be performed in red-cell alloimmunized pregnancies [105,106].

An important development was the determination of free foetal DNA from maternal plasma using PCR analysis, first introduced by Lo in 1998 [107]. Several studies have been performed in this field and at present this test is considered reliable for antenatal Rh(D) typing and is being introduced in most countries [108,109]. In future, apart from identifying foetuses at risk for alloimmune haemolytic disease, this test may also be used to select only those Rh(D) negative women that carry a Rh(D) positive foetus, for antenatal immunoprophylaxis [108].

Obstetric History

Haemolytic alloimmune disease appears to be a poorly predictable disorder. It has long been noticed, that the severity of the disease usually becomes progressively worse in subsequent pregnancies [110]. However, a similar or even a remarkable milder course than in a previous pregnancy may occur [110,111]. A protective effect of maternal FcR-blocking alloantibodies may be an explanation for the incidentally observed milder course of disease [90].

Management protocols usually consider it safe, to start the first intervention at approximately 10 weeks before the earliest previous foetal or neonatal death, foetal transfusion, or birth of a severely anaemic baby [112]. However, there is no good evidence to support this regimen. Moreover, relying on obstetric history carries the risk of underestimating the severity of the disease. It may therefore be wise, to start close foetal monitoring in all pregnancies of women with high antibody levels early in the second trimester, irrespective of the obstetric history [113].

Plasmapheresis

Plasmapheresis in red-cell alloimmunization, first introduced in 1970, has been used for many years in severely alloimmunized women with a poor obstetric history [114-116]. The aim of this treatment was to lower maternal circulating antibody levels. Initially, with this technique large volumes of plasma were removed and replaced with donor plasma. In later years, techniques were modified and a scheme of weekly small volume plasmapheresis was generally preferred [117]. The background of the weekly scheme was the finding of Rubinstein, that most sensitised individuals have clear-cut weekly cycles in which antibody levels vary [118]. The value of plasmapheresis in preventing severe foetal haemolysis has never been proven. Therefore, plasmapheresis is not implemented in the modern routine management of alloimmune haemolytic disease, although this method is still applied by some, usually in combination with immunoglobulin treatment [119,120].

Immunoglobulin in Red Cell Alloimmunization

Maternal intravenous immunoglobulin (IVIG) treatment is considered to be effective in the treatment of foetal alloimmune thrombocytopenia [121,122]. In the 1980s, immunoglobulin was also applied in red-cell alloimmunization, and although different results were reported, most studies suggested a positive effect [123-130]. Moreover, no adverse effects have been reported. The mode of action of IVIG in red-cell alloimmunization is hypothesized to be a combination of at first inhibition of antibody synthesis, at second Fc receptor blockade in reticuloendothelial tissues and at third blockade of Fc mediated placental transport of antibodies. Gottvall and Selbing concluded from their study, that IVIG mainly acts on red cell destruction by Fc receptor blockade [128]. The main reasons for the limited experience with immunoglobulin treatment in red-cell alloimmunization are the extremely high costs of this preparation and the fact that severe alloimmune fetal anaemia may nowadays be safely treated with intrauterine intravascular transfusions. However, though not routinely applied, intravenous immunoglobulin is still used by some in red-cell alloimmunization [128-130]. Voto et al. recently concluded, that maternal treatment with IVIG followed by intrauterine foetal transfusion resulted in a significantly less occurrence of foetal hydrops and in a higher perinatal survival rate, when compared to foetuses only treated with intrauterine transfusions [130]. Although the limited experience thus far suggests a beneficial effect of IVIG in red-cell alloimmunization, there is much doubt on the cost-effectiveness of this treatment. However, it may be hypothesized, that additional maternal IVIG treatment may be of benefit, to prevent the early onset of foetal haemolytic disease in those women with a poor obstetric history.

A study on IVIG administration directly to the foetus at intravascular transfusion, showed no beneficial effects, when compared with foetuses treated with transfusions only [131]. It was suggested that the IVIG dose, limited to prevent overload of the foetoplacental circulation, might have been too low to reveal a conceivable positive effect [131].

Foetal monitoring

Amniocentesis

The issue of chronic foetal haemolysis in red cell alloimmunization inspired Liley in 1961 to initiate amniotic fluid bilirubin measurements by spectrophotometry at 450 nm (ΔOD450) [8]. This concept was previously studied by Bevis in 1950 [132]. By measuring foetal haemolysis, the degree of foetal anaemia is estimated, and this was for many years the cornerstone for the management of red-cell alloimmunized pregnancies and an important tool for the most optimal timing of intrauterine transfusion therapy. Liley described in 1963 some pitfalls of the new technique, but he also estimated some years later that by the use of serial amniotic fluid bilirubin measurements, 70% of otherwise fatally affected erythroblastotic babies may survive, as hydrops is avoided by timely intrauterine transfusion [133, 134].

Originally, Liley described and interpreted amniotic fluid measurements from 27 weeks gestation onwards. Amniocenteses were performed serially with 2 to 3 weeks intervals [8]. The timing of the first amniocentesis depended on obstetrical history and maternal Rh(D) antibody titre. Results were plotted against gestational age in Liley's chart, of which the lower zone indicated absence or just mild anaemia, the middle zone suggested mild to moderate anaemia, and in the upper zone severe anaemia was assumed [8]. Intrauterine treatment by transfusion, in later years preceded by foetal blood sampling, was recommended if ΔOD450 measurements reached Liley's zone III or the upper-third of zone II. In later years, Liley and others performed amniocenteses for the assessment of the degree of foetal haemolysis, also in the second trimester of pregnancy, by extrapolating the original curves [134].

Though infrequently occurring, maternal diseases such as hepatitis and sickle cell disease are known to falsely elevate bilirubin optical density measurements in amniotic fluid, moreover, the results are also altered by exposure to light and the presence of meconium and red blood cells. The severity of foetal anaemia is the net result of both haemolysis and compensatory haematopoiesis. Therefore, the most important explanation for the sometimes disappointing predictive value of Liley's method for foetal anaemia, is the fact that this method merely indicates the amount of foetal haemolysis and not the foetal haematopoietic response. Given the fact that foetal anaemia in Kell alloimmunization predominantly results from suppression of erythroid progenitor cells, and to a lesser extent from haemolysis of peripheral red blood cells, bilirubin measurements in amniotic fluid are not assumed to be of value in estimating foetal anaemia in this alloimmune condition [77,78].

Since the introduction of amniotic fluid bilirubin measurements in red cell alloimmunization, many studies have been performed, to test both the accuracy of the technique in predicting fetal anaemia and its applicability in the second trimester of pregnancy [135-142]. More accurate studies on this subject could be performed after the introduction of foetal blood sampling in 1983, creating the opportunity to correlate Liley's method directly with the actual foetal haematocrit [26]. The clinical usefulness of amniotic fluid bilirubin measurements, studied by Nicolaides et al. in relation with cord blood haematocrit, appeared to be disappointing before 27 weeks gestation, as the severity of anaemia could not be reliably predicted by the trend in optical density [139]. Adjustments of the curves for use in the second trimester were suggested by Queenan et al. [143], but later studies showed no clear benefit over the original Liley chart [144]. A recently published study in this field showed encouraging results, regarding the ability of Liley's method to predict severe foetal anaemia in both the second and third trimester of pregnancy, with sensitivities of 95% and 98% respectively for values in zone III and the upper third of zone II [145].

Not only the reliability of the method but also the complication rate of amniocentesis is a reason of concern, since in red-cell alloimmunization this procedure is often serially performed, with intervals ranging from one to four weeks. Foetal loss after the early "genetic" amniocentesis was extensively studied and appears to be around 0.5% [146-149]. Moreover, there is the risk of enhanced sensitisation, especially after transplacental needling [102, 103]. Although Liley's method has at least appeared to be of great use in the past 40 years, non-invasive methods to accurately diagnose foetal anaemia are highly preferable, in order to eliminate all additional risks of amniocentesis.

Cordocentesis

Fetal blood sampling is without any doubt the most reliable method to assess foetal haematocrit in a situation at risk for foetal anaemia. Initially foetal blood was sampled by foetoscopy, but in later years the safer ultrasound guided percutaneous approach was preferred by most [26,150,151].

In the 1980s, several experienced clinicians have advocated the routine use of cordocentesis as the primary and only test to assess the degree of foetal anaemia, in pregnancies complicated by red-cell alloimmunization [152-154]. Not surprisingly, Nicolaides et al. concluded from their study on second trimester amniocenteses, that the only reliable method to determine the severity of rhesus alloimmunization was the direct measurement of foetal haemoglobin [139]. Weiner et al., who started performing serial diagnostic cordocenteses at indirect globulin titres of 1:8, also concluded that a foetal blood sample in haemolytic disease permits a reliable identification of the foetus at risk of having anaemia [153]. Despite the clear advantages of foetal blood sampling in the management of red-cell alloimmunization, there is also the indisputable risk of complications related to the procedure. Often transient foetal bradycardia is observed during or after 2.4 to 12% of cordocenteses [155-162]. Bleeding from the puncture site also frequently occurs, especially after transamniotic needling and in the presence of foetal thrombocytopenia [155,157, 160,161,163]. Although foetal bradycardia and bleeding are generally transient complications of cordocentesis, on occasion bleeding, infection, cord haematoma and premature rupture of membranes may result in foetal demise [155-167]. Reported foetal loss rates after ultrasound guided percutaneous foetal blood sampling, performed after 18 weeks of gestation in a low risk population, vary from 0 to 3.1% [44, 45,157-164]. Foetal losses significantly more often occur after puncturing the umbilical artery [164]. Maxwell et al. found foetal loss after cordocentesis to be clearly related to the indication of the procedure, with rates varying from 1.3% in unaffected low risk foetuses to 25% in pathological conditions [168]. Ghidini et al. reviewed the literature on cordocentesis, and reported a total foetal loss rate of

2.7%, consisting of a foetal loss of 1.4% before 28 weeks and an additional 1.4% risk on perinatal death after 28 weeks [44]. By correcting loss rates after foetal blood sampling for the background loss in a control group of healthy subjects, Tongsong et al. recently assessed a pure procedure-related foetal loss rate of the procedure of 1.4% [45].

Apart from acute complications that jeopardize the foetal condition, boosting of maternal antibody titres may result in an increase of the severity of foetal and neonatal disease, not only in the current but also in future pregnancies [169-173]. As serious complications do occur, cordocentesis in red-cell alloimmunization should nowadays only be performed, if foetal anaemia is seriously suspected and therefore with blood available to be able to perform a foetal transfusion in the same procedure.

Cardiotocography, Electrocardiography, Fetal Movements and Biophysical Profile Scoring

In the third trimester of pregnancy, cardiotocography (CTG) may show abnormal foetal heart rate patterns in the presence of foetal anaemia. In the 1980s a sinusoidal foetal heart rate pattern was described in relation to severe foetal anaemia [174-178]. In later years not only sinusoidal patterns, but also tachycardia, loss of baseline variability and decelerations were described in foetal heart rate tracings of foetuses with severe anaemia [178-182]. Nicolaides et al. studied foetal heart rate patterns in relation to foetal haemoglobin and oxygenation at cordocentesis, and found non-reactive, suboptimal or pathological foetal heart rate patterns more commonly in hypoxaemic and anaemic foetuses [180,181].

However, the sensitivity of these pathologic patterns in predicting moderate to severe hypoxaemia or anaemia was 45% and 33% respectively [181]. From their studies, Nicolaides et al. concluded that pathologic foetal heart rate patterns, occasionally observed in foetal anaemia, were more likely associated with a disturbance in foetal oxygenation than with the haemoglobin deficit [181]. Therefore, abnormal foetal heart rate tracings in red-cell alloimmunization may be expected particularly if foetal condition is seriously compromised. From these and other studies, it was concluded, that normal heart rate tracings may falsely reassure the clinician, and that cardiotocography is a poor predictor of the presence of foetal anaemia [180-182]. This is in accordance with the conclusion of a recent Cochrane review, implicating that in general there is no evidence that cardiotocography is useful for antenatal foetal assessment [183]. In addition, an important limitation of cardiotocography is the fact that it is impracticable in the second trimester of pregnancy.

An alternative method to predict foetal anaemia was evaluated by Economides et al. and consisted of the computerized measurement of foetal heart rate variation in relation to foetal haematocrit in Rh(D) alloimmunized pregnancies [184]. In this study, computerized foetal heart rate variation analysis appeared to be of limited value in the prediction of foetal anaemia, as not only positive predictive values of 85% to 90% were found, but also negative predictive values up to 57% [184].

Studying foetal electrocardiography in red cell alloimmunization, Brambati et al. found a clear correlation between ventricular depolarisation time and haemoglobin at birth, suggesting the early involvement of the foetal heart in anaemia [185]. However, the clinical usefulness of foetal electrocardiography in red-cell alloimmunization has not been established, since no further studies have been performed on this subject. Absent or diminished perception of foetal movements by the mother has also been reported in severely anaemic and hydropic foetuses [186,187]. Although abnormal movements may predict a poor perinatal outcome, absence of foetal movements is a late and ominous sign, often preceding foetal or neonatal demise [188]. Therefore the maternal perception of foetal movements is not eligible for the assessment of the degree of foetal anaemia, although diminished movements should be taken seriously, as this symptom may indicate an unexpected severely compromised foetal state.

Biophysical profile scoring (BPS) is advocated by some, in order to discriminate those severely hydropic foetuses having a seriously compromised condition, who may benefit of special precautions, such as limitating volume load at intrauterine transfusion [189]. However, in general there is no evidence from randomised trials to consider biophysical profile scoring as a reliable test of foetal well-being in high risk pregnancies [190].

Ultrasound and Doppler

Visualization of the foetus in red-cell alloimmunization was first experienced at the Leiden University Hospital in the late 1960s, by injecting fat-soluble and water-soluble contrast media in the amniotic cavity, followed by a roentgenogram 24 hours later [191]. This so called foetography was used to guide intrauterine intraperitoneal transfusions, first performed in Leiden in 1965 by Bennebroek Gravenhorst [22,192,193]. Although not meant for this purpose, by visualizing fetal contours and intestines, a gross impression of foetal condition and of the presence or absence of foetal hydrops could be gained by the use of foetography.

The first experience with ultrasonography in red cell alloimmunized pregnancies date from the early 1970s [31, 194]. Langezaal studied in Leiden placental thickness in a cohort of 42 red cell alloimmunized pregnancies, and found a significant correlation of placental thickness and amniotic fluid optical density [194]. In subsequent years, ultrasonography was predominantly applied to guide intrauterine intraperitoneal transfusions and to diagnose foetal hydrops [30, 195,196]. However, a large proportion of foetuses with severe anaemia appear to have no signs of hydrops, as was shown by both Nicolaides et al. and Chitkara et al. [197,198]. In order to diagnose foetal anaemia or early signs of foetal hydrops, ultrasound measurements such as: placental thickness, cardiac enlargement, liver size, abdominal circumference, umbilical vein diameter and spleen perimeter, have been studied and applied in pregnancies complicated by maternal red-cell alloimmunization [31,33,34,194, 107-204]. Unfortunately, studies on the correlation of sonographic findings with the actual degree of foetal anaemia, revealed that the value of most ultrasound measurements in predicting foetal anaemia appeared to be foetal liver length and spleen perimeter, as was found in several studies [34,203,204]. Although polyhydramnios was for many years considered to be an important symptom of severe red-cell alloimmunization, amniotic fluid measurements do not play a role in the management of red-cell alloimmunization, as most severely anaemic foetuses without hydrops and about 50% of those with hydrops have normal amniotic fluid volumes [197].

The use of Doppler in pregnancies complicated by red-cell alloimmunization is based on the assumption of a hyperdynamic circulation in foetal anaemia, resulting from the combination of decreased blood viscosity and increased cardiac output. The first experiences were published in the early 1980s [36,37,205]. After the introduction of cordocentesis, the value of Doppler measurements to predict foetal anaemia could be studied, by correlating the results with the actual foetal haematocrit. Doppler studies were performed and studied in several foetal vessels, such as: the umbilical vein, the thoracic aorta, the common carotid artery, the inferior vena cava, the ductus venosus, the splenic artery and the middle cerebral artery [38-43,204-212]. Although foetal haemoglobin appeared to be negatively correlated with blood flow velocities in most vessels, the accuracy and clinical usefulness of Doppler measurements often appeared to be disappointing [42, 206, 209]. The clinical value of some of the measurements is also limited by the fact that the feasibility and reproducibility not only depend on foetal position but also on training and expertise. Doppler blood flow velocity measurements in the intrahepatic umbilical vein and in the middle cerebral artery appeared to be better predictors of foetal anaemia than liver and spleen measurements [41,215,216]. By now, large prospective studies regarding this subject have shown that the peak systolic velocity in the middle cerebral artery appears to be the most reliable predictor of foetal anaemia, with reported sensitivities up to 100% [215-220]. Other studies revealed that middle cerebral artery peak systolic velocity tends to decrease immediately and significantly following correction of foetal anaemia by intrauterine transfusion [221,222]. Moreover, middle cerebral artery peak flow measurements may presumably also be applied for the optimal timing of subsequent intrauterine transfusions after intrauterine transfusion therapy was initiated [223]. However, despite the promising results of Doppler middle cerebral artery peak flow measurements in red cell alloimmunization, others conclude that rigorous prospective research is still imperative, in order to produce more valid and reliable estimates of diagnostic test accuracy and effectiveness [224,225]. Although further research is needed, it is not just hypothetical, that invasive foetal testing in red-cell alloimmunization may in the near future be completely replaced by non-invasive testing, carrying no additional risks.

Intrauterine Transfusion

Intraperitoneal Transfusion

In the first decade after the introduction of this technique, intraperitoneal foetal transfusions were performed by the use of X ray and amniography or foetography [19,191,193]. Reported survival rates in these years were approximately 50% (range 38%-71%) [22,134,226-233]. Foetuses with hydrops had significantly lower mean survival rates (32%; range 7%-57%), than those without hydrops (63%; range 44%-80%) [22,227-233]. A lesser absorption of erythrocytes from the foetal intraperitoneal cavity is one of the possible explanations of the poor outcome of alloimmune hydrops [234,235].

From 1980 onwards, most intraperitoneal transfusions were performed under ultrasound guidance. In these years, overall survival rates increased to about 70% (range 54%-92%) [22-24,228,229,236-240]. Again survival was highest in the absence of hydrops (mean 87%; range 69%-100%), whereas outcome remained disappointing in the presence of hydrops (mean 49%; range 36%-75%) [22,23,228,229,236-240]. Bennebroek Gravenhorst and others not only reported a lower survival of hydropic fetuses, but also of those needing intrauterine transfusion before 26 weeks of gestation [22,228].Nicolini et al. found that intraperitoneal pressure monitoring during the procedure reduced the risk on complications and therefore improved the outcome of intrauterine transfusion therapy [241].However, this method never became widely used.

In the first follow-up studies on the development of children, surviving after intrauterine intraperitoneal blood transfusions, minor and major handicap rates of respectively 17% and 5% were reported [242-244]. However, White et al., comparing the outcome after intrauterine intraperitoneal transfusions with controls, matched for gestational age, birth weight and mode of delivery, found no differences in developmental outcome [245]. Viëtor et al. found that donor cells in recipients of intraperitoneal transfusions may persist for over 20 years, without demonstrable immunological consequences [246].After the introduction of the intravascular transfusion technique, Harman et al. conducted a case control study, comparing outcome and complications of intraperitoneal versus intravascular transfusions [23]. As the intravascular approach performed better on almost every level studied, such as: procedural complications and traumatic death, the authors concluded that intraperitoneal transfusion should only be used in very limited circumstances [23].

Others combined the intravascular with the intraperitoneal approach and found a more stable haematocrit after transfusion, allowing longer intervals between the procedures [247-249]. Nicolini et al. performed intravascular transfusions in the intrahepatic part of the umbilical vein, and therefore the combined procedure in their study was carried out by a single needle insertion in the fetal abdomen [249]. Nowadays, this latter technique is by most assumed to be one of the few advisable applications of intraperitoneal transfusion. In addition, intraperitoneal transfusion may still be a reasonable alternative if all attempts to perform an intravascular transfusion fail.

Intravascular Transfusion

Technical aspects and foetal adaptation to transfusion – The first attempts to perform foetal exchange transfusions date from the 1960s [250-252]. As the procedures could only be performed by hysterotomy, loss rates were high and therefore these techniques were not applicable to clinical practise. It was not until 1981, that a safe intravascular transfusion technique was introduced [25]. Rodeck et al. published the first results of their foetoscopically guided intravascular technique in 1984, and reported an overall survival rate of 72% [253]. Survival of foetuses with hydrops was comparable to those without hydrops, and a survival rate of 84% was found when the initial transfusion was performed at or before 25 weeks of gestation [253].

Ultrasound-guided techniques were described soon after the first reports on direct intravascular foetal transfusion and soon became established practice, being less invasive and therefore safer [27,28]. Percutaneous foetal blood sampling is usually performed with the use of a 20 to 22 Gauge spinal needle [254]. Ultrasonography is not only indispensable for visualizing and guiding the needle tip at intrauterine transfusion, but also for monitoring both foetal condition and progress of the procedure by observing a continuous echogenic venous turbulence during transfusion [255].

Rodeck et al. first introduced a formula for calculating the volume of blood to be transfused to the fetus, based on the estimated foetoplacental volume (V), the actual foetal haematocrit (Ht_1), the donor blood haematocrit (Ht_2) as well as the desired haematocrit (Ht_3) [Transfusion volume=$V(Ht_3-Ht_1) / Ht_2$] [25]. Nowadays, this formula is still being used by many, performing intravascular transfusions. However, new formulas, generally based on different calculations of foetoplacental volume and occasionally on estimated foetal weight, have been designed by others [256-262]. The timing of a subsequent transfusion largely depends on the assumed haematocit decline after the procedure that, according to most studies, is estimated to be 1 to 2% per day [248,256,259,263-265]. Abdel-Fattah et al. found no difference in the daily decline of foetal haemoglobin after transfusion in the presence or absence of hydrops [266]. The limited experience with intravascular transfusion of maternal red blood cells suggests, that there may be less consumption of maternal than of donor red blood cells [267]. However, red cell decline after intrauterine transfusion not only depends on rate of destruction of erythrocytes, but also on changes in foetoplacental volume, predominantly resulting from fetal growth [268]. Moreover, the rate of decline of foetal red cells, usually disappearing during the interval between the first and second transfusion, is unpredictable. For the optimal timing of the next procedure or alternatively to plan delivery, apart from the expected haematocrit decline, close surveillance of the foetal condition by ultrasound and Doppler remains of utmost importance [223].

Direct intravascular foetal transfusions are not only being performed in the umbilical cord at the cord insertion, or alternatively in a free loop of cord, but also in the intrahepatic portion of the umbilical vein [27,28,269,270]. Intrauterine transfusions in the umbilical cord are preferably performed in the vein, as puncturing one of the umbilical arteries is associated with a higher complication and loss rate [271-273]. The intrahepatic approach may be considered as a safe alternative to cord needling, as was found by Nicolini et al. [270]. However, it was demonstrated by Giannakoulopoulos et al. that needling the foetal trunk for intrahepatic transfusion resulted in a significantly greater increase in foetal plasma noradrenalin levels, when compared to puncturing the placental cord insertion [274]. Foetal discomfort at intrahepatic procedures is also suggested by the finding of an acute cerebral haemodynamic response, that was not observed at cord punctures [275]. The safety of intracardiac fetal transfusions, performed in some centres, has not been proven, due to the limited experience of this technique [276-278].

Especially in the first years after the introduction of direct intravascular foetal transfusions, some choose to perform a foetal exchange transfusion instead of a simple transfusion [279-281]. Studies comparing different techniques revealed that the foetus generally may tolerate a bolus transfusion and that the procedure time of simple transfusions is shorter than for exchange transfusions [248,281]. Although theoretically exchange transfusion may result in a more stable haematocrit, allowing longer intervals between procedures, there is also a supposed increased risk of accidental needle displacement that may result in cord complications and bleeding [279]. Nowadays, exchange transfusions are reserved by most for those severely anaemic foetuses, assumed to have a compromised condition, in order to reduce the volume load administered [189]. Selbing et al. found a negative correlation between net transfusion volume and fetal survival in a series of 124 consecutive intravascular transfusions [282]. Radunovic et al. confirmed the poor tolerance of particularly severely anaemic and hydropic foetuses to large and acute increases in haematocrit [283]. Therefore, not only exchange transfusion, but also frequent small volume transfusions may alternatively benefit the outcome in severe foetal compromise [189]. Hallak et al. found adverse outcome at transfusion to be related to umbilical vein pressures exceeding 10 mm Hg [284]. From these results, and that of other studies, it was hypothesized that intravascular pressure monitoring at transfusion may increase the safety of the procedure [284-286]. However, this concept dates from over 10 years ago and there is no evidence from recent studies to support the clinical value and usefulness of pressure monitoring at intrauterine transfusion.

The striking foetal tolerance to volume expansion has been subject to many studies. It has been demonstrated in animal studies, that foetoplacental volume only moderately increases after transfusion, and also that afterwards this volume rapidly returns to pre-transfusion values [287]. Doppler studies in human foetuses showed a decrease in blood velocity in most vessels, immediately following transfusion, generally explained by the increase in blood viscosity resulting in a decrease in stroke volume and a fall in cardiac output [221,222, 288-293]. It has been postulated that the rapid adaptation of the foetus to volume load is mediated by vasoactive substances, such as: prostaglandins, vasopressin, atrial natriuretic peptide (ANP) and endothelin [294-300]. Studies on foetal oxygenation at intrauterine transfusion confirm foetal tolerance to volume load and transfusion with adult red blood cells [301,302]. Minor and generally transient changes in foetal blood gas and acid-base status were found after transfusion, consisting of a slight decrease in pH and base excess and an increase in pCO_2 [301-303]. However, foetuses with anaemic hypoxia appear to have elevated lactate levels and are unable to maintain adequate oxygenation to all tissues [304].

Foetal paralysis is frequently applied at intrauterine transfusion, in order to prevent complications resulting from foetal movements [305, 306]. Spencer et al. found a reduction in foetal heart rate variation of 60%, after the administration of pancuronium bromide at transfusion [307]. To diminish these side-effects on the foetal heart rate pattern, the use of other paralysing agents has been advocated in several studies [308,309]. There is no uniformity regarding the routine use of tocolysis or antibiotic prophylaxis at intrauterine transfusion, as evidence for the beneficial effect of these measures is lacking.

Complications of intravascular foetal transfusion – Foetal complications during or after an invasive procedure may either result from the procedure or from the underlying pathologic condition necessitating treatment. Cordocentesis is only followed by intravascular transfusion after the assessment of foetal anaemia. Tongsong et al. found a pure procedure-related foetal loss rate after cordocentesis of 1.4% [45]. However, it may be assumed that both the longer duration of intravascular transfusion and the volume administered to the foetus may result in a higher complication rate, when compared to diagnostic cordocentesis [310]. Important complications that may seriously jeopardize foetal condition, and even result in foetal demise, are premature rupture of membranes and preterm delivery, intrauterine infection and foetal distress, resulting from local cord complications or excessive bleeding [160].

Preterm delivery after intrauterine transfusion is observed by some after 2% of procedures and frequently appears to be related to the presence of intrauterine infection [160,279]. Bacterial and viral infections have been described after cordocentesis and intrauterine transfusion and may threaten both foetal and maternal condition [160,163,311,312]. Especially the exposure to viral infections is a known risk factor of blood transfusion. Additional risks, such as elevated plasma potassium levels, may result from the preparation and preservation of donor blood [313,314]. However, the most feared complication is acute foetal distress during or immediately following intrauterine transfusion. Foetal distress may, depending on the gestational age, result in emergency caesarean section or perinatal death. Foetal distress at transfusion most frequently originates from either local cord complications, such as haematoma or arterial spasm, or from excessive bleeding followed by exsanguination [189]. As cord haematoma and bleeding frequently result from needle dislodgement induced by foetal movements, foetal paralysis is assumed to reduce the risk on these life-threatening complications [305-309]. Arterial puncture, being a well-known risk factor for foetal distress resulting from vasospasm, is avoided by most [160, 273].

According to Harman, significant effects on the foetal cardiovascular state are to be expected if bleeding exceeds 300 seconds [189]. However, in vitro studies revealed that it impossible to accurately estimate the volume of blood loss by ultrasound observation [315]. Ney et al. found a beneficial effect of amniotic fluid compared to isotonic saline, on the duration of bleeding from cord puncture, and explained this finding by the coagulation properties of thromboplastins [316]. Excessive bleeding is more frequently observed after transamniotic cord needling and in the presence of foetal thrombocytopenia [189,315]. As thrombocytopenia is often observed in the hydropic and severely anaemic foetus, a routine platelet supplementation at intrauterine transfusion is implemented in some centres, in order to prevent prolonged bleeding of these foetuses [189,317]. Foetal loss due to haemopericardium was observed at 2.6% of intracardiac transfusion procedures [278]. Intrahepatic transfusions are considered as a safe alternative to umbilical cord needling, as even lower loss rates have been reported in studies comparing both techniques [270]. Although larger volume intrauterine transfusions benefit foetal outcome, by reducing the number of procedures, it was also found that large increases in haematocrit enhance the risk of adverse outcome in the presence of severe anaemia or foetal hydrops [283,318]. Welch et al. also found adverse outcome to be related to a massive rise in whole blood viscosity [318]. Therefore, limiting the volume load seems advisable, if the foetus is assumed to suffer from a compromised condition [189].

Schumacher and Moise reviewed the literature on intrauterine transfusions and found a mean procedure-related foetal loss rate of 2% in 708 procedures, performed in several centres [29]. This figure gives an impression of procedural loss in specialized centres, although complications were not uniformly defined and different techniques were used. By independent evaluation of all complications occurring during or after intrauterine transfusion, we found a procedure-related foetal loss rate of 1.6% per procedure [320].

Few case reports on the presence of porencephalic cysts, necrotising enterocolitis and graft versus host disease after intrauterine transfusion have been published, but evidence of a causal relationship of these complications with intrauterine treatment is lacking [321-323]. Diminished foetal growth in the presence of haemolytic disease was formerly suggested, but the birth weight of foetuses treated with intrauterine transfusions appeared comparable to control subjects [324,325].

Free radical cell damage due to iron overload and increased plasma haemoglobin is not only hypothesized to play a role in the pathogenesis of alloimmune hydrops and in the relatively short lifespan of donor red cells, but may according to some also lead to foetal hepatic and cardiac damage [326-330]. Neonatal liver function disorders due to iron overload have been reported after intrauterine transfusions [328,330]. More research is needed to elucidate these possible mechanisms.

Enhanced maternal sensitisation and the development of additional antibodies have been reported after intrauterine transfusions and may both result in a more severe foetal haemolytic disease in future pregnancies [169-173,331]. Finally,

Table 1. Summary of studies using intrauterine intravascular transfusions for foetal anaemia due to maternal red cell alloimmunization

		Survival n / total n (%)					
First author	**Year**	**Hydrops**		**No hydrops**		**Total**	
Rodeck [253]	1984	11/15	(73)	7/10	(70)	18/25	(72)
Nicolaides [269]	1986	10/11	(91)	10/10	(100)	20/21	(95)
Westgren [277]	1988	10/16	(63)	19/21	(90)	29/37	(78)
Barss [337]	1988	5/6	(83)	7/8	(88)	12/14	(85)
Berkowitz [338]	1988	3/5	(60)	10/12	(83)	13/17	(76)
Grannum [336]	1988	25/32	(78)	12/15	(80)	37/47	(79)
Parer [339]	1988	6/12	(50)	30/33	(91)	36/45	(84)
Orsini [340]	1988	4/8	(50)	6/7	(86)	10/15	(67)
Poissonnier [279]	1989	29/47	(62)	55/60	(92)	84/107	(79)
Lemery [341]	1989	2/4	(50)	8/11	(73)	10/15	(67)
Pattison [264]	1989	1/2	(50)	17/18	(94)	18/20	(90)
Nicolini [270]	1990	3/4	(75)	23/27	(85)	26/31	(84)
Weiner [342]	1991	11/13	(85)	35/35	(100)	46/48	(96)
Ney [343]	1991	6/7	(86)	16/19	(84)	22/26	(85)
Sampson [344]	1994	20/33	(61)	39/45	(87)	59/78	(76)
Plöckinger [345]	1994	5/7	(71)	13/14	(93)	18/21	(86)
Harman [189]	1995	36/49	(73)	78/80	(98)	114/129	(88)
Grab [346]	1999	7/11	(64)	28/32	(88)	35/43	(81)
Farina [347]	2000	30/38	(79)	47/48	(98)	77/86	(90)
van Kamp [348]	2003	62/80	(78)	119/130	(92)	181/210	(86)
Total	–	286/400	(72)	579/635	(91)	865/1035	(84)

more research seems to be needed on possible long-term immunological effects to both mother and child [332,333].

Outcome and follow-up after intravascular transfusion – Overall survival rates exceeding 80% have been reported since the introduction of intravascular intrauterine transfusion therapy in the 1980s [29,334,335]. Table 1, including series with at least 10 patients, shows the reported survival rates after treatment with foetal intravascular transfusions. Most procedures were plain umbilical cord transfusions, although intrahepatic, intracardiac and exchange transfusions, as well as combined intravascular and intraperitoneal procedures were also included in the table. Nevertheless, comparable results were reported for all techniques, with a significantly lower survival rate in the presence of foetal hydrops, compared to survival in the absence of hydrops.

Reversal of foetal alloimmune hydrops after correction of foetal anaemia is observed in about 60% of the cases, and generally results in a survival rate, that is comparable to those of foetuses without hydrops [334]. Persistence of foetal hydrops, despite successful intrauterine transfusions, results in a poor outcome with survival rates of on average 40% [334,336]. We also demonstrated a close correlation of the reversal of alloimmune hydrops to subsequent survival, and found that the severity of alloimmune foetal hydrops is highly predictive of foetal outcome [349]. Mild hydrops resolved in 88% and severe hydrops in only 39% of the cases [349]. After resolution of hydrops, 98% of foetuses survived, whereas persisting hydrops resulted in a survival rate of 55% [349]. It is hypothesized that the irreversibility of foetal hydrops in a substantial proportion of cases, is caused by massive injury of foetal vascular endothelium [329,350].

Late postnatal hyporegenerative anaemia is frequently observed in alloimune haemolytic disease, treated with intrauterine and neonatal simple or exchange transfusions [351-354]. Not only haemolysis of newly formed erythrocytes by circulating antibodies, but also suppressed erythropoiesis may explain the need for often repeated transfusions in the first months after birth [354,355]. Saade et al found the need for late transfusions to be related to the extent and duration of foetal bone marrow suppression [356]. Treatment with erythropoietin is assumed to be beneficial in severe and persisting cases of late hyporegenerative anaemia [357].Several studies on the long-term developmental outcome of children treated with intrauterine intravascular transfusions, for anaemia resulting from maternal alloimmunization, showed no differences when compared to control subjects [355-362].

Intrauterine transfusions at the Leiden University Medical Centre; 1988-1999. – Since 1965, the Leiden University Medical Centre is the single national referral centre for the management and intrauterine treatment of foetal anaemia [192, 193]. Our methods have been described in detail in former and recent publications [254,348].

In the period of 1988 to 1999, 210 foetuses from 208 pregnancies of 187 women, received intrauterine transfusion therapy for foetal anaemia due to red-cell alloimmunization. A total of 593 successful transfusions were performed (median 3; range 1-7), 528 (89%) of which in the umbilical cord and 61 (10%) in the intrahepatic part of the umbilical vein. In addition, there were three intraperitoneal transfusions as well as one intracardiac procedure. Hydrops was present in 38% of the foetuses. Anaemia resulted from maternal Rh(D) alloimmunization in 86% of the foetuses, Kell and Rh(c) immunization were present in 9% and 4% of the cases respectively. Rh(E), Rh(c) and Fy^a immunization were found in one case each. The median gestational age at the first transfusion was 27 weeks (range 17-35 weeks). Median foetal haemoglobin at the first proce-

Table 2. Survival of 210 foetuses classified according to type of maternal antibody and absence or presence of hydrops

	Hydrops					
	Absent (n=130)		**Present (n=80)**		**Total (n=210)**	
Rh(D) n (%)	**110/117**	**(94)a,b**	**50/63**	**(79)**	**160/180**	**(89)c**
Kell n (%)	5/9	(56)a	6/10	(60)	11/19	(58)c
Rh(c) n (%)	3/3	(100)	5/5	(100)	8/8	(100)
Total n (%)	119	(92)d	62	(78)d	181	(86)

a. p=0.003; b. p=0.003; c. p<0.001; d. p=0.004.

dure was 3.0 mmol/l (range 0.7-8.2). Haemoglobin at the initial transfusion appeared significantly lower in the presence than in the absence of foetal hydrops (2.0 versus 3.7 mmol/l; P<0.001).

Data on overall perinatal survival of foetuses with anaemia resulting from the most frequently observed alloimmunizations are summarized in Table 2.

Logistic regression analysis of the data revealed that survival was negatively associated with the presence of hydrops (P = 0.004), and with Kell immunization (P = 0.005). In addition both a younger gestational age at the first transfusion (P < 0.001) and a higher number of successful transfusions (P < 0.001) were positively and independently associated with survival. The poor foetal outcome of Kell immunization in our study, may be explained by the fact that foetal disease was often diagnosed late in gestation, resulting in a late referral and start of intrauterine treatment. The routine red cell antibody screening program, introduced in the Netherlands in 1998, may help to identify all pregnancies at risk for alloimmune foetal haemolytic disease early in gestation. We found the procedure-related fatal complication rate in a somewhat larger cohort (740 procedures) to be 1.6% per procedure [320]. A follow-up study on the developmental outcome of the first 77 surviving children shows no increase in minor and major handicaps, when compared to children that were born at comparable gestational ages [362].

In conclusion, our study, representing the outcome of intrauterine treatment for red-cell alloimmunization in the Netherlands, confirms that intravascular transfusion is a safe and effective method to treat foetal anaemia. Intrauterine treatment for foetal anaemia should preferably be started before the development of hydrops. Our results emphasize the importance of the early diagnosis of alloimmunization in pregnancy and of timely referral of women at risk to a centre specialized in the management of alloimmunized pregnancies.

References

1. Darrow RR. Icterus gravis (erythroblastosis) neonatorum; an examination of etiologic considerations. Arch Pathol 1934;56:378-417.

2. Levine P, Stetson RE. Unusual case of intra-group agglutination. J Amer Med Ass 1939;113:126-27.
3. Levine P. The discovery of Rh haemolytic disease. Vox Sang 1984;47: 187-90.
4. Landsteiner K, Weiner AS. An agglutinable factor in human blood recognized by immune sera for Rhesus blood. Proc Soc Exper Biol Med 1940; 43:223.
5. Kloosterman GJ. Over de polyletaliteit in verband met het vlokkenstroma en de rhesusfactor [thesis]. Amsterdam: University of Amsterdam; 1947.
6. Reepmaker J, Nijenhuis LE, van Loghem JJ. Note on the influence of ABO bloodgroup incompatibility on Rhesus immunization in pregnancy. Vox Sang 1954; 4:117.
7. Wallerstein H. Treatment of severe erythroblastosis by simultaneous removal and replacement of the blood of the newborn infant. Science 1946; 103:583-84.
8. Liley AW. Liquor amnii analysis in the management of the pregnancy complicated by rhesus sensitization. Am J Obstet Gynecol 1961;82: 1359-70.
9. Clarke CA, Donohoe WTA, McConnell RB, et al. Further experimental studies on the prevention of Rh haemolytic diseaese. Br Med J 1963;i: 979-84
10. Freda VJ, Gorman JG, Pollack W. Successful prevention of experimental RH sensitization in man with an RH gamma2-globin antibody preparation: A preliminary report. Transfusion 1964;4:26-32.
11. Hamilton EG. RH_0 (D) immunoglobulin (RHOGAM): How it came into being. Obstet Gynecol 1991;77:957.
12. Chown B, Duff AM, James J, et al. Prevention of primary Rh Immunization: First report of the Western Canadian Trial, 1966-1968. Can Med Assoc J 1968;100: 1021-24.
13. Clarke CA, Donohoe WTA, Finn R, et al. (Medical Research Council Party) Prevention of Rh-haemolytic disease: final results of the 'high risk' clinical trial. Br Med J 1971;2:607-09.
14. Ascari WG, Allen AE, Baker WJ, Pollack W. Rho(D) immune globulin (human) evaluation in women at risk of Rh immunization. JAMA 1968;205: 71-74.
15. Dudok de Wit C, Borst-Eilers E, van der Weerdt ChM, Kloosterman GJ. Preventie van rhesus-immunisatie met behulp van anti-rhesus(D)-immunoglobuline [Prevention of rhesus isoimmunization with anti-rhesus (D) immunoglobulin]. Ned Tijdschr Geneesk 1968;112:2345-51.
16. Mackenzie IZ, Bowell P, Gregory H, Pratt G, Guest C, Entwistle CC. Routine antenatal Rhesus D immunoprophylaxis: the results of a prospective 10 year study. Br J Obstet Gynaecol 1999;106:492-97.
17. Urbaniak SJ. The scientific basis of antenatal prophylaxis. Br J Obstet Gynaecol 1998;105:11-18.

18. Crowther CA, Keirse MJ. Anti-D administration in pregnancy for preventing rhesus alloimmunisation. Cochrane Database Syst Rev 2000;2: CD 000020.
19. Liley AW. Intrauterine transfusion of foetus in haemolytic disease. Br Med J 1963;ii:1107-09.
20. Liley AW. The administration of blood transfusions to the foetus in utero. Triangle 1966;7:184-89.
21. Harman CR,. Specialized applications of obstetric ultrasound: management of the alloimmunized pregnancy. Semin Perinatol 1985;9:184-97.
22. Bennebroek Gravenhorst J, Kanhai HH, Meerman RH, et al. Twenty-two years of intra-uterine intraperitoneal transfusions. Eur J Obstet Gynecol Reprod Biol 1989; 33:71-77.
23. Harman CR, Bowman JM, Manning FA, Menticoglou SM. Intrauterine transfusion-intraperitoneal versus intravascular approach: A case-control comparison. Am J Obstet Gynecol 1990;162:1053-59.
24. Pattison NS, Roberts AB, Mantell N. Intrauterine fetal transfusion, 1963-90. Ultrasound Obstet Gynecol 1992;2:329-32.
25. Rodeck CH, Kemp JR, Holman CA, Whitmore DN, Karnicki J, Austin MA. Direct intravascular fetal blood transfusion by fetoscopy in severe Rhesus isoimmunisation. Lancet 1981;1:625-27.
26. Daffos F, Capella-Pavlovski M, Forestier F. A new procedure for fetal blood sampling in utero: Preliminary results of fifty-three cases. Am J Obstet Gynecol 1983;146:985-87.
27. Bang J, Bock JE, Trolle D. Ultrasound-guided fetal intravenous transfusion for severe rhesus hemolytic disease. Br Med J 1982;284:373-74.
28. de Crespigny LCh, Robinson HP, Quinn M, Doyle L, Cauchi M. Ultrasound-guided fetal blood transfusion for severe Rhesus isoimmunization. Obstet Gynecol 1985; 66:529-32.
29. Schumacher B, Moise KJ. Fetal transfusion for red blood cell alloimmunization in pregnancy. Obstet Gynecol 1996;88:137-50.
30. Hofman D, Hollander HJ. Die intrauterine diagnostiek des hydrops fetalis universalis mittels ultraschal. Zentralbl Gynaekol 1968;90:667.
31. Jones M. Ultrasonic B scanning in rhesus incompatibility. J Clin Ultrasound 1974; 2:185.
32. Weiner S, Bolognese RJ, Librizzi RJ. Ultrasound in the evaluation and management of the isoimmunized pregnancy. J Clin Ultrasound 1981;9: 315-23.
33. Vintzileos AM, Campbell WA, Storlazzi E, Mirochnick MH, Escoto DT, Nochimson DJ. Fetal liver ultrasound measurements in isoimmunized pregnancies. Obstet Gynecol 1986;68:162-67.
34. Oepkes D, Meerman RH, Vandenbussche FPHA, van Kamp IL, Kok FG, Kanhai HHH. Ultrasonographic fetal spleen measurements in red cell alloimmunized pregnancies. Am J Obstet Gynecol 1993;169:121-28.
35. Manning FA, Platt LD, Sipos L. Antepartum fetal evaluation: Development of a fetal biophysical profile. Am J Obstet Gynecol 1980;136:787-95.

36. Kirkinen P, Jouppila P, Eik-Nes S. Umbilical venous flow as indicator of fetal anaemia. Lancet 1981;i(8227):1004-05.
37. Gill RW, Kossoff G, Warren PS, Garrett WJ. Umbilical venous flow in normal and complicated pregnancy. Ultrasound Med Biol 1984;10:349-63.
38. Copel JA, Grannum PA, Belanger K, Green J, Hobbins JC. Pulsed Doppler flow-velocity waveforms before and after intrauterine intravascular transfusion for severe erythroblastosis fetalis. Am J Obstet Gynecol 1988;158: 768-74.
39. Bilardo CM, Nicolaides KH, Campbell S. Doppler studies in red cell isoimmunization. Clin Obstet Gynecol 1989;32:719-27.
40. Rightmere DA, Nicolaides KH, Rodeck CH, Campbell S. Fetal blood velocities in Rh isoimmunization: relationship to gestational age and to fetal hematocrit. Obstet Gynecol 1986:68:223-26.
41. Oepkes D, Brand R, Vandenbussche FP, Meerman RH, Kanhai HHH. The use of ultrasonography and Doppler to predict the severity of fetal hemolytic anemia: a multivariate analysis. Br J Obstet Gynaecol 1994;101: 680-84.
42. Hecher K, Snijders R, Campbell S, Nicolaides K. Fetal venous, arterial and intracardiac blood flows in red blood cell isoimmunization. Obstet Gynecol 1995;85: 122-28.
43. Mari G, Adrignolo A, Abuhamad AZ, Pirhonen J, Jones DC, Ludomirsky A, Copel JA. Diagnosis of fetal anemia with Doppler ultrasound in the pregnancy complicated by maternal blood group immunization. Ultrasound Obstet Gynecol 1995;5:400-05.
44. Ghidini A, Sepulveda W, Lockwood CJ, Romero R. Complications of fetal blood sampling. Am J Obstet Gynecol 1993;168:1339-44.
45. Tongsong T, Wanapirak C, Kunavikatikul C, Sirirchotiyakul S, Piyamongkol W, Chanprapaph P. Fetal loss rate associated with cordocentesis at midgestation. Am J Obstet Gynecol 2001;184:719-23.
46. Charles AG, Blumethal LS. Promethazine hydrochloride therapy in severely Rh-sensitized pregnancies. Obstet Gynecol 1982;60:627-30.
47. Navot D, Rozen E, Sadovski E. Effect of dexamethasone on amniotic fluid absorbance in Rh-sensitized pregnancies. Br J Obstet Gynaecol 1982;89: 456-58.
48. Caudle MR, Scott JR. The potential role of immunosuppression, plasmapheresis and desensitization as treatment modalities for Rh immunization. Clin Obstet Gynecol 1982;25:313-19.
49. Gold WR, Queenan JT, Woody J, Sacher RA. Oral desensitization in Rj disease. Am J Obstet Gynecol 1983;146:980-81.
50. Clarke C. Rhesus haemolytic disease of the newborn and its prevention. Br J Haematol 1982;52:525-35.
51. Duerbeck NB, Seeds JW. Rhesus immunization in pregnancy: a review. Obstet Gynecol Surv 1993; 48: 801-10.
52. Pollock W, Ascari WQ, Kochesky RJ. Studies on Rh prophylaxis. Relationship between doses of anti Rh and size of antigen stimulus. Transfusion 1971;11:333.

53. Kumpel BM. On the mechanism of tolerance to the Rh D antigen mediated by passive anti-D (Rh D prophylaxis). Immunol Lett 2002;82:67-73.
54. Salama A, Kiefel V, Amberg R, Mueller-Eckhardt C. Treatment of autoimmune thrombocytopenic purpura with rhesus antibodies [anti-Rh0(D)]. Blut 1984;49:29-35.
55. Scaradavou A, Bussel JB. Clinical experience with anti-D in the treatment of idiopathic thrombocytopenic purpura. Semin Hemaltol 1998;35(1 suppl 1):52-57.
56. Moser AM, Shalev H, Kapelushnik J. Anti-D exerts a very early response in childhood acute idiopathic thrombocytopenic purpura. Pediatr Hematol Oncol 2002;19: 407-11.
57. Michel M, Novoa MV, Bussel JB. Intravenous anti-D as a treatment for immune thrombocytopenic purpura (ITP) during pregnancy. Br J Haematol 2003;123:142-46.
58. Borst-Eilers E. Rhesusimmunisatie: ontstaan en preventie [thesis]. Amsterdam: University of Amsterdam; 1972.
59. Lee D, Contreras M, Robson SC, Rodeck CH, Whittle MJ. Recommendations for the use of anti-D immunoglobulin for Rh prophylaxis. Transfus Med 1999;9:93-97.
60. van Dijk BA, Hirasing RA, Overbeeke MAM. Hemolytische ziekte van de pasgeborene en irregulaire-bloedgroepantagonisme in Nederland: prevalentie en morbiditeit [Hemolytic disease of the newborn and irregulair blood group antagonism in the Netherlands: prevalence and morbidity]. Ned Tijdschr Geneesk 1999;143:1465-69.
61. Bowman JM. The prevention of Rh immunisation. Transfus Med Rev 1988; 2:129-50.
62. Tovey LAD, Townley A, Stephenson BJ, Taverner J. The Yorkshire antenatal anti-D immunoglobulin trial in primigravidae. Lancet 1983;2: 244-46.
63. Huchet J, Dallamagne S, Huchet CI, Brossard M, Larsen M, Parnet-Mathieu F. Application ante-partum du traitment preventif d'immunisation RhD chez les femmes Rh negatif. J Gynecol Obstet Biol Reprod 1987;16: 101-11.
64. Vick S, Cairns J, Urbaniak S, Whitfield CR, Raafat A. Cost-effectiveness of antenatal anti-D prophylaxis. Health Economics 1996;5:319-28.
65. Statement from the consensus conference on Anti-D prophylaxis, 7 and 8 april 1997 (no authors listed). Vox Sang 1998;74:127-28.
66. Fung Kee Fung K, Eason E, Crane J, Armson A, De La Ronde S, Farine D et al. Prevention of Rh alloimmunization. J Obstet Gynaecol Can 2003;25: 765-73.
67. Kumpel BM. Monoclonal anti-D development progarmme. Transpl Immunol 2002;10:199-204.
68. Levine P. Hemolytic disease due to antibodies other than anti-D. Rev Hematol 1955;10:215-26.
69. Moise KJ,Jr. Non-anti-D antibodies in red-cell alloimmunization. Eur J Obstet Gynecol Reprod Biol 2000;92:75-81.

70. Bowell PJ, Brown SE, Dike AE, Inskip MJ. The significance of anti-c alloimmunization in pregnancy. Br J Obstet Gynaecol 1986;93:1044-48.
71. Freire-Lizama T, Oepkes D. Management of Kell alloimmunized pregnancies. Fetal Maternal Med Rev 2002;13:1-16.
72. Grant SR, Kilby MD, Meer L, Waever JB, Gabra GS, Whittle MJ. The outcome of pregnancy in Kell alloimmunisation. Br J Obstet Gynaecol 2000; 107:481-85.
73. Goodrick MJ, Hadley AG, Poole G. Hemolytic disease of the fetus and newborn due to anti-Fya and the potential clinical value of Duffy genotyping in pregnancies at risk. Transfus Med 1997;7:301-04.
74. Moran P, Robson SC, Reid MM. Anti-E in pregnancy. Br J Obstet Gynaecol 2000; 107:1436-38.
75. Bowman JM, Pollock JM, Manning FA, Harman CR. Severe anti-C hemolytic disease of the newborn. Am J Obstet Gynecol 1992;166:1239-43.
76. Babinsky A, Berkowitz RL. Haemolytic disease of the newborn caused by anti-c, anti-E and anti-Fya antibodies: report of five cases. Prenat Diagn 1999;19:533-36.
77. Weiner CP, Widness JA. Decreased fetal erythropoiesis and hemolysis in Kell hemolytic anemia. Am J Obstet Gynecol 1996;174:547-51.
78. Vaughan JI, Manning M, Warwick RM, Letsky EA, Murray NA, Roberts IAG. Inhibition of erythroid progenitor cells by anti-Kell antibodies in fetal alloimmune anemia. N Engl J Med 1998;338:798-803.
79. Gezondheidsraad. Preventie van zwangerschapsimmunisatie. Rapport 1992/ 08. Den Haag: Gezondheidsraad, 1992.
80. Bowell PJ, Wainscoat JS, Peto TEA, Gunson HH. Maternal anti-D concentrations and outcome in rhesus haemolytic disease of the newborn. BMJ 1982;285:327-29.
81. American College of Obstetricians and Gynecologists. Management of isoimmunization in pregnancy. Washington: ACOG 1996; technical bulletin no 227.
82. Nicolaides KH, Rodeck CH. Maternal serum anti-D antibody concentration and assessment of rhesus isoimmunization. BMJ 1992;304:1155-56.
83. Moise KJ, Perkins JT, Sosler SD, Brown SJ, Saade G, Carpenter RJ, et al. The predictive value of maternal serum testing for detection of fetal anemia in red blood cell alloimmunization. Am J Obstet Gynecol 1995;172:1003-09.
84. Oepkes D, van Kamp IL, Simon MJ, Mesman J, Overbeeke MA, Kanhai HH. Clinical value of an antibody-dependent cell-mediated cytotoxicity assay in the management of Rh D alloimmunization. Am J Obstet Gynecol 2001;184:1015-20.
85. van Dijk BA, Dooren MC, Overbeeke AM. Red cell alloantibodies in pregnancy: there is no 'critical titre'. Transfusion Med 1995;4:199-202.
86. Clarke DA. Red-cell antibodies in pregnancy: evidence overturned. Lancet 1996; 347: 485-86.

87. Taslimi MM, Sibai BM, Mason JM, Dacus JV. Immunoglobulin G subclasses and isoimmunized pregnancy outcome. Am J Obstet Gynecol 1986; 154:1327-32.
88. Weiner E, Atwal A, Thompson KM, Melamed MD, Gorick B, Hughes-Jones NC. Differences between the activities of human monoclonal IgG1 and IgG3 subclasses of anti-D(Rh) antibody in their ability to mediate red cell binding to macrophages. Immunology 1987;62:401-04.
89. Ouwehand WH. The activity of IgG1 and IgG3 antibodies in immune-mediated destruction of red cells; clinical significance in rhesus haemolytic disease of the newborn [thesis]. Amsterdam, University of Amsterdam; 1984.
90. Dooren MC, van Kamp IL, Kanhai HHH, Bennebroek Gravenhorst J, von dem Borne AEGKr, Engelfriet CP. Evidence of the protective effect of maternal FcR-blocking IgG alloantibodies in Rh D-haemolytic disease of the newborn. Vox Sang 1993; 65:55-58.
91. Urbaniak SJ, Greiss MA, Crawford RJ, Fergusson MC. Prediction of the severity of rhesus haemolytic disease of the newborn by an ADCC assay. Lancet 1981;2:142-43.
92. Engelfriet CP, Ouwehand WH. ADCC and other cellular bioassays for predicting the clinical significance of red cell alloantibodies. Balliere's Clin Haematol 1990;3:321-37.
93. Larson PJ, Thorp JM, Miller RC, Hoffman M. The monocyte monolayer assay: a noninvasive technique for predicting the severity of in utero hemolysis. Am J Perinat 1995;12:157-60.
94. Hadley AG, Wilkes A, Goodrick J, Penman D, Soothill P, Lucas G. The ability of the chemoluminescence test to predict clinical outcome and the necessity for amniocenteses in pregnancies at risk of haemolytic disease of the newborn. Br J Obstet Gynaecol 1998;105:231-34.
95. Mollison PL. Results of tests with different cellular bioassays in relation to severity of RhD haemolytic disease. Vox Sang 1991;60:225-29.
96. Chiu RW, Murphy MF, Fidler C, Zee BC, Wainscoat JS, Lo YM. Determination of RhD zygosity: comparison of a double amplification refractory mutation system approach and a multiplex real-time quantitative PCR approach. Clin Chem 2001;47: 667-72.
97. Philip J, Brandt NJ, Fernandes A, Freiesleben E, Trolle D. ABO and Rh phenotyping of fetal blood obtained by foetoscopy. Clin Gen 1974;14:324-29.
98. Kanhai HH. Bennebroek Gravenhorst J, Gemke RJ, Overbeeke MA, Bernini LF, Beverstock GC. Fetal blood group determination in first trimester pregnancy for the management of severe immunization. Am J Obstet Gynecol 1987;156:120-23.
99. Fisk NM, Bennett P, Warwick RM, et al. Clinical utility of fetal RhD typing in alloimmunized pregnancies by means of polymerase chain reaction on amniocytes or chorionic villi. Am J Obstet Gynecol 1994;17:50-54.

100. Bennett PR, Le Van Kim C, Colin Y, et al. Prenatal determination of fetal RhD type by DNA amplification. N Engl J Med 1993;329:607-10.
101. van den Veyver IB, Moise KJ,Jr. Fetal RhD typing by polymerase chain reaction in pregnancies complicated by rhesus alloimmunization. Obstet Gynecol 1996;88 :1061-67.
102. Lee S, Bennettt PR, Overton T, Warwick R, Wu X, Redman CM. Prenatal diagnosis of Kell blood group genotypes: Kel1 and Kel2. Am J Obstet Gynecol 1996;175:455-59.
103. Bowman JM. Transplacental fetal hemorrhage after amniocentesis. Obstet Gynecol 1985;66:749-54.
104. Lele AS, Carmody PJ, Hurd ME, O'Leary JA. Fetomaternal bleeding following diagnostic amniocentesis. Obstet Gynecol 1982;60:60-64.
105. Brambati B, Guercilena S, Bonacchi I, Oldrini A, Lanzani A, Piceni L. Feto-maternal transfusion after chorionic villus sampling: clinical implications. Hum Reprod 1986;1:37-40.
106. Moise KJ,Jr, Carpenter RJ,Jr. Increased severity of fetal hemolytic disease with known rhesus alloimmunization after first-trimester transcervical chorionic villus biopsy. Fetal Diagn Ther 1990;5:76-78.
107. Lo YM, Hjelm NM, Fidler C, Sargent IL, Murphy MF, Chamberlain PF et al. Prenatal diagnosis of fetal RhD status by molecular analysis of maternal plasma. N Engl J Med 1998;339:1734-38.
108. van der Schoot CE, Tax GH, Rijnders RJ, de Haas M, Christiaens GC. Prenatal typing of Rh and Kell blood group system antigens: the edge of a watershed. Transfus Med Rev 2003;17:31-44.
109. Finning KM, Martin PG, Soothill PW, Avent ND. Prediction of fetal D status from maternal plasma: introduction of a new non-invasive fetal RHD genotyping service. Transfusion 2002;42:1079-85.
110. Bowman JM. The management of Rh-isoimmunization. Obstet Gynecol 1978;52:1-16.
111. Drew JH, Mountain KR, Beischer NA. Spontaneous improvement in severity of erythroblastosis with advancing parity. Austr N Z J Obstet Gynaec 1977;117:229-31.
112. Rodeck CH, Deans A. Red cell alloimmunisation. In: Rodeck CH, Whittle MJ eds. Fetal medicine: Basic Science and Clinical Practice. London, Churchill Livingstone; Harcourt Brace and Company, 1999:785-809.
113. Oepkes D. The modern management of red cell alloimmunization. The Obstetrician & Gynaecologist 2003;5:35-40.
114. Powell LC,Jr. Intense plasmapheresis in the pregnant Rh-sensitized woman. Am J Obstet Gynecol 1968;101:153-70.
115. Clarke CA, Bradley J, Elson CJ, Donohoe WTA. Intensive plasmapheresis as a therapeutic measure in Rhesus immunized women. Lancet 1970;i:793-99.
116. Fraser ID, Bennet MO, Bohamley JE, Airth GR. Intensive antenatal plasmapheresis in severe rhesus isoimmunization. Lancet 1976;i:6-9.

117. Rubinstein P. Repeated small volume plasmapheresis in the management of haemolytic disease of the newborn. In: Frigoletto, Jewet, Konugres eds. Rh haemolytic disease: new strategy for eradication. Hall, Boston, 1982: 89-93.
118. Rubinstein P. Cyclical variations in anti-Rh titer detected by automatic quantitative haemagglutination. Vox Sang 1972;23:508-22.
119. Collinet P, Subtil D, Puech F, Vaast P. Successful treatment of extremely severe fetal anemia due to Kell alloimmunization. Obstet Gynecol 2002; 100:1102-05.
120. Fernandez-Jimenez MC, Jimenez-Marco MT, Hernandez D, Gonzalez A, Omenaca F, de la Camara C. Treatment with plasmapheresis and intravenous immunoglobulin in pregnancies complicated with anti-PP1Pk or anti-K immunization: a report of two patients. Vox Sang 2001;80:117-20
121. Radder CM, Brand A, Kanhai HH. A less invasive treatment strategy to prevent intracranial hemorrhage in fetal and neonatal alloimmune thrombocytopenia. Am J Obstet Gynecol 2001; 185:683-88.
122. Bussel JB. Alloimmune thrombocytopenia in the fetus and newborn. Semin Thromb Hemost 2001;27:245-52.
123. Berlin G, Selbing A, Ryden G. Rhesus haemolytic disease treated with high-dose intravenous immunoglobulin. Lancet 1985;i:1153.
124. De la Cámara C, Arrieta R, González A, Iglesias E, Omenaca F. High-dose intravenous immunoglobulin as the sole prenatal treatment for severe Rh immunization. N Engl J Med 1988;318:519-20.
125. Sacher RA, King JC. Intravenous gammaglobulin in pregnancy: a review. Obstet Gynecol Surv 1988;44:25-33
126. Chitkara U, Bussel J, Alvarez M, Lynch L, Meisel RL, Berkowitz RL. High-dose intravenous gammaglobulin: does it have a role in the treatment of severe erythroblastosis fetalis? Obstet Gynecol 1990;76:703.
127. Margulies M, Voto LS, Mathet E, Margulies M. High-dose intravenous IgG for the treatment of severe rhesus alloimmunization. Vox Sang 1991; 61:181-89.
128. Gottvall T, Selbing A. Alloimmunization during pregnancy treated with high dose intravenous immunoglobulin: effects on fetal haemoglobin concentration and anti-D concentrations in the mother and fetus. Acta Obstet Gynecol Scand 1995;74:777-83.
129. Porter TF, Silver RM, Jackson GM, Branch DW, Scott JR. Intravenous immune globulin in the management of severe haemolytic disease, Obstet Gynecol Surv 1997;52:193-97.
130. Voto LS, Mathet ER, Zapaterio JL, Lede RL, Margulies M. High-dose gammaglobulin (IVIG) followed by intrauterine transfusions (IUTs): a new alternative for the treatment of severe haemolytic disease. J Perinat Med 1997;25:85-88.
131. Dooren MC, van Kamp IL, Scherpenisse JW, et al. No beneficial effect of intravenous gammaglobulin in combination with intravascular fetal transfusion in severe Rh D-haemolytic disease. Vox Sang 1994;66:253-57.

132. Bevis DC. Blood pigments in haemolytic disease of the newborn. J Obstet Gynaecol Br Emp 1956;63:68-75.
133. Liley AW. Errors in the assessment of haemolytic disease from amniotic fluid. Am J Obstet Gynecol 1963;86:485-94.
134. Liley AW. The use of amniocentesis and fetal transfusion in erythroblastosis fetalis. Pediatrics 1965;35:836-47.
135. Freda VJ. The Rh problem in obstetrics and a new concept of its management using amniocentesis and spectrophotometric scanning of amniotic fluid. Am J Obstet Gynecol 1965;92:341-73.
136. Alpern WM, Charles AG, Friedman EA. Amniocentesis in the management of Rh-sensitized pregnancies. Am J Obstet Gynecol 1966;95: 11238.
137. Pridmore BR, Robertson EG, Walker W. Liquor bilirubin levels and false prediction of severity in rhesus haemolytic disease. BMJ 1972;3:136-69.
138. Fairweather DVI, Whyley GA, Miller MD. Six years experience of the prediction of severity in rhesus haemolytic disease. Br J Obstet Gynaecol 1976;83:698-706.
139. Nicolaides KH, Rodeck CH, Mibashan MD, Kemp JR. Have Liley charts outliced their usefulness? Am J Obstet Gynecol 1986;155:90-94.
140. Ananth U, Warsof SL, Coulehan JM, Wolf PH, Queenan JT. Midtrimester amniotic fluid delta optical density at 450 nm in normal pregnancies. Am J Obstet Gynecol 1986;155:664-66.
141. Ananth U, Queenan JT. Does midtrimester ΔOD450 of amniotic fluid reflect severity of Rh disease? Am J Obstet Gynecol 1989;161:47-49.
142. Spinnato JA, Ralston KK, Greenwell ER, Marcell CA, Spinnato JAIII. Amniotic fluid bilirubin and fetal haemolytic disease. Am J Obstet Gynecol 1991;165:1030-35.
143. Queenan JT, Tornai TP, Ural SH, King JC. Deviation in the amniotic fluid optical density at a wave length of 450 nm in Rh-immunized pregnancies from 14-40 weeks gestation: a proposal for clinical management. Am J Obstet Gynecol 1993;168:1370-76.
144. Spinnato JA, Clark AL, Ralston KK, Greenwell ER, Goldsmith LJ. Hemolytic disease of the fetus: a comparison of the Queenan and extended Liley methods. Obstet Gynecol 1998;92:441-45.
145. Sikkel E, Vandenbussche FP, Oepkes D, Meerman RH, Le Cessie S, Kanhai HH. Amniotic fluid delta OD 450 values accurately predict severe fetal anemia in D-alloimmunization. Obstet Gynecol 2002;100:51-57.
146. Tongsong T, Wanapirak C, Sirivatanapa P, Piyamongkol W, Sirichotiyakul S, Yampochai A. Amniocentesis-related fetal loss: a Cohort study. Obstet Gynecol 1998;92:64-67.
147. Antsaklis A, Papantoniou N, Xygakis A, Mesogitis S, Tzortzis E, Michalas S. Genetic amniocentis in women 20-34 years old: associated risks. Prenat Diagn 2000;20:247-50.
148. Wilson RD. Amniocentesis and chorionic villus sampling. Curr Opin Obstet Gynecol 2000;12:81-86.

149. Eisenberg B, Wapner RJ. Clinical procedures in prenatal diagnosis. Best Pract Clin Obstet Gynaecol 2002;16:611-27.
150. Rodeck CH, Campbell S. Sampling pure fetal blood by fetoscopy in second trimester of pregnancy. Br Med J 1978;ii;728-30.
151. Rodeck CH. Fetoscopy guided by real-time ultrasound for pure fetal blood samples, fetal skin samples, and examination of the fetus in utero. Br J Obstet Gynecol 1980;87:449-56.
152. Mackenzie IZ, Bowell PJ, Castle BM, Selinger M, Ferguson JF. Serial fetal blood sampling for the management of pregnancies complicated by severe rhesus(D) isoimmunization. Br J Obstet Gynecol 1988;95:753-58.
153. Weiner CP, Williamson RA, Wenstrom KD, Sipes SL, Grant SS, Widness JA. Management of fetal hemolytic disease by cordocentesis I. Prediction of fetal anaemia. Am J Obstet Gynecol 1991;165:546-53.
154. Nicolaides KH, Clewell WH, Mibashan RS, Soothill PW, Rodeck CH, Campbell S. Fetal haemoglobin measurement in the assessment of red cell isoimmunization. Lancet 1988;*i*:1073-75.
155. Daffos F, Capella-Pavlovsky M, Forestier F. Fetal blood sampling during pregnancy with the use of a needle guided by ultrasound: A study of 606 consecutive cases. Am J Obstet Gynecol 1985;153:655-60.
156. Benacerraf BR, Barss VA, Saltzman DH, Greene MF, Penso CA, Frigoletto Jr FD,. Acute fetal distress associated with percutaneous umbilical blood sampling. Am J Obstet Gynecol 1987;156:1218-20.
157. Ludomirsky A, Weiner S. Percutaneous fetal umbilical blood sampling. Clin Obstet Gynecol 1988;31:19-26.
158. Orlandi F, Damiani G, Jakil C, Lauricella S, Bertolino O, Maggio A. The risks of early cordocentesis (12-21 weeks): analysis of 500 procedures. Prenat Diagn 1990;10:425-28.
159. Boulot P, Deschamps F, Lefort G, et al. Pure fetal blood samples obtained by cordocentesis: technical aspects of 322 cases. Prenat Diagn 1990;10:93-100.
160. Weiner CP, Wenstrom KD, Sipes SL, Williamson RA. Risk factors for cordocentesis and fetal intravascular transfusion. Am J Obstet Gynecol 1991;165:1020-25.
161. Donner C, Simon P, Karioun A, Avni F, Rodesch F. Experience of a single team of operators in 891 diagnostic funipunctures. Obstet Gynecol 1994; 84:827-31.
162. Nicolaides KH. Cordocentesis. Clin Obstet Gynecol 1988;31:123-35.
163. Pielet BW, Socol ML, MacGregor SN, Ney JA, Dooley SL. Cordocentesis: an appraisal of risks. Am J Obstet Gynecol 1988;159:1497-500.
164. Weiner CP, Okamura K. Diagnostic fetal blood sampling – technique related losses. Fetal Diagn Ther 1996;11:169-75.
165. Wilkins I, Mezrow G, Lynch L, Bottone EJ, Berkowitz RL. Amnionitis and life-threatening respiratory distress after percutaneous umbilical blood sampling. Am J Obstet Gynecol 1989;160:427-28.

166. Jauniaux E, Donner C, Simon P, Vanesse M, Hustin J, Rodesch F. Pathologic aspects of the umbilical cord after percutaneous umbilical blood sampling. Obstet Gynecol 1989;73:215-18.
167. McColgin SW, Wayne Hess L, Martin RW, Martin JN, Morrison JC. Group B streptococcal sepsis and death in utero following funipuncture. Obstet Gynecol 1989;74:464-65.
168. Maxwell DJ, Johnson P, Hurley P, Neales K, Allan L, Knott P. Fetal blood sampling and pregnancy loss in relation to indication. Br J Obstet Gynaecol 1991;98:892-97.
169. Bowell PJ, Selinger M, Ferguson J, Giles J, Mackenzie IZ. Antenatal fetal blood sampling for the management of alloimmunized pregananzies: effect upon maternal anti-D potency levels. Br J Obstet Gynecol 1988;95:759-64.
170. Weiner C, Grant S, Hudson J, Williamson R, Wenstrom K. Effect of diagnositic and therapeutic cordocentesis on maternal serum α-fetoprotein concentration. Am J Obstet Gynecol 1989;161:706-08.
171. MacGregor SN, Silver RK, Sholl JS. Enhanced sensitization after cordocentesis in a rhesus-isoimmunized pregnancy. Am J Obstet Gynecol 1991; 165:382-83.
172. Bowman JM, Pollock JM, Peterson LE, Harman CR, Manning FA, Menticoglou SM. Fetomaternal hemorrhage following funipuncture: increase in severity of maternal red-cell alloimmunization. Obstet Gynecol 1994;84: 839-43.
173. van Selm M, Kanhai HHH, van Loo. Detection of fetomaternal haemorrhage associated with cordocentesis using serum α-fetoprotein and the kleihauer technique. Pren Diagn 1995;15:313-16.
174. Modanlou HD, Freeman RK, Ortiz O, Hinkes P, Pillsbury Jr G,. Sinusoidal fetal heart rate pattern and severe fetal anemia. Obstet Gynecol 1977; 49:537-41.
175. Verma U, Tejani N, Chatterjee S, Halitsky V. Sinusoidal fetal heart rate patterns in severe Rh disease. Obstet Gynecol 1980;55:666-69.
176. Katz M, Meizner I, Shani N, Insler V. Clinical significance of sinusoidal fetal heart rate pattern. Br J Obstet Gynaecol 1983;90:832-36.
177. Sigurd J, Joelsson I. Sinusoidal fetal heart rate pattern. An indicator of fetal anemia in iso-immunization. Acta Obstet Gynecol Scand 1984;63:463-66.
178. Visser GH. Antepartum sinusoidal and decelerative heart rate patterns in Rh disease. Am J Obstet Gynecol 1982;143:538-44.
179. Sadovsky G, Visser GH, Nicolaides KH. Heart rate patterns in fetal anemia. Fetal Ther 1988;3:216-23.
180. Nicolaides KH, Sadovsky G, Cetin E. Fetal heart rate patterns in red blood cell isoimmunized pregnancies. Am J Obstet Gynecol 1989;161:351-56.
181. Nicolaides KH, Sadovsky G, Visser GH. Heart rate patterns in normoxemic, hypoxemic, and anemic second-trimester fetuses. Am J Obstet Gynecol 1989;160: 1034-37.

182. Olofsson P, Stangenberg M, Selbing A, Rahman F, Westgren M. Fetal heart rate responses to anaemia in Rh isoimmunization. J Perinat Med 1990;18:187-94.
183. Pattison P, McCowan L. Cardiotocography for antepartum fetal assessment. Cochrane Database Syst Rev 2000;(2):CD001068
184. Economides DL, Selinger M, Ferguson J, Bowell PJ, Dawes GS, Mackenzie IZ. Computerized measurement of heart rate variation in fetal anemia caused by rhesus alloimmunization. Am J Obstet Gynecol 1992; 167:689-93.
185. Brambati B, Pardi G. The intraventricular conduction time of fetal heart in pregnancies complicated by rhesus haemolytic disease. Br J Obstet Gynaecol 1981;88:1233-40.
186. Shelley-Jones D, Beischer N, de Crespigny L, Chew F. Severe rhesus iso-immunization detected by cardiotocography performed for diminished fetal movements. Aust N Z J Obstet Gynaecol 1991;31:362-65.
187. Sadovsky E, Laufer N, Beyth Y. The role of fetal movements: assessment in cases of severe Rh immunized patients. Acta Obstet Gynecol Scand 1979;58:313-16.
188. Leader LR, Baillie P, Schalkwyk DJ. Fetal movements and fetal outcome: a prospective study. Obstet Gynecol 1981;57:431-36.
189. Harman CR. Invasive techniques in the management of Alloimmune anemia. In: Harman CR, ed. Invasive fetal testing and treatment. Boston: Blackwell Scientific Publications, 1995:107-91.
190. Alfirevic Z, Neilson JP. Biophysical profile for fetal assessment in high risk pregnancies. Cochrane Database Syst Rev 2000;(2):CD000038.
191. Wiesenhaan PF. Fetography. Am J Obstet Gynecol 1972;113:819-22
192. Bennebroek Gravenhorst J. Intrauterine transfusion: a therapeutic intervention in erythroblastosis foetalis [thesis]. Leiden, Leiden University 1968.
193. Bennebroek Gravenhorst J. Intrauterine blood transfusion of the fetus. Ned Tijdschr Geneeskd 1970;114:822-28.
194. Langezaal CFM. Echografie in de verloskunde [thesis]. Leiden University; 1971.
195. Buscaglia M, Ferazzi E, Zuliani G, Caccamo ML, Pardi G. Ultrasound contributions to the management of the severely isoimmunized fetus. J Perinat Med 1986;14:51-58.
196. Salzman DH, Frigoletto FD, Harlow BL, Barss VA, Benacerraf BR. Sonographic evaluation of hydrops fetalis. Obstet Gynecol 1989;71:106-11.
197. Chitkara U, Wilkins I, Lynch L, Mehalek K, Berkowitz RL. The role of sonography in assessing severity of fetal anemia in Rh- and Kell-iso-immunized pregnancies. Obstet Gynecol 1988;71:393-98.
198. Nicolaides KH, Fontanarosa M, Gabbe SG, Rodeck CH. Failure of ultrasonographic parameters to predict the severity of fetal anemia in rhesus isoimmunization. Am J Obstet Gynecol 1988;158:920-26.
199. Benacerraf BR, Frigoletto FD,Jr. Sonographic sign for the detection of early fetal ascites in the management of severe isoimmune disease without intrauterine transfusion. Am J Obstet Gynecol 1985;152:1039-41.

200. Roberts AB, Mitchell JM, Pattison NS. Fetal liver length in normal and isoimmunized pregnancies. Am J Obstet Gynecol 1989;161:42-46.
201. DeVore GR, Mayden K, Tortara M, Berkowitz RL, Hobbins JC. Dilatation of the fetal umbilical vein in rhesus haemolytic anemia: a predictor of severe disease. Am J Obstet Gynecol 1981;141:464-66.
202. Witter FR, Graham D. The utility of ultrasonically measured umbilical vein diameters in isoimmunized pregnancies. Am J Obstet Gynecol 1983;146: 225-26.
203. Bahado-Singh R, Oz U, Mari G, Jones D, Paidas M, Onderoglu L. Fetal splenic size in anemia due to Rh-alloimmunization. Obstet Gynecol 1998; 92:828-32.
204. Roberts AB, Mitchell JM, Lake Y, Pattison NS. Ultrasonographic surveillance in red blood cell alloimmunization. Am J Obstet Gynecol 2001;184: 1251-55.
205. Kirkinen P, Jouppila P, Eik-Nes S. Umbilical vein blood flow in rhesus-isoimmunization. Br J Obstet Gynaecol 1983;90:640-43.
206. Copel JA, Grannum PA, Green JJ, Belanger K, Hobbins JC. Pulsed Doppler flow-velocity waveforms in the prediction of fetal hematocrit of the severely isoimmunized pregnancy. Am J Obstet Gynecol 1989;161:341-44.
207. Jouppila P, Kirkinen P, Puukka R. Correlation between umbilical vein blood flow and umbilical blood viscosity in normal and complicated pregnancies. Arch Gynecol 1986;237:191-97.
208. Favre Y, Vetter K, Huch R, Huch A. Doppler flow velocity measurement of the aorta when there is incompatibility of blood between the mother and the fetus. J Gynecol Obstet Biol Reprod 1989:18:740-46.
209. Nicolaides KH, Bilardo CM, Campbell S. Prediction of fetal anaemia by measurement of the mean blood velocity in the fetal aorta. Am J Obstet Gynecol 1990;162:209-12.
210. Vyas S, Nicolaides KH, Campbell S. Doppler examination of the middle cerebral artery in anemic fetuses. Am J Obstet Gynecol 1990;162:1066-68.
211. Kanzaki T, Chiba Y. Evaluation of the preload condition of the fetus by inferior vena caval blood flow patterns. Fetal Diagn Ther 1990;5:168-74.
212. Oepkes D, Vandenbussche FPHA, van Bel F, Kanhai HHH. Fetal ductus venosus blood flow velocities before and after transfusion in red cell alloimmunized pregnancies. Obstet Gynecol 1993;82:237-41.
213. Bahado-Singh R, Oz U, Deren O, et al. A new splenic artery Doppler velocimetric index for prediction of severe fetal anemia associated with Rh alloimmunization. Am J Obstet Gynecol 1999;180:49-54.
214. Bahado-Singh RO, Oz AU, Hsu C, Kovanci E, Deren O, Onderoglu L, Mari G. Middle cerebral artery Doppler velocimetric deceleration angle as a predictor of fetal anemia in Rh-alloimmunized fetuses without hydrops. Am J Obstet Gynecol 2000;183:746-51.
215. Iskaros J, Kingdom J, Morrison JJ, Rodeck C. Prospective non-invasive monitoring of pregnancies complicated by red cell alloimmunization. Ultrasound Obstet Gynecol 1998;11:432-37.

216. Dukler D, Oepkes D, Seaward G, Windrim R, Ryan G. Noninvasive tests to predict fetal anemia: a study comparing Doppler and ultrasound parameters. Am J Obstet Gynecol 2003;188:1310-14.
217. Mari G, Deter RL, Carpenter RL, et al. Noninvasive diagnosis by Doppler ultrasonography of fetal anemia due to maternal red-cell alloimmunization. Collaborative Group for Doppler Assessment of the Blood Velocity in Anemic Fetuses. N Engl J Med 2000;342:9-14.
218. Teixeira JM, Duncan K, Letsky E, Fisk NM. Middle cerebral artery peak systolic velocity in the prediction of fetal anemia. Ultrasound Obstet Gynecol 2000;15:205-08.
219. Zimmerman R, Carpenter RJ,Jr, Duerig P, Mari G. Longitudinal measurement of peak systolic velocity in the fetal middle cerebral artery for monitoring pregnancies complicated by red cell alloimmunisation: A prospective multicentre trial with intention-to-treat. Brit J Obstet Gynecol 2002:109:746-52.
220. Mari G, Detti L, Oz U, Zimmerman R, Duerig P, Stefos T. Accurate prediction of fetal hemoglobin by Doppler ultrasonography. Obstet Gynecol 2002;99:589-93.
221. Stefos T, Cosmi E, Detti L, Mari G. Correction of fetal anemia on the middle cerebral artery peak systolic velocity. Obstet Gynecol 2002;99:211-15.
222. Sikkel E, Vandenbussche FP, Oepkes D, et al. Effect of increase of the hematocrit on middle cerebral artery peak and umbilical vein maximum velocities in anemic fetuses. Fetal Diagn Ther 2003;18:472-78.
223. Detti L, Oz U, Guney I, Ferguson JE, Bahado-Singh RO, Mari G; Collaborative Group for Doppler Assessment of the Blood Velocity in Anemic Fetuses. Doppler ultrasound velocimetry for timing the second intrauterine transfusion in fetuses with anemia from red cell alloimmunization. Am J Obstet Gynecol 2001;185:1048-51.
224. Whitecar PW, Moise KJ,Jr. Sonographic methods to detect fetal anemia in red blood cell alloimmunization. Obstet Gynecol Surv 2000;55:240-50.
225. Divakaran TG, Waugh J, Clark TJ, Khan KS, Whittle MJ, Kilby MD. Noninvasive techniques to detect fetal anemia due to red blood cell alloimmunization: a systemic review. Obstet Gynecol 2001;98:509-17.
226. Holt EM, Boyd IE, Dewhurst CJ, Murray J, Naylor CH, Smitham JH. Intrauterine transfusion: 101 consecutive cases treated at Queen Charlotte's Maternity Hospital. BMJ 1973;3:39-43.
227. Robertson EG, Brown A, Ellis MI, Walker W. Intrauterine transfusion in the management of severe rhesus isoimmunization. Br J Obstet Gynecol 1976;83:694-97.
228. Frigoletto FDJ, Umansky I, Birnholz J, Acker D, Easterday CL, Harris GB et al. Intrauterine transfusion in 365 fetuses during 15 years. Am J Obstet Gynecol 1981; 139:781-90.
229. Scott JR, Kochenour NK, Larkin JM, Scott MJ. Changes in the management of severely Rh-immunized patients. Am J Obstet Gynecol 1984;149: 336-41.

230. Berkowitz RL, Hobbins JC. Intrauterine transfusion utilizing ultrasound. Obstet Gynecol 1981;33-36.
231. Harman CR, Manning FA, Bowman JM, Lange IR. Severe Rh disease – poor outcome is not inevitable. Am J Obstet Gynecol 1983;145:823-29.
232. Hamilton EG. Intrauterine transfusion: safeguard or peril. Obstet Gynecol 1977;50:255-60.
233. Clewell WH, Dunne MG, Johnson ML, Bowes WA,Jr. Fetal transfusion with real-time ultrasound guidance. Obstet Gynecol 1981;57:516-20.
234. Taylor WW, Scott DE, Pritchard JA. Fate of compatible adult erythrocytes in the fetal peritoneal cavity. Obstet Gynecol 1966;28:175-78.
235. Hashimoto B, Filly RA, Callen PW, Parer JT. Absorption of fetal intraperitoneal blood after intrauterine transfusion. J Ultrasound Med 1987;6: 421-23.
236. Larkin RM, Knochel JQ, Lee TG. Intrauterine transfusions: new techniques and results. Clin Obstet Gynecol 1982;25:303-12.
237. Bowman JM, Manning FA. Intrauterine fetal transfusions: Winnipeg 1982. Obstet Gynecol 1983;61:203-09.
238. Buscaglia M, Ferrazzi E, Zuliani G, Caccamo ML, Pardi G. Ultrasound contributions to the management of the severely isoimmunized fetus. J Perinat Med 1986;14:51-58
239. Watts DH, Luthy DA, Benedetti TJ, Cyr DR, Easterling TR, Hickok D. Intraperitoneal fetal transfusion under direct ultrasound guidance. Obstet Gynecol 1988;71:84-88.
240. Parer JT, Callen PW, Creasy RK, Filly RA. Intrauterine transfusion under sonographic guidance. J Reprod Med 1981;26:551-54.
241. Nicolini U, Talbert DG, Fisk NM, Rodeck CH. Pathophysiology of pressure changes during intrauterine transfusion. Am J Obstet Gynecol 1989; 160:1139-45.
242. Hardyment AF, Salvador HS, Towell ME, Carpenter CW, Jan JE, Tingle AJ. Follow-up of intrauterine transfused surviving children. Am J Obstet Gynecol 1979; 133:235-41.
243. Ellis MI. Follow-up study of survivors after intrauterine transfusion. Dev Med Child Neurol 1980;22:48-54.
244. Phibbs RH, Harvin BA, Jones MA, et al. Development of children who had received intra-uterine transfusions. Pediatrics 1971;47:689-97.
245. White CA, Goplerud CP, Kisker CT, Stehbens JA, Kitchell M, Taylor JC. Intrauterine fetal transfusion, 1965-1976, with an assessment of the surviving children. Am J Obstet Gynecol 1978;130:933-42.
246. Viëtor HE, Hallensleben E, van Bree SP, et al. Survival of donor cells 25 years after intrauterine transfusion. Blood 2000;95:2709-14.
247. Santaloya J, Warsof SL. Combined intravascular-intraperitoneal transfusions in hydropic twins due to Rh (D) alloimmunization. Fetal Diagn Ther 1990;5:70-75.

248. Moise KJ,Jr, Carpenter RJ,Jr, Kirshon B, Deter RL, Sala JD, Cano LE. Comparison of four types of intrauterine transfusion: effect on fetal hematocrit. Fetal Ther 1989;4:126-37.
249. Nicolini U, Kochenour NK, Greco P, Letsky E, Rodeck CH. When to perform the next intra-uterine transfusion in patients with R hallo-immunization: combined intravascular and intraperitoneal transfusion allows longer intervals. Fetal Ther 1989; 4:14-20.
250. Freda VJ, Adamsons K. Exchange transfusion in utero: report of a case. Am J Obstet Gynecol 1964;89:817-21.
251. Asensio SH, Figueroa-Longo JG, Pelegrina IA. Intrauterine exchange transfusion. Am J Obstet Gynecol 1966;95:1129-33.
252. Seelen J, van Kessel H, van Leusden H, Eskes T, Been J, Evers J. A new method of exchange transfusion in utero. Cannulation of vessels on the fetal side of the human placenta. Am J Obstet Gynecol 1966;95:872-76.
253. Rodeck CH, Nicolaides KH, Warsof SL, Fysh WJ, Gamsu HR, Kemp JR. The management of severe rhesus isoimmunization by fetoscopic intravascular transfusions. Am J Obstet Gynecol 1984;150:769-74.
254. Kanhai HH, Bennebroek Gravenhorst J, van Kamp IL, et al. Management of severe hemolytic disease with ultrasound-guided intravascular fetal transfusions. Vox Sang 1990;59:180-84.
255. Seeds JW, Bowes Jr WA, Chescheir NC. Echogenic venous turbulence is a critical feature of successful intravascular transfusion. Obstet Gynecol 1989;73:488-90.
256. Plecas DV, Chitkara U, Berkowitz GS, Lapinski RH, Alvarez M, Berkowitz RL. Intrauterine intravascular transfusion for severe erythroblastosis fetalis: how much to transfuse. Obstet Gynecol 1990;75:965-69.
257. MacGregor SN, Socol ML, Pielet BW, Sholl JT, Minogue JP. Prediction of fetoplacental blood volume in isoimmunized pregnancy. Am J Obstet Gynecol 1988;159: 1493-97.
258. Mandelbrot L, Daffos F, Forestier F, MacAleese J, Descombey D. Assessment of fetal blood volume for computer-assisted management of in utero transfusion. Fetal Ther 1988;3:60-66.
259. Nicolaides KH, Clewell WH, Rodeck CH. Measurement of human fetoplacental blood volume in erythroblastosis fetalis. Am J Obstet Gynecol 1987; 157:50-53.
260. Leduc L, Moise KJ,Jr, Carpenter RJ,Jr, Cano LE. Fetoplacental blood volume estimation in pregnancies with Rh alloimmunization. Fetal Diagn Ther 1990;5:138-46.
261. Hoogeveen M, Meerman RH, Pasman S, Egberts J. A new method to determine fetoplacental volume based on dilution of fetal haemoglobin and an estimation of plasma fluid loss after intrauterine intravascular transfusion. Br J Obstet Gynaecol 2002;109:1132-36.
262. Giannina G, Moise KJ,Jr, Dorman K. A simple method to estimate volume for fetal intravascular transfusions. Fetal Diagn Ther 1998;13:94-97.

263. MacGregor SN, Socol ML, Pielet BW, Sholl JS, Silver RK. Prediction of hematocrit decline after intravascular transfusion. Am J Obstet Gynecol 1989;161:1491-93.
264. Pattison N, Roberts A. The management of severe erythroblastosis fetalis by fetal transfusion: survival of transfused adult erythrocytes in the fetus. Obstet Gynecol 1989;74:901-04.
265. Jones HM, Linch DC, Nicolaides K, Rodeck CH. Survival of transfused adult cells in the fetus. Fetal Ther 1986;1:193-95.
266. Abdel-Fattah SA, Carroll SG, Kyle PM, Soothill PW. The effect of fetal hydrops on the rate of fall of haemoglobin after intravascular transfusion for red cell alloimmunization. Fetal Diagn Ther 2000;15:262-66.
267. El-Azeem SA, Samuels P, Rose RL, Kennedy M, O'Shaughnessy RW. The effect of the source of transfused red blood cells in pregnancies affected by red blood cell alloimmunization. Am J Obstet Gynecol 1997;177:753-57.
268. Egberts J, van Kamp IL, Kanhai HHH, Meerman RH, Giordano PC, Bennebroek Gravenhorst J, The disappearance of fetal and donor red blood cells in alloimmunised pregnancies: a reappraisal. Br J Obstet Gynaecol 1997;104:818-24.
269. Nicolaides KH, Soothill PW, Rodeck CH, Clewell W. Rh disease: intravascular fetal blood transfusion by cordocentesis. Fetal Ther 1986;4: 185-92.
270. Nicolini U, Nicolaidis P, Fisk NM, Tannirandorn Y, Rodeck CH. Fetal blood sampling from the intrahepatic vein: Analysis of safety and clinical experience with 214 procedures. Obstet Gynecol 1990;76:47-53.
271. Weiner CP, Okamura K. Diagnostic fetal blood sampling-technique related losses. Fetal Diagn Ther 1996;11:169-75.
272. Bernaschek G, Yildiz A, Kolankaya A, Stuempflen I, Duetinger J. Complications of cordocentesis in high-risk pregnancies: effects on fetal loss or preterm delivery. Prenat Diagn 1995;15:995-1000.
273. Goodrum LA, Moise KJ, Saade GR, Belfort MA, Ayres NA, Carpenter RJ. Effects of intravascular transfusion for red cell alloimmunization on fetal arterial blood pressure. Fetal Diagn Ther 1997;12:149-52.
274. Giannakoulopoulos X, Teixeira J, Fisk N, Glover V. Human fetal and maternal noradrenaline responses to invasive procedures. Pediatr Res 199;45: 494-99.
275. Teixeira JM, Glover V, Fisk NM. Acute cerebral redistribution in response to invasive procedures in the human fetus. Am J Obstet Gynecol 1999; 181:1018-25.
276. Antsaklis AI, Papantoniou NE, Mesogitis SA, Koutra PT, Vintzileos AM, Aravantinos DI. Cardiocentesis : an alternative method of fetal blood sampling for the diagnosis of hemoglobinopathies. Obstet Gynecol 1992;79: 630-33.
277. Westgren M, Jabbar F, Larsen JF, Rahman F, Selbing A, Stangenberg M. Introduction of a programme for intravascular transfusions at severe rhesus isoimmunization. J Perinat Med 1988;16:417-22.

278. Westgren M, Selbing A, Stangenberg M. Fetal intracardiac transfusions in patients with severe rhesus isoimmunization. Br Med J 1988;296:885-86.
279. Poissonnier MH, Brossard Y, Demedeiros N, et al. Two hundred intra-uterine exchange transfusions in severe blood incompatibilities. Am J Obstet Gynecol 1989; 161:709-13.
280. Grannum PA, Copel JA, Plaxe SC, Scioscia Al, Hobbins JC. In utero exchange transfusion by direct intravascular injection is severe erythroblastosis fetalis. New Engl J Med 1986;314:1431-34.
281. Ronkin S, Chayen B, Wapner RJ, et al. Intravascular exchange and bolus transfusion in the severely isoimmunized fetus. Am J Obstet Gynecol 1989; 160:407-11.
282. Selbing A, Stangenberg M, Westgren M, Rahman F. Intrauterine intravascular transfusions in fetal erythroblastosis: the influence of net transfusion volume on fetal survival. Acta Obstet Gynecol Scand 1993;72: 20-23.
283. Radunovic N, Lockwood CJ, Alvarez M, Plecas D, Chitkara U, Berkowitz RL. The severely anemic and hydropic isoimmune fetus: changes in fetal hematocrit associated with fetal death. Obstet Gynecol 1992;79:390-93.
284. Hallak M, Moise KJ,Jr, Hesketh DE, Cano LE, Carpenter RJ,Jr. Intravascular transfusion of fetuses with rhesus incompatibility: prediction of fetal outcome by changes in umbilical venous pressure. Obstet Gynecol 1992; 80:286-90.
285. Nicolini U, Talbert DG, Fisk NM, Rodeck CH. Pathophysiology of pressure changes during intrauterine transfusion. Am J Obstet Gynecol 1989; 160:1139-45.
286. Weiner CP, Peltzer GD, Heilskov J, Wenstrom KD, Williamson RA. The effect of intravascular transfusion on umbilical venous pressure in anemic fetuses with and without hydrops. Am J Obstet Gynecol 1989;161:1498-501.
287. Brace RA. Ovine fetal cardiovascular responses to packed red blood cell transfusions. Am J Obstet Gynecol 1989;161:1367-74.
288. Moise KJ, Mari G, Fisher DJ, Huhta JC, Cano LE, Carpenter Jr RJ. Acute fetal hemodynamic alterations after intrauterine transfusion for the treatment of severe red blood cell alloimmunization. Am J Obstet Gynecol 1990;163:776-84.
289. Copel JA, Grannum PA, Belanger K, Green J, Hobbins JC. Pulsed Doppler flow-velocity waceforms befora and after intrauterine intravascular transfusion for severe erythroblastosis fetalis. Am J Obstet Gynecol 1988;158:768-74.
290. Weiner CP, Anderson TL. The acute effect of cordocenteses with or without fetal curarization and of intravascular transfusion upon umbilical artery waveform indices. Obstet Gynecol 1989;73:219-24.
291. Bilardo CM, Nicolaides KH, Campbell S. Doppler studies in red cell isoimmunization. Clin Obstet Gynecol 1989;32:719-27.
292. Hanretty KP, Whittle MJ, Gilmore DH, McNay MB, Howie CA, Rubin PC. The effect of intravascular transfusion for rhesus haemolytic disease on um-

bilical artery Doppler flow velocity waveforms. Br J Obstet Gynaecol 1989;96:960-63.
293. Mari G, Moise KJ,Jr, Deter RL, Carpenter Jr RJ. Flow velocity waveforms of the umbilical and cerebral arteries before and after intravascular transfusion. Obstet Gynecol 1990;75:584-89.
294. Weiner CP, Robillard JE. Effect of acute intravascular volume expansion on human fetal prostaglandin concentrations. Am J Obstet Gynecol 1989; 161:1494-97.
295. Weiner CP, Smith F, Robollard JE. Arginine vasopressin and acute, intravascular volume expansion in the human fetus. Fetal Ther 1989;4:69-72.
296. Ross MG, Ervin G, Lam RW, Castro L, Leake RD, Fisher DA. Plasma atrial natriuretic peptide response to volume expansion in the ovine fetus. Am J Obstet Gynecol 1987;157:1292-97.
297. Panos MZ, Nicolaides KH, Anderson JV, Economides DL, Rees L, Williams R. Plasma atrial natriuretic peptide in human fetus: response to intravascular blood transfusion. Am J Obstet Gynecol 1989;161:357-61.
298. Bennett TL, Rose JC. Atrial natriuretic factor responses to volume expansion in pregnant and nonpregnant sheep. Am J Obstet Gynecol 1991;165: 1627-34.
299. Walther T, Stephan H, Faber R. Dual natriuretic peptide response to volume load in the fetal circulation. Cardiovasc Res 2001;49:817-19.
300. Radunovic R, Nastic D, Rebarber A, Kuczynski E, Lockwood CJ. The effect of fetal intravascular blood transfusion on plasma endothelin levels in fetuses with rhesus alloimmunization. Obstet Gynecol 1998;91:956-60.
301. Nicolini U, Santolaya J, Fisk NM, Hubinont C, Kochenour NK, Greco P, Rodeck CH. Changes in fetal acid base status during intravascular transfusion. Arch Dis Child 1988;63:710-14.
302. Soothill PW, Nicolaides KH, Rodeck CH, Bellingham AJ. The effect of replacing fetal haemoglobin on blood gas and acid-base parameters in human fetuses. Am J Obstet Gynecol 1988;158:66-69.
303. Vandenbussche FPHA, van Kamp IL, Oepkes D, Hermans J, Bennebroek Gravenhorst J, Kanhai HHH. Blood gas and pH in the human fetus with severe anemia. Fetal Diagn Ther 1998;13:115-22.
304. Soothill PW, Nicolaides KH, Rodeck CH, Clewell WH, Lindridge J. Relationship of fetal haemoglobin and oxygen content to lactate concentration in Rh isoimmunized pregnancies. Obstet Gynecol 1987;69:268-71.
305. Copel JA, Grannum PA, Harrison D, Hobbins JC. The use of pancuronium bromide to produce fetal paralysis during intravascular transfusion. Am J Obstet Gynecol 1988;158:170-71.
306. Moise KJ,Jr, Deter RL, Kirshon B, Adam K, Patton DE, Carpenter RJ,Jr. Intravenous pancuronium bromide for fetal neuromuscular blockade during intrauterine transfusion for red-cell alloimmunization. Obstet Gynecol 1989;74:905-08.

307. Spencer JA, Ryan G, Ronderos-Dumit D, Nicolini U, Rodeck CH. The effect of neuromuscular blockade on human fetal heart rates and its variation. Br J Obstet Gynaecol 1994;101:121-24.
308. Watson WJ, Atchison SR, Harlass FE. Comparison of pancuronium and vecuronium for fetal neuromuscular blockade during invasive procedures. J Matern Fetal Med 1996;5:151-54.
309. Mouw RJC, Klumper F, Hermans J, Brandenburg HCR, Kanhai HHH. Effect of atracurium or pancuronium on the anemic fetus during and directly after intravascular intrauterine transfusion; a double blind randomized study. Acta Obstet Gynecol Scand 199;78:763-67.
310. Bournazeau JA, Aublet-Cuvellier B, Raiga J, Jacquetin B, Lemery D. Complications of cordocentesis associated fetal therapy. J Gynecol Obstet Biol Reprod 1999;28:24-30.
311. Geulen O, Hansmann M, Offergeld R, Kaiser R, Dame C, Hoch J. Maternal and fetal hepatitis C virus exposure by intrauterine transfusion. Lancet 2000;355:1887-88.
312. Evans DGR, Lyon AJ. Fatal congenital cytomegalovirus infection acquired by an intra-uterine transfusion. Eur J Pediatr 1991;150:780-81.
313. Galligan BR, Cairns R, Schifano JV, Selbing A, Bernvil SS. Preparation of packed red cells suitable for intravascular transfusion in utero. Transfusion 1989;29:179-81.
314. Thorp JA, Plapp FV, Cohen GR, Yeast JD, O'Kell RT, Stephenson S. Hyperkalemia after irradiation of packed red blood cells: possible effects with intravascular fetal transfusion. Am J Obstet Gynecol 1990;163:607-09.
315. Segal M, Manning FA, Harman CR, Menticoglu S. Bleeding after intravascular transfusion: experimental and clinical observations. Am J Obstet Gynecol 1991; 165:1414-18
316. Ney JA, Fee SC, Dooley SL, Socol ML, Minogue J. Factors influencing hemostasis after umbilical vein puncture in vitro. Am J Obstet Gynecol 1989;160:424-26.
317. Saade GR, Moise KJ,Jr, Copel JA, Belfort MA, Carpenter Jr RJ. Fetal platelet counts correlate with the severity of the anemia in red-cell alloimmunization. Obstet Gynecol 1993;82:987-91.
318. Inglis SR, Lysikiewicz A, Sonnenblick AL, Streltzoff JL, Bussel JB, Chervenak FA. Advantages of larger volume, less frequent intrauterine red blood cell transfusions for maternal red cell alloimmunization. Am J Perinatol 1996;13:27-33.
319. Welch R, Rampling MW, Anwar A, Talbert DG, Rodeck CH. Changes in hemorheology with fetal intravascular transfusion. Am J Obstet Gynecol 1994;170:726-32.
320. van Kamp IL, Klumper FJCM, Oepkes D, et al. Complications of intrauterine intravascular transfusion for fetal anemia duet o maternal red-cell alloimmunizatiuon. Am J Obstet Gynecol 2003; submitted for publication.

321. Dildy GA, Smith LG, Jr, Moise KJ, Jr, Cano LE, Hesketh DE. Porencephalic cyst: a complication of fetal intravascular transfusion. Am J Obstet Gynecol 1991;165:76-78.
322. Musemeche CA, Reynolds M. Necrotizing enterocolitis following intrauterine blood transfusion. J Pediatr Surg 1991;26:1411-12.
323. Harte G, Payton D, Carmody F, O'Regan P, Thong YH. Graft versus host disease following intrauterine and exchange transfusions for rhesus haemolytic disease. Aust N Z J Obstet Gynaecol 1997;37:319-22.
324. Utter GO, Socol ML, Dooley SL, MacGregor SN, Millard DD. Is intrauterine transfusion associated with diminished fetal growth? Am J Obstet Gynecol 1990; 163:1781-84.
325. Roberts A, Grannum P, Belanger K, Pattison N, Hobbins J. Fetal growth and birthweight in isoimmunized pregnancies after intravenous intrauterine transfusion. Fetal Diagn Ther 1993;8:407-11.
326. Berger HM, Lindeman JH, van Zoeren Grobben D, Houdkamp E, Schrijver J, Kanhai H.H. Iron overload, free radical damage, and rhesus hemolytic disease. Lancet 1990;335:933-36.
327. Nasrat HA, Nicolini U, Nicolaidis P, Letsky EA, Gau G, Rodeck CH. The effect of intrauterine intravascular blood transfusion on iron metabolism in fetuses with Rh alloimmunization. Obstet Gynecol 1991;77:558-62.
328. Egberts J, Luykx LM, Berger HM. Antioxidant protection against free radicals is reduced in fetal plasma after intrauterine red blood cell transfusion. Biol Neonate 2003;83:188-90.
329. de Groot CJM, Oepkes D, Egberts J, Kanhai HHH. Evidence of endothelium involvement in the pathophysiology of hydrops fetalis. Early Hum Dev 2000;57: 205-09.
330. Lasker MR, Eddleman K, Toor AH. Neonatal hepatitis and excessive hepatic iron deposition folowing intrauterine blood transfusion. Am J Perinatol 1995;12:14-17.
331. Viëtor HE, Kanhai HHH, Brand A. Induction of additional red cell alloantibodies after intrauterine transfusions. Transfusion 1994;34:970-74.
332. Viëtor HE, Hawes GE, van den Oever C, et al. Intrauterine transfusions affect fetal T-cell immunity. Blood 1997;90:2492-501.
333. Viëtor HE. Immunomodulation induced by intrauterine transfusions. Eur J Obstet Gynecol Biol 1998;78:33-35.
334. Tannirandorn Y, Rodeck CH. New approaches in the treatment of haemolytic disease of the fetus. Baillieres Clin Haematol 1990;3:289-320.
335. Ryan G, Morrow RJ. Fetal blood transfusion. Clin Perinatol 1994;21:573-89.
336. Grannum PAT, Copel JA, Moya FR, et al. The reversal of hydrops fetalis by intravascular intrauterine transfusion in severe isoimmune fetal aemia. Am J Obstet Gynecol 1988;158:914-19.
337. Barss VA, Benacerraf BR, Frigoletto FD, et al. Management of isoimmunized pregnancy by use of intravascular techniques. Am J Obstet Gynecol 1988;159:291-93.

338. Berkowitz RL, Chitkara U, Wilkins IA, Lynch L, Plosker H, Bernstein HH. Intravascular monitoring and management of erythroblastosis fetalis. Am J Obstet Gynecol 1988;158:783-95.
339. Parer JT. Severe Rh isoimmunization – current methods of in utero diagnosis and treatment. Am J Obstet Gynecol 1988;158:1323-29.
340. Orsini LF, Pilu G, Calderoni P, et al. Intravascualr intrauterine transfusion for severe erythroblastosis fetalis using different techniques. Fetal Ther 1988;3:50-59.
341. Lemery D, Urbain MF, Van Lieferinghen P, Micorek JC, Jacquetin B. Intrauterine exchange transfusion under ultrasound guidance. Eur J Obstet Gynecol Reprod Biol 1989;33:161-68.
342. Weiner CP, Williamson RA, Wenstrom KD, et al. Management of fetal haemolytic disease by cordocenteses. II. Outcome of treatment. Am J Obstet Gyneco; 1991; 165:1302-07.
343. Ney JA, Socol ML, Dooley SL, MacGregor SN, Silver RK, Millard DD. Perinatal outcome following intravascular transfusion in severely isoimmunized fetuses. Int J Gynaecol Obstet 1991;35:41-46.
344. Sampson AJ, Permezel M, Doyle LW, de Crespigny L, Ngu A, Robinson H. Ultrasound-guided fetal intravascular transfusions for severe erythroblastosis, 1984-1993. Aust N Z J Obstet Gynaecol 1994;34:125-30.
345. Plöckinger B, Strümpflen I, Detinger J, Bernaschek G. Diagnosis and treatment of fetal anemia due to isoimmunization. Arch Gynecol Obstet 1994;225:195-200.
346. Grab D, Paulus WE, Bommer A, Buck G, Terinde R. Treatment of fetal erythroblastosis by intravascular transfusions: outcome at 6 years. Obstet Gynecol 1999;93:165-68.
347. Farina A, Calderoni P, Simonazzi G, Carinci P, Rizzo N. Survival analysis of transfuserd fetuses affected by Rh-alloimmunization. Prenat Diagn 2000; 20:881-85.
348. van Kamp IL, Klumper FJCM, Meerman RH, Oepkes D, Scherjon SA, Kanhai HH. Treatment of fetal anemia due to red-cell alloimmunization with intrauterine transfusions in the Netherlands, 1988 – 1999. Acta Obstet Gynecol Scand 2004,83: (in press).
349. van Kamp IL, Klumper FJCM, Bakkum RSLA, et al. The severity of immune fetal hydrops is predictive of fetal outcome after intrauterine treatment. Am J Obstet Gynecol 2001;185:668-73.
350. Smoleniec JS, Fraser I. Refractory rhesus (D) disease. Br J Obstet Gynaecol 1993; 100:955-57.
351. al-Alaiyan S, Omran A. Late hyporegenerative anemia in neonates with rhesus hemolytic disease. J Perinat Med 1999;27:112-15.
352. Thorp JA, O'Connor T, Callenbach J, Cohen GR, Yeast JD, Albin J. Hyporegenerative anemia associated with intrauterine transfusion in rhesus haemolytic disease. Am J Obstet Gynecol 1991;165:79-81.
353. Greenough A. Rhesus disease: postnatal management and outcome. Eur J Pediatr 1999;158:689-93.

354. Millard DD, Gidding SS, Socol ML, MacGregor SN, Dooley SL, Ney JA et al. Effects of intravascular, intrauterine transfusion on prenatal and postnatal hemolysis and erythropoiesis in severe fetal isoimmunization. J Pediatr 1990;117:447-54.
355. Dallacasa P, Ancora G, Miniero R, Gavella B, Brondelli L, Conte R et al. Erythropoietin course in newborns with Rh hemolytic disease transfused and not transfused in utero. Pediatr Rev 1996;40:357-60.
356. Saade GR, Moise KJ, Belfort MA, Hesketh DE, Carpenter RJ. Fetal and neonatal hematologic parameters in red cell alloimmunization: predicting the need for late neonatal transfusions. Fetal Diagn Ther 1993;8:161-64.
357. Nicaise C, Gire C, Casha P, d'Ercole C, Chau C, Palix C. Erythropoietin as treatment for late hyporegenerative anemia inneonates with Rh haemolytic disease after in utero exchange transfusion. Fetal Diagn Ther 2002;17:22-24.
358. Doyle LW, kelly EA, Rickards AL, Ford GW, Callanan C. Sensorineural outcome at 2 years for survivors of eythroblastosis treated with fetal intravascular transfusions. Obstet Gynecol 1993;81:931-35.
359. Stewart G, Day RE, Del Priore C, Whittle MJ, Turner TL, Holland BM. Developmental outcome after intravascular intrauterine transfusion for rhesus haemolytic disease. Arch Dis Child Fetal Neonatal Ed 1994;70:F52-53.
360. Farrant B, Battin M, Roberts A. Outcome of infants receiving in-utero transfusions for haemolytic disease. N Z Med J 2001;114:400-03.
361. Hudon L, Moise KJ, Hegemier SE, et al. Long-term neurodevelopmental outcome after intrauterine transfusion for the treatment of fetal hemolytic disease. Am J Obstet Gynecol 1998;179:858-63.
362. Janssens HM, de Haan MJJ, van Kamp IL, Brand R, Kanhai HHH, Veen S. Outcome for children treated with fetal intravascular transfusions because of severe blood group antagonism. J Pediatr 1997;131:373-80.

NEW TREATMENT OPTIONS IN NEONATAL HYPERBILIRUBINAEMIA

P.T. Pisciotto[1]

Introduction

Jaundice is one of the most common problems encountered in the newborn period. It has been estimated that in the United States over 60% of the 4 million newborns born each year develop clinical jaundice with bilirubin levels greater than 5 mg/dL (86 μmol/L) in the first week of life. Bilirubin encephalopathy, known pathologically as kernicterus for the yellow staining of the subthalmic nuclei (kerns), has been recognized for a long time. The degree to which bilirubin may cause more subtle neurologic abnormalities remains controversial [1]. While clinical jaundice is commonly encountered in the newborn, kernicterus is a rare occurrence. Factors that affect bilirubin toxicity are complex and incompletely understood. These include; the serum albumin concentration and available binding sites on albumin for bilirubin, the integrity of the blood brain barrier and therefore ability for bilirubin to enter the brain, the duration of bilirubin exposure and the type and stage of development of the cells being exposed [2]. The relationship between increasing total serum bilirubin (TSB) levels, particularly greater then 20 mg/dL (344 μmol/L), and the risk of developing kernicterus in infants with Rh haemolytic disease of the newborn (HDN) was observed in the late 1940s and early 1950s [3]. This led to an aggressive approach to the treatment of jaundice in these patients with exchange transfusion being the predominant mode of therapy to maintain bilirubin levels below 20 mg/dL (344 μmol/L). In 1958 it was observed that premature infants exposed to sunlight or blue fluorescent light experienced a decrease in TSB levels [4]. This prompted the recognition of the possible use of phototherapy as adjunct therapy to exchange. The use of phototherapy as part of the management of hyperbilirubinaemia for infants has remained a standard of care for the past four decades. The use of more effective phototherapy over time has significantly decreased the need for exchange transfusions [5].

1. Department of Laboratory Medicine, University of Connecticut Health Center, Farmington, CT, USA.

Aggressive management strategies based on observations in infants with Rh HDN extended to neonates with hemolytic disease from other causes as well as to infants with hyperbilirubinaemia without evidence of haemolysis. The relationship however, between non-haemolytic hyperbilirubinaemia and developmental outcome in healthy term infants is not well defined [6]. The risk of bilirubin encephalopathy in healthy term infants is believed to be relatively small, even at bilirubin levels of 25 mg/dL (430 µmol/L) [7]. In the late 1980's and early 1990's concern was raised about the risks versus the benefits of treating high bilirubin levels in full term infants who were otherwise healthy. Based on a review of the literature at the time and expert opinion, the American Academy of Pediatrics (AAP) issued the first practice parameter on the management of non-haemolytic hyperbilirubinaemia in healthy newborns in 1994 [8]. Infants with HDN and premature infants are believed to be at increased risk for bilirubin toxicity and therefore it is generally recommended to treat hyperbilirubinaemia at lower levels then healthy term infants [9,10]. It is common to initiate phototherapy in low-birth weight infants based on a sliding scale; the lower the birth weight and sicker the infant the lower the level of TSB at which phototherapy is instituted. With the advent of early hospital discharge for term and often near term healthy infants, prior to peak bilirubin levels being reached, hyperbilirubinemia requiring phototherapy has become the most common readmission diagnosis of newborn infants [11,12]. Recent reports have also suggested that there may be an increase in the frequency of kernicterus, which has prompted a re-evaluation of the approaches to the prevention, detection and treatment of hyperbilirubinaemia [13-15].

Pathophysiology

The predominant source of bilirubin is from the breakdown of haemoglobin. The breakdown of 1g of haemoglobin produces approximately 35 mg of bilirubin.

Haeme (iron protoporphyrin) is degraded by the enzyme haeme oxygenase (HO) into iron, which is conserved; carbon monoxide (CO), which is exhaled; and biliverdin. Biliverdin is further metabolised to bilirubin by the enzyme biliverdin reductase. Since bilirubin and CO are produced in equimolar amounts when haeme is degraded the measurement of CO in exhaled air (measured as end title CO [ETCO]) has served as an index of bilirubin production [16]. The bilirubin that is formed is then transported tightly bound to albumin to the liver. When the complex comes in contact with the hepatocyte, only bilirubin is transported into the cell where is it bound to ligandin (bilirubin-binding protein) and transported to the endoplasmic reticulum to be converted to its water-soluble conjugate. This reaction is catalyzed by the enzyme uridine diphosphate glucuronyl transferase (UDPGT). A single form of this enzyme (UDPGT1) accounts for almost all of the bilirubin glucuronide in the liver [17]. The conjugated bilirubin is excreted through the bile into the intestine where, in the presence of normal gut flora that are capable of converting bilirubin to nonresorbable derivatives, it is further metabolised to stercobilins and excreted in the stool.

Jaundice is seen in a high proportion of neonates resulting from a combination of mechanisms. As a result of the shortened life span of neonatal red cells, newborns normally have a rate of bilirubin production (approximately 6 to 8 mg/kg/day) that is approximately 2 to 3 times the rate of production in an adult [16]. The clearance of bilirubin is decreased as a result of a deficiency in ligandin and a deficiency in the enzyme UDPGT, which has approximately 1% of the activity in the adult [9]. The activity is lower in premature infants. Finally, unlike adults, newborns have fewer bacteria in the small and large intestine to reduce bilirubin, slow intestinal motility and a greater degree of the deconjugating enzyme β-glucuronidase. The conjugated bilirubin is hydrolysed to unconjugated bilirubin and reabsorbed (enterohepatic circulation) increasing the bilirubin load to the liver.

Risk of Severe Hyperbilirubinaemia

The natural history of neonatal jaundice in normal term infants in the U.S. has changed over the past decade with peak levels obtained later then previously observed (4th-5th day vs. 3rd day) and frequently no significant decline starting before the 6th or 7th day.[18] The 95th percentile for peak TSB levels presently approaches approximately 15 to 17.5 mg/dL (258-301 μmol/L) versus 12 to 13 mg/dL (206-224 μmol/L) observed several decades ago [18-20]. There are mul-

Table 1. Causes of unconjugated hyperbilirubinaemia

Overproduction/ increased load to liver	
Haemolysis	
Immune	Rh, ABO, other
Non-immune	Membrane defect (i.e. spherocytosis) Enzyme defect (i.e. G6PD deficiency) Infection
Non-haemolytic	Polycythaemia Extravasated blood (i.e. cephalohaematoma)
Increased enterohepatic	Breast feeding
Circulation	Pyloric stenosis Ileus Cystic fibrosis
Decreased elimination	
Decreased uptake	Inadequate perfusion Ligandin deficiency
Decreased conjugation	Enzyme deficiency (Crigler-Najjar, Gilbert) Enzyme inhibition Breast milk jaundice
Miscellaneous	Hypothyroidism Infection

tiple factors that may be contributing to this exaggerated form of jaundice including: the increase in the number of breastfed infants in the past few decades (30% at discharge in the 1960's vs. 60% in 1997) [21], an increase in the number of East Asian infants born in some regions of the U.S. and shorter hospital stays [15]. It has been postulated that increased incidence of neonatal unconjugated hyperbilirubinemia in certain ethnic and geographic populations may be attributed to environmental influences (i.e. herbal medications, food) or genetic predisposition to slower maturation of bilirubin metabolism and transport [22]. The severity of hyperbilirubinemia depends on the degree of imbalance between the infant's bilirubin production and ability to eliminate bilirubin. There are various epidemiological and clinical conditions (Table 1) that can alter this balance and increase the risk of developing severe unconjugated hyperbilirubinaemia. Several strategies have been utilized to evaluate the ability to predict which infants may develop severe hyperbilirubinaemia [20,23]. Cord bilirubin and the rate of rise of TSB concentration have played an important role in evaluating which infants may be at risk for hyperbilirubinaemia. A nested case control study looking at the predictors for extreme hyperbilirubinaemia ($\geq$25 mg/L [$\geq$430 μmol/L]) in infants born at 36 weeks or later and weighing $\geq$2000g term found the following biological variables: jaundice within 24 hours (odds ration [OR]=7.3), previous sibling with jaundice (OR = 6.0), exclusive breastfeeding (OR = 5.7), bruising (OR = 4.0), Asian race (OR = 3.5), cephalohaematoma (OR = 3.3) maternal age > 25 years (OR = 3.1) and lower gestational age (OR = 0.6/week) [24]. Recently the use of an hour specific TSB concentration plotted against a percentile nomogram for term and near-term infants has been evaluated to help predict infants at risk for subsequent development of hyperbilirubinaemia. One study involving 2840 healthy term and near term infants showed that infants whose TSB level fell in the 95th percentile at 18 to 72 hours after birth (n = 172) had a 40% probability of developing severe hyperbilirubinaemia ($\geq$17 mg/dL [293 μmol/L]) whereas infants with concentrations less than the 40th percentile (n = 1756) had a probability of zero [20].

Measurement of ETCO in conjunction with TSB has not been found to improve the predictability of the hour-specific TSB value but it provides insight into the processes that contribute to hyperbilirubinaemia [25].

Treatment of Unconjugated Hyperbilirubinaemia

The decision as to the intensity and invasiveness of therapy that is initiated in a neonate will be determined by many factors including the gestational and chronological age, relative health of the neonate, level of TSB and estimation of the rate of rise and the nature of bilirubin metabolism in the newborn. Treatment will usually be modified based on the perceived risk for kernicterus with infants often being placed into four categories: healthy term ($\geq$ 37 weeks gestation), sick term, healthy premature and sick premature. Bilirubin levels rising faster than 0.5 mg/dL (8.6 μmol/L) per hour are usually indicative of haemolysis. In these situations estimation of the anticipated peak may result in a course of phototherapy or exchange transfusion at a lower bilirubin level than a similar level achieved at a later time. Once therapy is started it is continued until the TSB concentration is reduced to levels considered safe in view of the infant's age and clinical condition

Phototherapy

Cremer introduced phototherapy as a means of reducing unconjugated hyperbilirubinaemia in 1958, but it was not widely adopted for nearly a decade later when further studies showed its safety and efficacy in neonates [4,26].

Since that time it has become the most widely used treatment for hyperbilirubinaemia. It was originally used prophylactically in order to reduce the need for exchange transfusion and prevent kernicterus. This could be accomplished with a relatively low dose of phototherapy. In the Collaborative Study on the Effectiveness and Safety of Phototherapy under the auspices of the National Institute of Child Health and Human Development (NICHHD) phototherapy was found to be effective in preventing hyperbilirubinaemia in both low birth weight and larger infants [27]. Of the 462 low birth weight infants treated with phototherapy only 17.7% had bilirubin levels higher then 10 mg/dl (172 μmol/L) versus 62.8% of 460 controls with 4.1% of the infants in the phototherapy group requiring exchange transfusion versus 24.4% of the control infants. In the larger group of infants (≥2500 gm; ≥ 34 weeks gestation) studied, 140 in the treatment group and 136 in the control group, it was found that the use of phototherapy was effective in decreasing the rate of exchange transfusion in those infants with hyperbilirubinaemia secondary to non-haemolytic causes or with negative Coomb's test [27,28]. Decreases in the use of exchange transfusion in term infants since the introduction of phototherapy, independent of the effect of Rh immune globulin use, have been reported in other populations even in infants with ABO haemolytic disease of the newborn [5,29]. Neurologic, psychometric, behavioral and auditory evaluation at 1 and 6 years in infants who had participated in the randomised control collaborative study of phototherapy indicated that this therapy was not associated with an excess or a decrease in long-term morbidity [30]. Recently, with shorter hospitalisation stays for term infants and re-admission of infants with already high levels of bilirubin, the objective of phototherapy has been to reduce the bilirubin concentration as fast as possible requiring a more intensive or therapeutic dose to be delivered [5].

Mechanism of Action

In order for phototherapy to have a biologic effect the light must be absorbed by a photoreceptor molecule which leads to transient excitation of the molecule to a higher energy level and in turn leads to a useful photochemical reaction. Bilirubin absorbs light and undergoes photoisomerization and photooxidation. It is converted to photoisomers (geometric and structural) that are more polar and can be excreted from liver into bile without undergoing conjugation and do not require the presence of the canalicular multispecific organic anion transporter (cMoat) for excretion [31]. The geometric isomers (4Z15E) are formed almost immediately, accounting for approximately 20% of the TSB concentration where as the structural isomer (lumirubin) is formed more slowly accounting for approximately 2% to 6% of the TSB. The formation of lumirubin, however, is not reversible and is cleared much more rapidly than the 4Z15E isomer (half life of 2 hours versus 15 hours) being excreted both through bile and in the urine [32].

Therefore it is believed that lumirubin formation may be the main reason for the observed phototherapy decline in TSB in infants [18,32]. Geometric isomers will also revert to natural unconjugated bilirubin in the intestine which in turn contribute to the bilirubin load via the enterohepatic circulation and may account in part for why phototherapy is most effective during the first 24 hours [18]. The photooxidative products that are formed are believed to play a minor role in this pathway.

Techniques

There is no standardized technique for delivering phototherapy. A recent international survey which included 108 neonatal units (NICU) from 22 countries spanning 4 continents showed great variability not only in practice criteria for initiation of phototherapy but considerable diversity in the type of phototherapy unit used with fluorescent lamps being used most frequently [33]. According to the AAP guidelines to deliver intensive phototherapy the method used must be able to reduce the bilirubin concentration by 1 to 2 mg/dL over 4 to 6 hours with a continuous and steady decline thereafter [8]. There is a direct relationship between the dose of phototherapy and the decrease in the measured TSB concentration [34]. The dose of phototherapy will depend on the spectrum or wavelength of the light source, the energy output or irradiance of the light source, the distance of the light from the infant and the surface area of the infant exposed to light. Irradiance is the radiant power (energy output) on a surface per unit area of surface expressed as watts per square centimeter (W/cm^2) whereas spectral radiance is the irradiance in a certain wavelength band and is expressed as microwatts per square centimeter per nanometer ($\mu W/cm^2/nm$). Since the radiometers used take measurements across a band of wavelengths (i.e. 425-475 nm or 400 to 480 nm) the spectral irradiance is determined by dividing the irradiance by the width of the interval of the bands (i.e. irradiance of 500 $\mu W/cm^2$ in 425 to 475 nm would equal 500/50 or 10 $\mu W/cm^2/nm$). The irradiance is directly related to the distance between the light and infant, the closer the lamp the more effective it is. The spectral power then is the product of the spectral irradiance across the surface area being exposed [5]. The more surface area exposed the more effective the treatment. Most infants are placed naked under the lights, with a small diaper, if necessary, and with shielding over their eyes. The infant's position should also be changed frequently to increase skin exposure.

There have been several sources of light that have been used in phototherapy devices. (Table 2) Probably the most important variable of the efficacy of phototherapy is the wavelength of the light used to induce photoisomerisation. Bilirubin, which is a yellow pigment, absorbs light maximally in the blue-green

Table 2. Light sources of phototherapy

Fluorescent lamps
– White
– Blue
– Special blue (emits narrow spectrum)
– Green
Halogen lamps
Fiberoptic systems
Light emitting diodes (LEDs)

ranges (from 420 to 500 nm). The peak absorption for albumin-bound bilirubin, which most likely is the bilirubin that is being affected by phototherapy, is at 460 nm and that for unbound bilirubin is 440 nm. Daylight and cool white fluorescent lamps are broad spectrum with a spectral peak between 550 and 660 nm therefore only a fraction of the light is acting on the bilirubin. Blue light (approximately 450 nm) is most readily absorbed. Special blue lamps, which emit a narrower spectrum (420 – 480 nm) of light then blue lamps, are most effective. Green light has a longer wavelength (peak at 525 nm) and therefore penetrates the skin more deeply but may not be as effective as special blue lights. A study evaluating the efficacy of daylight, special blue and green lamps in the management of non-haemolytic hyperbilirubinaemia showed that the rate of decline in bilirubin levels with special blue lamps was twice that with green lamps despite comparable irradiance measurements in their respective wavelengths [35]. Both the blue and green lamps caused side effects of dizziness, headache and nausea in the nursing staff. To decrease this effect phototherapy units will often consist of a combination of white and blue lights. Mercury vapour halogen lamps have a broad emission but do have a significant output in the blue spectrum. They are more compact then fluorescent systems. However, they cannot be brought close to the infant without putting the infant at risk of a burn, therefore limiting the ability to increase the irradiance. The surface area of infant exposure is also usually less than that of a bank of fluorescent lamps. Fibre-optic phototherapy systems were introduced in the 1980's and consist of a halogen lamp with attached fibre-optic cables containing fibres that end spread out in a flat mat. The light is transmitted via the fibres to the mat, which is placed in direct contact with the skin. There are several advantages to this system since no eye patches are necessary, it is more portable and convenient for mothers and for home therapy. While the irradiance generated is comparable to other forms of phototherapy the spectral power is low since they cover a small surface area. Therefore, in general, they have been found to be less effective then conventional therapy for term infants [36,38]. One study evaluating the use of fibre-optic phototherapy in full term infants showed that the use of a double mat resulted in a 24 hour decline rate and overall decline rate that was comparable to conventional phototherapy and significantly better then the use of either a single standard sized or large sized mat [39]. However, fibre-optic therapy has been an efficient way to deliver both single and double phototherapy in preterm infants [38,40]. The newest light sources are high-intensity gallium nitride light emitting diodes (LEDs). They are more efficient then fluorescent tubes or incandescent filament devices at converting electrical energy to light energy and emit narrow bands of light in the wavelength region that is best for phototherapy. They have a long halftime, emit little heat, and are lightweight and portable. The power output is low but groups can be wired together. Since they do not emit infrared or ultraviolet radiation they can also be placed close to the infant. A prototype has been designed consisting of 6 focused arrays each with 100 3-mm blue LEDs. When placed at a distance of 20 cm this system can generate >100 $\mu W/cm^2/nm$. The prototype unit has been tested in clinical trial showing that when used at a low irradiance (5 to 8 $\mu mol/cm^2/nm$) it was as effective as conventional therapy [41].

Standard or conventional phototherapy, in which infants are exposed to between 7 to 10 $\mu W/cm^2/nm$, result in decreases of 6% to 20% of the initial bilirubin level over the first 24 hours, which is sufficient for prophylactic use [5]. For term and near term infants who are readmitted to the hospital on days 4 to 7 with bilirubin levels $\geq$ 20 mg/dL more intensive therapy is required. Using special blue lamps and bringing them as close to the infant as possible, necessitating having the infant in a bassinet, can accomplish this. Special blue lights that are placed no further then 10 cm from the infant can generate a spectral irradiance greater than 50 $\mu W/cm^2/nm$ [5]. The use of double phototherapy which results in a larger surface area being exposed to a constant irradiance has proved to be an effective way of increasing efficacy of therapy. Double phototherapy has been achieved either by using fibre-optic pads in combination with lights, or a combination of lights distributed around the infant [40,42]. The use of fibre-optic pads is more effective in low birth weight then full-term infants since they can cover more surface area in the low birth weight infant [38]. The use of a reflecting material (white sheet, aluminum) has been another method of increasing the surface area exposed. The various techniques used to alter the delivery of phototherapy to give maximum efficacy have resulted in a decrement in initial bilirubin concentration of 30% to 50% within 24 hours [5]. There have been several retrospective studies looking at rebound levels both in term and preterm infants, as well as infants receiving intensive phototherapy. These studies have shown that significant rebound following discontinuation of phototherapy is rare [43,44].

Phototherapy is usually well tolerated by infants. There is an increase in body temperature and insensible water loss therefore fluid balance and management is extremely important. Stools are also often slightly looser and more frequent which can be managed by feeding a non-lactose formula. Since the effect of high-intensity light exposure on the eyes is unknown the newborn's eyes should be well covered during treatment. Haemodynamic affects have been seen in preterm infants association with phototherapy including an increase in cerebral blood flow and a re-opening of patent ductus arteriosus [45]. Rashes have been observed and infants who have cholestasis undergoing phototherapy may develop dark gray-brown discoloration of the skin described as bronze baby syndrome. The latter may be related to accumulation of porphyrins in the plasma [18].

Exchange Transfusion

While exchange transfusion remains the most rapid way to reduce bilirubin levels the frequency of exchange transfusion in the postnatal period has decreased significantly [5]. This is the result of several factors including the use of Rh immune globulin to prevent Rh isoimmunization, approaches to prenatal management of haemolytic disease and more aggressive phototherapeutic management of jaundice in the newborn as described above. Prior to performing an exchange transfusion it is important to balance the risk of the procedure to the benefit of potentially preventing kernicterus. As with phototherapy the factors that are considered in the decision to perform an exchange transfusion include: gestational age, evidence of haemolysis, degree of anaemia, rate of rise of bilirubin and concurrent clinical conditions, such as asphyxia, acidosis and hypoalbuminaemia that may exacerbate bilirubin entry and toxicity to the CNS. A double volume exchange (85 mL/kg x 2 for term infants up to 100 mL/kg x 2 for very low birth weight infants) should remove approximately 90% of the fetal circulating red cells and a single volume exchange between 70 to 75%. The bilirubin level however is only decreased by approximately 50% due to tissue re-equilibration with a rebound in bilirubin level to approximately 60% of the pre-exchange level [46].

The commonly used method for exchange transfusion is the discontinuous technique described by Diamond in 1951 [47]. Small aliquots of blood are withdrawn and replaced through a single catheter with a special 4-way stopcock. Usually no more than 5 mL/kg body weight or 5% of the infant's blood volume are removed and replaced during a 3 to 5 minute cycle. The total time duration for a double volume exchange is 90 to 120 minutes or 45 to 60 minutes for a single volume exchange. It is important to assure that the infant is stable prior to initiating an exchange transfusion. The infant should be under a warmer for ready accessibility and needs to be monitored closely throughout the procedure. This should include temperature monitoring, cardiopulmonary and pulse-oximetry monitoring to evaluate pressure fluctuations as well as laboratory monitoring (complete blood counts, electrolytes, glucose, calcium) to avoid potential metabolic complications or coagulopathies. In the NICHHD collaborative phototherapy study, they demonstrated a mortality rate associated with exchange transfusion of 0.5% and a rate of adverse clinical problems of 6.7% [48]. Jackson et al. [49] in a review of 106 infants undergoing exchange transfusion during a more recent time period (15 year span from 1980 to 1995) reported an incidence of procedure-related complications leading to death of 2% and the rate of severe complications of 4%. Therefore it is important to have a good understanding of the dynamics of this procedure when weighing the risks versus the benefits.

Pharmacological Approach

Pharmacological approaches have centered on either reducing bilirubin production or enhancing bilirubin conjugation and excretion. Synthetic metalloporphyrins, in which other metals replace the central iron, inhibit the activity of HO, the rate-limiting enzyme for the degradation of heme to bilirubin.

There are two primary isoforms of HO, the inducible form (HO-1) and the constitutive form (HO-2). Several compounds are being evaluated as potential inhibitors of HO [50]. Compounds that would be the most appealing are ones that have a low I_{50}, are not a photosensitizer, do not cross the blood-brain barrier, are orally absorbable, short acting and easily excretable and do not substantially upregulate HO-1 mRNA or affect other enzyme systems (i.e. nitrous oxide synthase). Animal studies of tin-protoporphyrin (SnPP) demonstrated reduction in endogenonous bilirubin formation without impairing hepatic uptake, excretion or enteric resorption of bilirubin [51]. Since the meso derivative (SnMP) had comparable efficacy in adult rodents at a 10-fold lower dose, this is the drug that seemed to be favoured and has gone to clinical trials [50]. An early clinical trial was conducted in preterm infants to assess the effectiveness of increasing doses of SnMP in moderating hyperbilirubinaemia and decreasing the need for phototherapy. A dose of 6 μmol/kg BW administered within 24 hours of birth was found to reduce TSB by 41% and phototherapy by 76% compared to controls [52]. A light-induced erythaema which was mild and self limited occurred in some infants who received the combination of SnMP and phototherapy. A comparison study of the effectiveness of administering a single dose of SnMP (6 μmol/kg BW) versus the use of phototherapy (12 to 14 $\mu W/cm^2/nm$) in term and near term infants to control hyperbilirubinaemia showed that the time to achieve the stated endpoint was reduced by >30 hours in the SnMP treated infants compared with infants receiving phototherapy. None of the 44 SnMP treated infants needed supplemental phototherapy [53]. A more recent study of a single intramuscular dose of SnMP (6 μmol/kg BW) in full term breast fed infants with bilirubin levels of $\geq$15 mg/dL ($\geq$256 μmol/L) and $\leq$ 18 mg/dL ($\leq$308 μmol/L) reached between 48 to 96 hours was effective in controlling hyperbilirubinaemia, with no infants requiring phototherapy in contrast to 27% of control patients [54]. While SnMP has been shown to be effective in suppressing bilirubin production it does not possess all the qualities of the ideal compound since it is not orally absorbable, possesses photosensitizer properties and moderately upregulates HO-1. At present it is a desirable haeme-oxygenase inhibitor and is the only currently approved compound for investigational use.

Summary

Phototherapy is a simple and relatively safe method for managing neonatal hyperbilirubinaemia. An improved understanding about the mechanism of phototherapy and factors that affect the dose delivered has resulted in efficient and rapid reduction in bilirubin levels and marked decrease in the need for exchange transfusions. The development of new phototherapy techniques that are in process should increase the versatility and portability of this treatment. Studies evaluating the effectiveness of metalloporphyrin compounds to inhibit bilirubin production have been underway. Early clinical results using Sn-MP look promising. Follow-up surveillance studies are sill in progress and additional compounds are also being investigated.

References

1. Maisels MJ, Newman TB. Bilirubin and neurological dysfunction – do we need to change what we are doing? Pediatr Res 2001;50:677-78.
2. Dennery PA, Seidman DS, Stevenson DK. Drug therapy: Neonatal hyperbilirubinemia. N Engl J Med 2001:344:581-90.
3. Hsia DYY, Allen FH, Gellis SS, Diamond LK. Erythroblastosis fetalis. VIII. Studies of serum bilirubin in relation to kernicterus. N Engl J Med 1952;247: 668-71.
4. Cremer RJ, Perryman PW, Richards DH. Influence of light on the hyperbilirubinemia of infants. Lancet 1958;1:1094-97.
5. Maisels MJ. Phototherapy – Traditional and nontraditional. J Perinatol 2001;21(suppl):93-97.
6. Soorani-Lunsing I, Woltil HA, Hadders-Algra M. Are moderate degrees of hyperbilirubinemia in healthy term neonates really safe for the brain? Pediatr Res 2001;50: 701-05.
7. Newman TB, Maisels MJ. Evaluation and treatment of jaundice in the term newborn. A kinder, gentler approach. Pediatrics 1992;89:809-18.
8. AAP Provisional committee for Quality Improvement and Subcommittee on Hyperbilirubinemia. Practice parameter: Management of hyperbilirubinemia in the healthy term newborn. Pediatrics 1994;94:558-62.
9. Hanson TWR. Fetal and neonatal bilirubin metabolism. In Maisels MJ, Watchko JF, eds. Neonatal Jaundice. London: Harwood Academic, 2000 pp3-22.
10. Cashore WJ. Bilirubin and jaundice in the micropremie. Clin Perinatol 2000;27:171-79.
11. Seideman DS, Stevenson DK, Ergaz Z, Gale R. Hospital readmission due to neonatal hyperbilirubinemia. Pediatrics 1995;96:727-29.
12. Maisels MJ, King E. Length of stay, jaundice, and hospital readmission. Pediatrics 1998;101:995-98.
13. Johnson L, Brown AK. A pilot registry for acute and chronic kernicterus in term and near-term infants. Pediatrics 1999;104:(suppl):736a.
14. Ebbesen F. Recurrence of kernicterus in term and near-term infants in Denmark. Acta Paediatr 2000;89:1-5.
15. AAP Subcommittee on Neonatal Hyperbilirubinemia. Neonatal jaundice and kernicterus. Pediatrics 2001;108:763-65.

16. Maisels MJ, Pathak A, Nelson NM, et al. Endogenous production of carbon monoxide in normal and erythroblastotic newborn infants. J Clin Invest 1971;50:1-9.
17. Bosma PJ, Seppen J, Goldhoorn B, et al. Bilirubin UDP-glucuronyl transferase 1 is the only relevant bilirubin glucuronodating isoform in man J Biol Chem 1994;269:17960-64.
18. Maisels MJ. Neonatal hyperbilirubinemia. In Klaus MH, Fanaroff AA, eds. Care of the high risk neonate. Philadelphia: WB Saunders, 2001 pp324-62.
19. Hardy JB, Drage JS, Jackson EC. The first year of life: The Collaborative Perinatal Project of the National Institutes of Neurologic and Communicative Disorders and Stroke. Baltimore; Johns Hopkins University Press 1979.
20. Bhutani VK, Johnson L, Siveri EM. Predictive ability of a predischarge hour-specific serum bilirubin for subsequent significant hyperbilirubinemia in healthy term and near-term newborns. Pediatrics 1999;103:6-14.
21. Ryan AS. The resurgence of breastfeeding in the United States. Pediatrics 99:E12, 1997.
22. Beutler E, Gelbart T, Demina A. Racial variability in the UDP-glucuronosyl transferase (UGT1A1) promotor: a balanced polymorphism for regulation of bilirubin metabolism? Proc Natl Acad Sci USA 1998;95: 8170-74.
23. Bhutani VK, Johnson LH. Jaundice technologies: Prediction of hyperbilirubinemia in term and near-term newborns. J Perinatol 2001; 21:(suppl): 76-82.
24. Newman TB, Xiong B, Gonzales VM, Escobar GJ. Prediction and prevention of extreme neonatal hyperbilirubinemia in a mature health maintenance organization. Arch Pediatr Adolesc Med 2000;154:1140-47.
25. Stevenson DK, Fanaroff A, Maisels J. et al. Prediction of hyperbilirubinemia in term and near-term newborn infants. Pediatrics 2001;108:31-39.
26. Lucey J, Ferreiro M, Hewitt J. Prevention of hyperbilirubinemia of prematurity by phototherapy. Pediatrics 1968;41:1047-54.
27. Brown AK, Kim MH, Wu PYK, et al. Efficacy of phototherapy in prevention and management of hyperbilirubinemia. Pediatrics 1985;75:393-400.
28. Maurer HM, Kirpatrick BV, McWilliams NB et al. Phototherapy for hyperbilirubinemia of hemolytic disease of the newborn. Pediatrics 1985;75: 68-76.
29. Valaes T, Koliopoulos C, Koiopoulos A. The impact of phototherapy in the management of neonatal hyperbilirubinemia. Comparison of historical cohorts. Acta Paediatr 1996;85:273-76.
30. Scheidt PC, Bryla DA, Nelson KB, Hirtz DG, Hoffman HJ. Phototherapy for neonatal hyperbilirubinemia; six year follow-up of the national institute of child health and human development clinical trial. Pediatrics 1990; 85:455-63.
31. McDonagh AF. Phototherapy: From ancient Egypt to the new millennium. J Perinatol 2001;21:(suppl):7-12.

32. Ennever JF, Costarino AT, Polin RA, Speck WT. Rapid clearance of a structural isomer of bilirubin during phototherapy. J Clin Invest 1987;79: 1674-78.
33. Hanson TWR. Therapeutic approaches to neonatal jaundice: an international survey. Clin Pediatr 1996;75:393-400.
34. Tan KL. The pattern of bilirubin response to phototherapy for neonatal hyperbilirubinemia. Pediatr Res 1982;16:670-74.
35. Tan KL. Efficacy of fluorescent daylight, blue, and green lamps in the management of nonhemolytic hyperbilirubinemia. J Pediatr 1989;114:132-37.
36. Mills JF, Tudehope D. Fiberoptic phototherapy for neonatal jaundice. In: The Cochrane Library, Issue 1. Oxford: Update Software;2001.
37. Holtrop PC, Madison K, Maisels MJ. A clinical trial of fiberoptic phototherapy vs conventional phototherapy. AJDC 1992;146:235-37.
38. Tan KL. Comparison of the efficacy of fiberoptic and conventional phototherapy for neonatal hyperbilirubinemia. J Pediatr 1994;125:607-12.
39. Tan KL. Efficacy of bi-directional fiber-optic phototherapy for neonatal hyperbilirubinemia. Pediatrics 1997;99:e13.
40. Holtrop PC, Ruedisueli K, Maisels MJ. Double versus single phototherapy in low birth weight newborns. Pediatric 1992; 90:674-77.
41. Seidman DS, Moise J, Ergaz Z et al. A new blue light-emitting phototherapy device: A prospectiverandomized controlled study. J Pediatr 2000; 136:771-74.
42. Garg AK, Prasad RS, Hifzi IA. A controlled trial of high-intensity double-surface phototherapy on a fluid bed versus conventional phototherapy in neonatal jaundice. Pediatrics 1995;95:914-16.
43. Yetman RJ, Parks D, Huseby V, Mistry K, Garcia J. Rebound bilirubin levels in infants receiving phototherapy. J Pediatr 1998;133:705-07.
44. Maisels MJ, Kring E. Rebound in serum bilirubin level following intensive phototherapy. Arch Pediatr Adolesc Med. 2002;669-72.
45. Benders MJNL, van Bel F, van de Bor. The effect of photottherapy of cerebral blood flow velocity in preterm infants. Acta Paediatr 1998;87:786-91
46. Valaes, T. Bilirubin distribution and dynamics of bilirubin removal by exchange transfusion. Acta. Paediatr. Scand. 1963;52(suppl 149).
47. Diamond LK, Allen FH, Thomas WO Erythroblastosis fetalis. VII. Treatment with exchange transfusion. N Engl J Med. 1951;244:39.
48. Keenen WJ, Novak KK, Sutheralns JM, Bryla DA, Fetterly KL. Morbidity and mortality associated with exchange transfusion. Pediatrics 1985;75: (suppl):422-26.
49. Jackson JC. Adverse events associated with exchange transfusion in healthy and ill newborns. Pediatrics 1997;99:e7.
50. Vreman HJ, Wong RJ, Stevenson DK. Alternative metalloporphyrins for the treatment of neonatal jaundice. J Perinatol 2001;21:(suppl):108-13.
51. Whitington PF et al The effect of tin (IV)-protoporphyrin-IX on bilirubin production and excretion in the rat. Pediatr Res 1987;21:487-91.

52. Valaes T, Petmezaki, S, Henschke C, Drummond GS, Kappas A. Control of jaundice in preterm newborns by an inhibitor of bilirubin production: Studies with tin-mesoporphyrin. Pediatrics 1994;93:1-11.
53. Kappas A, Drummond GS, Henschke C, Valaes T. Direct comparison of Sn-Mesoprphorin, an inhibitor of bilirubin production and phototherapy in controlling hyperbilirubinemia in term and near-term newborns. Pediatrics 1995;95:468-74.
54. Martinez JC, Garcia HO, Otheguy LE, Drummonds GS, Kappas A. Control of severe hyperbilirubinemia in full-term newborns with the inhibitor of bilirubin production Sn-mesoporphyrin. Pediatrics 1999;103:1-5.

CONSENSUS AND CONTROVERSY IN FOETAL AND NEONATAL ALLOIMMUNE THROMBOCYTOPENIA

J.B. Bussel[1]

Foetal and neonatal alloimmune thrombocytopenia (AIT) is a disease in which there are a number of important controversies. These range from which neonates the diagnosis should be entertained in to what testing the laboratory should perform (especially if the first round of testing is not clearly diagnostic) to what treatment should be given. Increasingly there is consensus in broad areas but considerable variability in the details and in certain specific situations. Prior to discussing the controversies, it would be appropriate to first summarize the areas of consensus.

Areas of Consensus

There is a summary manuscript (submitted to the Journal of Thrombosis and Haemostasis) which will cover these major areas of consensus in detail and discuss some others as well, i.e. when to suspect AIT in a foetus [1]. What areas have achieved reasonable consensus among leading practitioners?

First, there is good consensus that one of the keys for diagnosis in the newborn is severe, isolated thrombocytopenia. This has been demonstrated in several studies in the past 10 years [2-4] including our recent one [5] involving direct comparison of babies with alloimmune thrombocytopenia (AIT) to those with thrombocytopenia who did not have AIT. This may change again in the future however in light of the studies of prospective screening which suggest that babies who "fly under the radar" do so because they are sufficiently mild as to be asymptomatic [6]. The "classical" criterion for diagnosis of AIT in the neonate was, and still is, unexplained thrombocytopenia. Recent data on the other side however is that, not surprisingly, patients with AIT can have other medical conditions that one might have assumed were the cause of the thrombocytopenia. Hence even "explained" thrombocytopenia deserves a work up especially if the thrombocytopenia is severe or if there is a family history of transient neonatal thrombocytopenia.

1. Weill Cornell Medical Center, New York, NY, USA.

Table 1. Consensus in diagnosis and treatment of AIT

- Severe thrombocytopenia in the first 24 hours of life, unexplained thrombocytopenia and familial transient neonatal thrombocytopenia all suggest AIT
- Any significant degree of neonatal thrombocytopenia mandates a radiologic investigation, i.e. cranial ultrasound or better CT or MRI, of the neonate no matter how well they appear clinically
- Clinical suspicion of AIT mandates both appropriate serologic/molecular testing as well as treatment of the affected neonate
- Serologic/Molecular Diagnosis of AIT requires a platelet specific antigen incompatibility between the parents and demonstration of maternal antibody whose specificity matches the incompatibility
- In general, laboratory testing in a suspected case of neonatal or foetal AIT should include typing for HPA-1, HPA-3, and HPA-5. In Asian populations, HPA-4 testing is required. Antibody determination should include glycoproteins IIB/IIIA, IB/IX, and IA/IIA as well as the father's platelets. Further testing depends upon the initial results and the clinical setting. In most cases, the parents alone need to be tested
- When AIT is suspected, platelet antigen typing and antibody testing should be performed by an experienced, reference laboratory
- Almost always, the next affected sibling in the family will be at least as severely affected as the first affected sibling and will have a significant chance of having severe foetal thrombocytopenia which may start by 20 weeks of gestation
- If the first affected sibling has an antenatal intracranial haemorrhage, the next affected sibling in the family is highly likely to have one as well

A second area of consensus is that when substantial thrombocytopenia is identified, even an asymptomatic baby requires a cranial radiologic study. The standard of care is an ultrasound but the consensus of Pediatric Neurologists is that either a head CT or an MR is better. Even remarkably well-appearing neonates can have clinically silent ICH [7]. This ICH needs to be detected because it would alter the management of the thrombocytopenia and also because it would have implications for the next sibling in the family [8, 9]. The latter is particularly true if the thrombocytopenia is the result of a condition that might recur in the next sibling.

Third, suspecting the diagnosis of AIT in the neonate entails two steps. One step is to initiate treatment consistent with the diagnosis of AIT i.e. IVIG and antigen-negative platelets as needed; the second step is laboratory testing to confirm the diagnosis. Treatment would generally be initiated in all neonates with AIT and a platelet count < 20,000/μl although many centres would use a higher cut off i.e. 30,000/μl. If there is an ICH, then the general consensus to maintain the platelet count at > 50-100,000/μl for at least 1-4 weeks.

A fourth consensus point is that laboratory testing to confirm the diagnosis requires demonstrating a platelet-specific antigen incompatibility between the parents and that the mother make an antibody that corresponds specifically to the incompatibility [10]. With improved testing and the discovery of many new platelet antigen systems in the past 5 years, it is increasingly likely that an antigen incompatibility will be discovered between any parents depending upon which and how many platelet antigens are tested. Similarly there is "false positive" antibody from a number of causes such that there may not rarely be an antigen incompatibility and anti-platelet antibody demonstrated. However if the antibody is not specific for the antigen incompatibility in question, then the diagnosis of AIT is not confirmed. This specificity ideally requires demonstration, for a specific platelet antigen, that the antibody binds to antigen-positive but not antigen-negative controls and also that it binds only to the specific platelet glycoprotein on which the polymorphism is located.

Fifth, there is a consensus among leading, reference laboratories that the specific antigens to test for include HPA-1, HPA-3, and HPA-5 [1]. Other platelet antigens may need to be added depending on the ethnic background, i.e. inclusion of HPA-4 in Asian families. An important part of testing is to screen maternal antibody against paternal platelets. This will explore the possibility of a rare or private platelet antigen and potentially allow its identification by determining to which platelet glycoprotein the antibody binds. HLA antibody can be confusing in this assay if specific glycoprotein determination is not performed.

Sixth, the laboratory, in order to be able to do the testing correctly, must have experience with the diagnosis, must have the appropriate controls, and must have the ability to do DNA-based typing depending on the requirements of the individual patient. This means that they need to be an experienced reference laboratory which takes part in regular workshops to validate their diagnostic skills and demonstrate their ability to diagnose cases with multiple antibodies, i.e. anti-HLA and anti-platelet specific glycoprotein, and a variety of platelet antigen incompatibilities.

Table 2. Consensus of antenatal treatment of the second affected sibling with AIT

- Be based upon serologic and/or molecular diagnosis from an experienced reference laboratory. In many cases, if the father is a homozygote for the antigen in question, i.e. HPA-1A, this is sufficient to mark the next foetus as affected if an unequivocal diagnosis of AIT has been made previously and if there is no doubt regarding paternity. Foetal platelet typing can be performed by amniocentesis if required
- Be under direction of experienced clinicians
- Minimize foetal blood sampling
- Use maternally-administered therapy as first-line for an affected foetus before the administering weekly foetal platelet transfusion
- Fetal blood sampling should be accompanied by a fetal platelet transfusion if there is severe thrombocytopenia (or platelet dysfunction)

Antenatal Management

Currently antenatal management focuses on the subsequent affected foetus in the family because there is no routine antenatal screening. In almost all instances this sibling will be more severely affected than the previous sibling. This was first formally documented when 40-50% of foetuses in a series of initial foetal blood samplings demonstrated that the platelet count was already lower in the subsequent sibling (foetus) than it had been in the previous sibling at birth [8].

Furthermore in the same study of almost 100 sibling pairs affected with AIT, having an antenatal haemorrhage predicted a lower platelet count on initial fetal sampling but the neonatal platelet count did not [8]. A smaller second study found that the neonatal platelet count of the first sibling did predict the severity of the next sibling [11]. The predictive value of antenatal ICH is consistent with reports in the literature in which > 80-90% of subsequent siblings who did not have antenatal treatment themselves essentially all had recurrent antenatal ICH although the numbers are small and there may have been a bias in the reporting [12]. Treatment is controversial in many specific issues (see later) but not in general. Table 2 lists the areas of consensus.

The use of an experienced, reference laboratory has been discussed above and is crucial to any endeavour in this area. It is very important that the foetus be shown to be affected prior to initiation of treatment. Since treatment is difficult, not risk free, takes time to administer, and is costly if IVIG is utilized, it is important not to use it blindly but rather to ensure that the foetus being treated is known to be affected.

The consensus to try to minimize foetal blood sampling has arisen out of the foetal losses in the cooperative European study that was just published [11] and the multi-centre American study that was recently completed [13]. Recognition of the complications of sampling, beyond the bleeding from the sampling that was seen prior to institution of foetal platelet transfusions at the time of sampling, has lead to agreement on the need to minimize sampling. How to accomplish this is controversial (see below). If foetal blood sampling is to be performed, there is consensus that it should be performed by a practitioner experienced in foetal blood sampling because of the risk of the procedure. There is no question that there is an experience curve suggesting that it should be restricted to a limited number of centres. For example in the Netherlands, the foetal medicine unit at Leiden is responsible for all IUT's for the country, i.e. for Rh and for AIT. With a population of 15 million, this is bigger than almost all states in the USA but the larger states in the US all have multiple centres which perform sampling and transfusion.

There is consensus that platelet transfusion should be given if sampling is performed in a patient with severe thrombocytopenia (or platelet dysfunction). At least one study has shown this by pointing out the high morbidity and mortality of foetal blood sampling (FBS) in thrombocytopenic foetuses [14]. The use of foetal platelet transfusions has appeared to be effective in eliminating bleeding complications of FBS. How to perform this is controversial, has risks of its own, and will be considered near the end of this manuscript.

Maternally-administered Intravenous (IV) Gammaglobulin (IVIG)

In regard to the initial use of maternally-administered treatment, intravenous (IV) gammaglobulin (IVIG) has become the standard of care. There is considerable debate and no clear consensus on how to monitor treatment, when to start it, and concomitant prednisone use, all of which will be discussed in this review. There is a consensus dose of 1 gm/kg/week of IVIG that is used by virtually everyone who uses IVIG for AIT. Even the definition of a "high risk" patient is in doubt. It ranges from one with a very low foetal or neonatal platelet count to one who has had a sibling with an ICH to one who has had a sibling with an early (in utero) ICH. The discussion of controversial topics in AIT will focus on specific areas, highlighting both major as well as minor controversies. Table 3 lists the areas to be reviewed. Since there is now considerable consensus on when the diagnosis of neonatal AIT should be suspected (see below Table 1, #1), the controversy arises when clinically one or more of the criteria for the diagnosis of AIT are met and testing is sent but the laboratory has equivocal or negative findings. For example, a term baby is born and noted to have petecchiae and ecchymoses. A blood count sent at 1-3 hours of age reveals a platelet count of 14,000/μl and is otherwise normal (Hb, WBC, and smear). This is easily recognized as the classical presentation for AIT. Typically one might expect that the testing for AIT would reveal Pl^{A1} incompatibility.

Table 3. Controversial topics in AIT

- Diagnosis in the Neonate: if one or more of the criterion listed in Table 1 are met but the initial laboratory work up of AIT is non-confirmatory (not diagnostic of AIT)
- Antenatal Management:
  - maternally administered therapy
  - foetal blood sampling (how minimal is minimal
  - preparation of platelets for transfusion to the foetus
  - which foetus should be transfused and when
- Routine antenatal Screening:
  - should it be performed

if it is worthwhile, how should it be performed

The controversy or confusion arises if the testing in such a case does not confirm AIT. The figure comprises 4 reports from the Blood Center of SouthEastern Wisconsin (BCSEW). They illustrate: a) classical AIT as a result of Pl^{A1} incompatibility; b) an equivocal case with anti-HLA antibodies alone; c) antibody to glycoprotein IIB/IIIA that is not directed against either $Pl^{A1/A2}$ or Bak a/b; and d) completely negative testing.

Panel A revealing classical AIT as a result of HPA-1a incompatibility is straightforward and not controversial. The father is a homozygote, essentially guaranteeing that all subsequent fetuses in the family will be at least as severely affected. If the father were a heterozygote, it is still not possible to identify the foetal $Pl^{A1/A2}$ platelet type in maternal blood. Therefore diagnosis would proceed most likely through amniocentesis, rather than either CVS or FBS, because of their greater risks. If there had been a very early antenatal CNS haemorrhage in the previous sibling, this might suggest that CVS be used so that therapy could be started earlier in gestation i.e. at 12 weeks of gestation.

Panel B testing reveals only anti-HLA antibody. It is controversial in that it is not known if anti-HLA ever causes AIT. It has not ever been conclusively proven that it actually did cause a case of AIT although there are cases of AIT with multiple affected (thrombocytopenic) children in which it is the only platelet-binding antibody detected. However as many as 25% or more of multiparous women have HLA antibodies and very, very few have thrombocytopenic foetuses and neonates. Recent work has demonstrated that "rare" platelet antigens such as Max may be involved (see discussion of Part D) in cases of apparent AIT. Since an intensive work up would be required to verify that none of the known platelet antigens are involved and no hidden antibodies are present, the significance of HLA antibodies in neonatal thrombocytopenia remains highly controversial.

Panel C is intended to illustrate a situation in which there is a possibility that a novel (rare) platelet-specific antigen may explain the incompatibility. If there is maternal platelet glycoprotein specific antibody detected which reacts with paternal platelets, then the likelihood is increased that a platelet specific antigen may be involved even if it is a "rare" one. The antibody specificity encourages exploration of a group of potential antigens which would not normally be tested.

Panel D illustrates negative testing. An issue here is that if the mother has the "common" allele and the father has the "rare" allele, then platelet antibody testing may not reveal maternal antibody because it is directed against the rare allele which is not represented in the normal controls. This setting is where testing against paternal platelets is crucial. The test must ideally be able to discriminate anti-HLA antibody so that, if present, antibody to a platelet specific antigen can be distinguished and a decision made to pursue further testing of rare antigens (or not).

The bottom line is that testing is clear and unequivocal (non-controversial) only if it is positive i.e. Panel A. If it is "negative" as it is in Panels B-D, this is less clear even though the finding of a "rare" antigen is likely to be uncommon at best. The clinical findings therefore should play an important role in determining how far a case of neonatal thrombocytopenia should be pursued in the laboratory. The clinical diagnosis of AIT has been covered above. What is controversial is which additional features should determine additional work up. In practice, if the thrombocytopenia is severe (< 20,000/µl on the first count obtained) and if there is an ICH, especially an antenatal one, then additional investigation more likely needs to be pursued. Many novel antigens have been

Table 4. Clinical features

Clinical features in the thrombocytopenic neonate which suggest that further work up for AIT may be warranted when the initial work up is negative:
– response to treatments: NO (confusing) to random platelets, YES to IVIG, and YES to matched platelets
– birth platelet count < 10-20,000/µl
– an intraparenchymal ICH occurring in a term neonate of > 2200 gms
– complete absence of any other findings that could explain thrombocytopenia including: 1 and 5 minute APGARs of at least 7, no evidence of respiratory distress, no evidence of sepsis, no haemangioma or other vascular malformation on exam, no other findings on exam i.e. normal radial rays, no recent maternal use of aspirin; and an otherwise normal CBC
If obtained, a normal PT and PTT.

characterized by work up of very severe index cases. Table 4 lists possible features, in addition to the two listed above (low platelet count, ICH) which suggest that further testing might be fruitful. If these features are present as well as the three cardinal features (Table 1, #1), and standard testing for HPA1, 3, and 5 incompatibilities are negative then the laboratory should be requested to add the full range of testing possible to diagnose AIT. As indicated above an important focus (albeit technically a difficult one) would be to determine whether there was non-HLA, maternal antibody against paternal platelets.

Overall, in a competent and experienced reference laboratory that participates in yearly international workshops and maintains a full range of controls and diagnostic PCR primers, the vast majority of cases will be diagnosed correctly. This will be facilitated if the ethnic background of the parents is provided. If the testing remains ambiguous, there are several approaches to take during a second pregnancy. However there is not a consensus on any one approach and this area remains controversial. The policy that our centre employs continues to evolve. One approach would be to retest sera for platelet specific antibody at 4-12 week intervals throughout gestation to see if a more informative (platelet antigen specific) antibody could be identified. This would then allow determination, including by inference if the father is homozygous, of the foetal status for the antigen in question and also contribute to assessment of prognosis.

Another approach would be to perform foetal blood sampling at 26-34 weeks to determine if the foetus was affected; we would almost always choose 32-34 weeks as long as there had not been an intracranial haemorrhage in the previous affected sibling. If there was, then the timing of the ICH would become paramount in deciding management. Another approach would be to test for antibody only (no FBS) as above along with appropriate NST's and foetal sonos (additional non-invasive monitoring). Finally one could opt for "blind" treatment with or without a later FBS. The presumed solution to this controversy would be more informative testing that would be "definitively" positive or negative in as high a percentage of prospective AIT cases as possible. This would seem to mandate testing for rare antigens early in the work up process of a high percentage of cases.

Antenatal Treatment

The most publicized area of major controversy is Antenatal Treatment. The approach to antenatal treatment can be divided into several categories, each of which is at least somewhat controversial in its own right. These include who should be treated, when they should be treated, and what they should be treated with.

Who: Which patient should receive antenatal treatment, and if being treated, with what, is open to a high degree of debate and uncertainty. On one end of the patient severity spectrum, there is consensus that if there is an antenatal intracranial haemorrhage in the previous sibling and confirmed AIT, then the possibility that an antenatal intracranial haemorrhage will recur in the next affected sibling is high, > 80-90% [12, 13, 15]. Therefore there is no debate about the need for treatment (see discussion about which treatment below). On the opposite end of the spectrum, if there was not an antenatal haemorrhage in the previous sibling but there is a documented platelet antigen incompatibility and corresponding antibody confirming the diagnosis of AIT, then there are many uncertainties. These include when treatment should be initiated, what form it should take, how it should be monitored (if at all), and how delivery should be undertaken. The specific antigen incompatibility is important, i.e. Br a incompatibility has been shown to be less severe than that of Pl^{A1} [16]. In general however all foetuses known to be affected by AIT will probably be treated, the intensity of the treatment being the area of variability.

When: Hypothetically the earlier treatment is started, the more likely it is that maternal antibody will be trapped on the maternal side of the placenta, the presumed mechanism of effect of IVIG. Although this is controversial, in large part because it is unproven, the data supporting it as a potential mechanism of treatment effect is derived from studies of placental perfusion [17]. In the absence of a previous ICH, it would seem highly unlikely (virtually unheard of) that an antenatal ICH would occur before 32 weeks of gestation, even without administration of treatment to the mother. Therefore if treatment is to be initiated, it should be started somewhat before then to be safe. However the range of "before then" is wide, from 12 to 20 to 30 weeks, without clear guidance as to which it should be. If there is an antenatal or "uncertain" hemorrhage, then treatment should be started early i.e. by 20 weeks of gestation depending upon the timing of the ICH in the first child.

What: this is the area in which there is the most data and therefore the greatest degree of consensus although considerable controversy still exists. Table 5

Table 5. Treatments of foetal AIT

Active:
– IVIG 1-2 gm/kg/wk/infusion
– Prednisone 10-20mg/day to 1.0 mg/kg/d
– Combination treatments i.e. prednisone and IVIG together
– In utero weekly platelet transfusion
Discontinued:
– Dexamethasone
– Inutero IVIG

lists the therapeutic regimens that have been tested as therapy for foetal AIT: Considerable data supports the use of IVIG administered to the mother as 1 gm/kg/infusion. There appears to be lesser efficacy in the highest risk cases, i.e. those with sibling antenatal haemorrhage; at least two cases of the latter have been known to develop recurrent antenatal ICH despite IVIG treatment [13, 18]. Recent data also suggests that IVIG at this dose is less efficacious if the initial foetal platelet count. Nonetheless alternative treatments are clearly less efficacious and/or more toxic. The data regarding the use of steroids alone is limited and involves only "low" risk cases [13, 19]. While oral prednisone has an effect, the role of steroids is best established as an adjunct to IVIG. Doses from 0.5 mg/kg to 20 mg/day of prednisone have been tried as sole treatment; other steroids i.e. dexamethasone, have not been extensively tried past 5 cases. In utero treatment has essentially been restricted to weekly platelet transfusion to the foetus. This appears to be effective but, even in experienced hands, there is a high morbidity and mortality with this approach if transfusions are given from 24 to 36 weeks of gestation [11, 20]. There is however a clear consensus that platelet transfusions should be given to the thrombocytopenic (or thrombocytopathic) fetus who is undergoing FBS (see discussion below). Other promising treatment options include: a) the combination of IVIG and steroids; and b) IVIG as 2 infusions of 1 gm/kg/infusion per week. The former is clearly superior to IVIG alone and to prednisone alone; only the former has been proved in a randomised trial [13]. IVIG 2 gm/kg, in preliminary data is as good as IVIG 1 gm/kg plus 0.5 mg/kg/day of oral prednisone. The 2 gm/kg dose has been successfully used following failure of IVIG 1 gm/kg as "salvage" or "rescue" therapy but has not been compared head to head with IVIG 1 gm/kg. Currently, a case of foetal AIT unresponsive to IVIG 2 gm/kg/wk combined with prednisone 1 mg/kg/day is unknown but this combination has only been used in a limited number of cases as "salvage" when the initial treatment has failed to increase the foetal platelet count. In summary, there is consensus that medical treatment (IVIG and/or prednisone) should be used first in the treatment of "standard risk" (no antenatal ICH in a previous sibling). The exact details of dosing, when to use combination IVIG and steroids, and which dose and schedule of each should be employed remain to be clarified.

A recent development has been discussion regarding the role of FBS in the management of foetal AIT. The initial studies all used FBS before and after treatment to learn more about the natural history of foetal AIT and to understand more about the effects of treatment. As treatment strategies became better developed, it became clear over time that FBS contributed too much morbidity (premature delivery) and mortality, especially as therapeutic efficacy improved [11, 13, 14]. It therefore became clear than an important component of a successful protocol was to minimize the use of FBS. How to do this without compromising treatment? One proposal is to eliminate FBS altogether and just to "blindly" treat affected foetuses (determined by antigen incompatibility with amniocentesis for foetal platelet type in cases of paternal heterozygosity or unavailability) with 1 gm/kg of IVIG. This clearly would work in the great majority of cases since they would not suffer an ICH in any event but it remains controversial if this would be sufficiently effective in higher risk cases [21].

Our current approach is to divide cases into 3 risk groups. The 2 higher risk groups (with antenatal ICH in a previous sibling) receive treatment with IVIG 1 or 2 gm/kg/wk beginning at 12 weeks of gestation. Their initial FBS is in the vicinity of 20-24 weeks so that treatment can be intensified if it is insufficiently effective in these very high risk cases (steroids, platelet transfusions). However the standard risk cases initiate treatment at 20 weeks of gestation (or at referral) and do not undergo FBS until 32 weeks. This is thought to be late enough to have a relatively healthy foetus (premature neonate) in the very unlikely event of a complication of sampling. Yet it would be early enough to avoid a potential ICH in an unresponsive foetus by intensifying therapy and considering early delivery. Thus far, at least 80 if not 90% of the foetuses had good counts at sampling and there have not been complications of FBS in the 30-40 patients entered thus far. Clearly the optimal resolution would be a test derived from maternal plasma that would predict foetal risk so that FBS could be eliminated in a population of "good foetal responders" and utilized in those who are predicted to have higher risk.

Foetal Platelet Transfusions

The last major controversy to be discussed in this overview involves how to handle foetal platelet transfusions. There is now general consensus that FBS in a severely thrombocytopenic foetus carries an increased risk of exsanguination and other complications. Once this was established the thought was that fetal platelet transfusions could be administered as part of an FBS in patients with AIT. In this case, the platelet transfusion would not be administered for general disease management but rather for specific "coverage" of the FBS procedure. There are several controversial areas within this domain. The first is who should be the donor. A second linked issue is how to prepare the platelets for transfusion to the foetus. The third is which foetus should receive a platelet transfusion i.e. anyone undergoing an FBS for AIT or only selected cases.

Donor selection involves primarily two possibilities: the mother's "automatically-matched" platelets and antigen-negative "random donor" platelets. Note there has never been a formal comparison of unmatched to matched platelets in either the foetus or the neonate to demonstrate the superiority of matched platelets although this is generally accepted. The advantages of maternal platelets are clear: 1) automatic match regardless of the specific antigen incompatibility and without any requirement for testing to demonstrate compatibility; 2) limited additional risk of infection transmission or foetal sensitisation; and 3) general availability. The primary negative has been the need to "handle" the maternal platelets, i.e. decrease the amount of maternal plasma transfused with the maternal platelets. Another potential problem is that the mother may have just delivered and be at a community hospital, removed from the tertiary centre to which the neonate has been transferred, and may not feel up to immediately donating platelets. However, even if all the anti-platelet antibody contained in the maternal plasma could be eliminated, the antibody contained within platelet alpha granules may represent as much as 25% of all anti-platelet antibody in platelet rich plasma which may be significant, although it has never been studied. A random never pregnant matched donor who had no antibody to the antigen in question would not have this drawback.

An important issue is the handling of the platelets. It had been proposed that the newer plateletapheresis machines would result in platelets sufficiently concentrated that they would not require additional washing (to remove platelet antibody in plasma) of maternal platelets. If platelets require concentration past collection, "washing" being too damaging, then they can be "gently" spun down and the plasma supernatant aspirated off. Even this may damage the platelets resulting in either shortened lifespan and/or impaired function. This could be performed even on unrelated donor matched platelets to reduce the volume of transfusion to the foetus, if desired. Finally there is uncertainty regarding with which solution to reconstitute the concentrated platelets: plasma versus buffered solution i.e. saline. Only one thing is clear in current clinical practice: there is no universal protocol. If one prefers to use unrelated antigen negative platelets, the time needed to perform the testing may be a factor. Since testing is not usually immediately available, it is hard to be certain what antigen negative is exactly unless the need for the platelets can be anticipated days to weeks ahead of their use. It has been estimated that HPA-1a, HPA-5b negative platelets would be effective in 80-90% of AIT patients and could be obtained by/stored in regional Blood Centres for emergent use. However this has not been systematically evaluated. Furthermore there has been no comparison between "concentrated" maternal and unrelated antigen negative platelets. In summary the absence of platelet antibody makes matched unrelated donor platelets more desirable. However the ready availability of maternal platelets is very useful.

Which foetus undergoing sampling for AIT should receive platelets? Ideally only the foetus who is known to be thrombocytopenic i.e. < 30-50,000/μl should receive platelets at the time of FBS. However, this is often not a practical approach. Because in almost all cases, the sampling cannot ascertain the platelet count quickly enough. Unless there is an automated platelet counter in the room where the sampling is being performed, there is an automatic delay of 3-5 minutes to take the blood to the lab and at least another minute to have it run. This is a long time to leave a needle in a foetal blood vessel in the umbilical cord and to hope that it will not be dislodged. Therefore whether platelets need to be given in all cases of sampling, at least a certain amount i.e. 3 ml, while waiting the results of the foetal platelet count is uncertain. The general practice is to do so and then to complete the 10 or more ml transfusion of "concentrated" platelets if the foetal count is indeed low.

Management of the Neonate

Finally there is controversy on management of the neonate. The questions are if random platelets are sufficiently effective to be used while matched platelets (maternal or unrelated) are being obtained and when platelet transfusion, as compared to IVIG, should be administered. One set of anecdotal cases implied that not only are unmatched platelets ineffective but they may actually worsen the situation [22]. On the other hand, one study found that they were effective in neonatal AIT approximately 2/3 of the time, at least in the short term [5]. IVIG, with or without (our centre prefers with) "low dose" i.e. 1 mg/kg/day of IV methylprednisolone, seems to be effective in the great majority of cases but the uncertainty regarding its use is that it may take 1-3 days to increase the platelet count. In the setting of ongoing or high risk of ICH or other serious neonatal haemorrhage, this is too long. Therefore one set of guidelines would support platelet transfusion, especially matched platelet transfusion, if the neonatal platelet count is < 30-50,000/μl and certainly in the setting of any haemorrhage. This clearly mandates immediately obtaining a cranial ultrasound or (better if possible per recommendation of the neonatal neurology stroke committee) a head CT [23]. A case series demonstrated that clinically-silent ICH may occur and suggested that aggressive treatment of neonatal ICH will limit the extent of the ICH and improve the long term outcome of the survivors [24]. Therefore it seems appropriate to provide the best platelets available if there is either ongoing haemorrhage or suspected haemorrhage. In the setting of a negative radiologic study of the head and no other ongoing haemorrhage, the administration of platelets depends upon a number of factors which have not been well-defined. These include the platelet count, the age of the patient both gestational in weeks and post-natal in days, and the APGAR scores as a measure of vulnerability to ICH. In all cases in which there is any likelihood of treatment being required, it would seem prudent to obtain matched platelets as soon as possible and to administer IVIG both for its primary platelet effects and because it may serve to protect transfused platelets (another not well-documented area) [25].

Conclusion

In summary, there has been considerable progress in the diagnosis and management of AIT. There are probably more cases of ICH caused by thrombocytopenia in AIT than by thrombocytopenia from all other causes combined. Diagnosis has improved considerably but the identification of many new antigen systems has resulted in greater difficulty in of serologic diagnosis at this time (unless there is a standard antigen incompatibility i.e. Pl^{A1} (HPA-1A) and the corresponding specificity of maternal antibody). Management of the neonate involves immediately obtaining a head sono or CT and rapid and effective treatment with matched or unmatched platelets and/or IVIG with low dose steroids. Management of the foetus has improved to the point that the question is how little intervention can be used. Only in the highest risk cases is the use of repeated FBS justified.

References

1. Bussel JB, Kaplan C, Murphy M, Kroll H. Recommendations for the evaluation and treatment of fetal and neonatal alloimmune thrombocytopenia. J Thromb Haemostasis 1991;65:631-34.
2. Dreyfus M, Kaplan C, Verdy E, Schlegel N, Durand-Zaleski I, Tchernia G. Screening primiparous women and newborns for fetal/neonatal alloimmune thrombocytopenia: a prospective comparison of effectiveness and costs. Immune Thrombocytopenia Working Group. Am J Perinatol 1996;13:423-31.
3. de Moerloose P, Boehlen F, Extermann P, Hohfeld P. Neonatal thrombocytopenia: incidence and characterization of maternal antiplatelet antibodies by MAIPA assay. Br J Haematol 1998;100:735-40.
4. Sainio S, Jarvenpaa AL, Renlund M, Riikonen S, Teramo K, Kekomaki R. Thrombocytopenia in term infants: a population-based study. Obstet Gynecol 2000;95:441-46.
5. Bussel JB, Zacharoulis S, Kramer K, McFarland J, Pauliny J, Kaplan C, and the Neonatal Alloimmune Thrombocytopenia Registry Group. Clinical and diagnostic features of neonatal alloimmune thrombocytopenia: Comparison to non-immune cases of thrombocytopenia. Ped Blood Cancer 2005; (in press).
6. Williamson LM, Hackett G, Rennie J, et al. The natural history of fetomaternal alloimmunization to the platelet-specific antigen HPA-1a PlA1, Zwa) as determined by antenatal screening. Blood 1998;92:2280-87.
7. Bussel JB, Tanli S, Peterson HC. Favorable neurological outcome in 7 cases of perinatal intracranial hemorrhage due to immune thrombocytopenia. Amer J Ped Hem Onc 1991;13:156-59.
8. Bussel, JB, Zabusky MR, Berkowitz RL, McFarland JG: Fetal alloimmune thrombocytopenia. N Engl J Med 1997;337:22-26.

9. Herman J, Jumbelic M, Ancona R, Kickler T. In utero cerebral hemorrhage in alloimmune thrombocytopenia. Am J Ped Hematol Oncol 1986;8:32-37.
10. Bussel JB, Kaplan C, McFarland JG, and the Working Party on Neonatal Immune Thrombocytopenia of the Neonatal Hemostasis Subcommittee of the Scientific and Standardization Committee of the ISTH. Recommendations for the evaluation and treatment of neonatal autoimmune and alloimmune thrombocytopenia. Thromb Haemostasis 1991;65:631-34.
11. Birchall JE, Murphy MF, Kaplan C, Kroll H. European collaborative study of the antenatal management of feto-maternal alloimmune thrombocytopenia. Br J Haem 2003;122:275-88.
12. Radder CM, Brand A, Kanhai HHH. Will it ever be possible to balance the risk of intracranial hemorrhage in fetal or neonatal alloimmune thrombocytopenia against the risk of treatment strategies to prevent it? Vox Sang 2003;84:318-25.
13. Berkowitz RL, Kolb EA, McFarland JG, Wissert M, Primiani A, Bussel JB. Prospective, Randomized Trial Evaluating the Safety and Efficacy of Risk-Based Therapy for Fetal Alloimmune Thrombocytopenia. In preparation.
14. Paidas MJ, Berkowitz RL, Lynch L, et al.. Alloimmune thrombocytopenia: fetal and neonatal losses related to cordocentesis. Am J Obstet Gynecol 1995;172:475-79.
15. Herman J, Jumbelic M, Ancona R, Kickler T. In utero cerebral hemorrhage in alloimmune thrombocytopenia. Am J Ped Hematol Oncol, 1986;8:32-37.
16. Kaplan C, Morel-Kopp MC, Kroll H et al. HPA-5b (Bra) neonatal alloimmune thrombocytopenia: clinical and immunological analysis of 39 cases. Br J Haematol 1991;78:425-29.
17. Urbaniak SJ, Duncan JI, Armstrong-Fisher SS, Abramovich DR, Page KR. Variable inhibition of placental IgG transfer in vitro with commercial IVgG preparations. Br J. Haem 1999;107:815-17.
18. Kroll H, Kiefel V, Giers G, et al. Maternal intravenous immunoglobulin treatment does not prevent intracranial hemorrhage in fetal alloimmune thrombocytopenia. Transfus Med 1994;4:293-96.
19. Daffos F, Forestier F, Kaplan C. Prenatal treatment of fetal alloimmune thrombocytopenia. Lancet 1988;2:90c.
20. Murphy MF, Metcalfe P, Waters AH, Ord J, Hambley H, Nicolaides K. Antenatal management of severe feto-maternal alloimmune thrombocytopenia: HLA incompatibility may affect responses to fetal platelet transfusions. Blood 1993;81: 2174-79.
21. Radder CM, Brand A, Kanhai HHH. A less invasive treatment strategy to prevent intracranial hemorrhage in fetal and neonatal alloimmune thrombocytopenia. Am J Obstet Gynecol 2001;185:683-88.
22. Kaplan C. Immune thrombocytopenia in the fetus and the newborn: diagnosis and therapy. Transfus Clin Biol 2001;8:311-14.
23. Ment LR, Bada HS, Barnes P, et al: Practice parameter: Neuroimaging of the neonate: report of the Quality Standards Subcommittee of the American

Academy of Neurology and the Practice Committee of the Child Neurology Society. Neurology 2002;58:1726-38.

24. Bussel JB, Tanli S, Peterson HC. Favorable neurological outcome in 7 cases of perinatal intracranial hemorrhage due to immune thrombocytopenia. Amer J Ped Hem Onc 1991;13:156-59.
25. Baumann MA, Menitove JE, Aster RH, Anderson T. Urgent treatment of idiopathic thrombocytopenia purpura with single-dose gamma-globulin infusion followed by platelet transfusion. Ann Internal Med 1988;108:560-63.

THE BLEEDING INFANT

H.M. van den Berg[1]

Introduction

A rare complication in infants is an increased bleeding tendency. The incidence of bleeding in infants is not well known and depends very much on the age of gestation and which symptoms are considered. The human haemostatic system is dynamic and largely influenced by age. It is considered immature in the new-born, however it is a physiological system which results in few problems in the term neonate. In the preterm and sick neonate the haemostatic system can be largely out of balance and as a result cause a high bleeding tendency. Many of the procoagulants, anticoagulants and proteins involved in the haemostatic system are dependent on the age of gestation. The new-born's haemostatic system matures in the weeks after delivery to become fully mature after 6 months. The preterm infant has much lower values, although they appear to normalise after

Table 1. An overview of the basic screening tests and clotting factors in preterm and term infants at delivery and during the first 6 months of their life

Test	**Adult**	**Preterm (25-32 wks)**	**Term infant**	**Infant (6 months)**
PT (ratio)	1.0	1.3	1.1	1.0
APTT (ratio)	1.0	3.0	1.3	1.1
TCT (ratio)	1.0	1.3	1.1	1.0
Fibrinogen (g/L)	2.78 (0.61)	2.50 (1.00)	2.40 (1.50)	2.51 (1.60)
Factor VII (U/mL)	1.00 (0.60)	0.37 (0.24)	0.57 (0.35)	0.87 (0.50)
Factor VIII (U/mL)	1.00 (0.60)	0.75 (0.40)	1.50 (0.55)	0.90 (0.50)
VWF (U/mL)	1.00 (0.60)	1.50 (0.90)	1.60 (0.84)	1.07 (0.60)

1. Paediatric haematologist, Van Creveldkliniek, University Medical Centre Utrecht, Urecht, NL.

delivery in the same 6 months period. It is important to realise this age-dependent changes and for the most important coagulation tests and clotting factors they can be found in Table 1. Data on haemostatic values in healthy neonates are scarce, the data in this chapter originate from the studies performed by Dr Andrew [1,2].

In the following paragraphs the diagnostic procedures necessary for a correct diagnosis will be further explained for the most important clinical diagnosis. More information can be obtained from the literature [3-5].

Investigation of the Neonate

It is very important to make a correct diagnosis as soon as possible in a bleeding infant. Bleeding is often severe and life threatening. When a bleeding is suspected at delivery or a child is born from a family with a positive family history, the diagnosis can be made from blood of a cord blood sample. Two techniques have proven adequate for collection of cord blood to be used for coagulation assays. As soon as the child has been delivered, the cord is clamped between two clamps and cut. When the infant is removed, and before separation from the placenta, the umbilical vein is punctured and the sample is withdrawn. Another technique is that a segment of cord is double-clamped with four clamps, this long segment of cord is than used to obtain blood with a system that contains citrate as anticoagulant. It is very important to emphasis that the results of a coagulation test or assay are very dependent on the sample collection [3]. This is both true for samples obtained from the cord or from a peripheral vein. Samples should not contain any intravenous fluids, particularly heparin has to be prevented. Activation of clotting is likely because of the slow sampling in neonates. Also platelet clumping is common, therefore blood samples should be inspected for fibrin strands and platelet clumps. Nowadays it is possible to perform the basic screening test with 1 ml tube that contains 3.2 % buffered sodium citrate [3]. Overfilled or underfilled samples should not be analysed. The basic screening tests will include a platelet count, activated protrombine time (APTT) and protrombine time (PT).

In order to make a diagnosis, it is important to differentiate between the "well" infant and the "sick" infant.

Well Infant

A decreased platelet count as the only abnormality in an infant with petechiae requires the differential diagnosis for thrombocytopenia. Prolongation of the PT (slight) and APTT (marked) with failure of correction of APTT with 1:1 mixing suggests heparin effect. If the PT can be corrected by mixing with vitamin K, a deficiency of vitamin K is likely. Prolongation of the APTT alone and correction with 1:1 mixing with normal plasma suggests haemophilia A or B. Isolated prolongation of the PT suggests hereditary factor VII deficiency. In the case that all screening tests are normal in a "well" appearing infant with bleeding, rare conditions like factor XIII deficiency should be considered, clinically a persistent bleeding of the umbilical cord is suspect for this condition.

Sick Infant

The sick appearing infant who displays evidence of a bleeding tendency is usually either a preterm infant or a term infant with evidence of CNS bleeding or sepsis. The only sign of bleeding may be shock or pallor. The screening test are usually abnormal. If only the platelet count is reduced consider sepsis or massive thrombosis. Dissiminated intravascular coagulation (DIC) mostly is diagnosed by a reduced platelet count, an increased PT and increased FDP. The same abnormalities can be found in patients with severe liver disease.

Gastrointestinal Bleeding

Infants with signs of gastrointestinal bleeding may have swallowed maternal blood during delivery. This can be diagnosed by the use of the Apt test on the presence of adult haemoglobin. The addition of 1% sodium hydroxide to a pink solution containing adult blood will result in a colour change form pink to yellow-brown [3]. When the pink colour remains it is quite likely that the solution contains mostly foetal blood and further investigation for the origin of the blood should be performed

Intracranial Haemorrhage

Intracranial haemorrhage is often seen in preterm infants . The incidence is around 15-20% for infants less than 32 weeks gestation [6]. The aetiology is multifactorial with alterations in cerebral blood flow, fragility of the vessels probably being more important than an impaired haemostasis. Therapeutic intervention with FFP and /or platelets are not undoubtedly beneficially [6]. However, most people will advise to infuse platelets when the count is below $30\text{-}50x10^9$ /l. Also in term neonates with an ICH clotting should be optimised and platelet kept above $50x10^9$ /l.

Vitamin K Deficiency

A generalised bleeding tendency can be caused by vitamin K deficiency. Vitamin K deficiency is an essential cofactor for the synthesis of the coagulation factors II, VII, IX, X protein C, and protein S. The primary haemostatic function of vitamin K is to mediate the carboxylation of selected 9 to 12 glutamates located near the NH2 terminus of the protein of to Gla residues used to bind calcium to phospholipid membranes, thus allowing formation of important coagulation complexes. The cycle is interrupted by warfarin-type compounds and causes than an increase of "proteins induced by vitamin K absence" or PIVKAs [3]. There exist three syndromes of haemorrhagic disease in infants caused by vitamin K deficiency Table 2.

Early haemorrhagic syndrome is most likely to occur in newborn infants whose mothers have been on anticonvulsant therapy. Up to 50% of the infants will show evidence of vitamin K deficiency, which can be prevented by the administration of daily 10 mg vitamin K orally to the mother from 2 weeks before delivery [7]. Late haemorrhagic syndrome occurs mainly in exclusively breast fed infants who received and inadequate prophylaxis with vitamin K. The presentation is often an intracranial haemorrhage, which can be prevented by the administration of 1 mg vitamin K directly after birth and vitamin K orally [8,9]. Some confusion still exist whether vitamin K administrated intramuscular increased the risk for childhood cancer. In further studies this has never been proven [5]. Infants of mothers that use oral anticoagulant should be given a weekly orally supplement of 1 mg vitamin K. Vitamin K deficiency may occur at any age and can be the first symptom of major pathology like cholestatic liver disease. Vitamin K is a fat-soluble vitamin and malabsorption is possible in a large variety of causes [3].

Congenital Hereditary Syndromes

A meticulous family history is mandatory. Patients with a positive family history for congenital hereditary syndromes should preferable already be recognised during pregnancy. In the case of haemophilia, families should be counselled already before pregnancy to inform them of the inheritance of the disease and the complications to be expected [10]. With counselling potential or obligate carriers should be recognised. In most families it is possible to perform genetic analysis. When a male child is expected, further prenatal diagnosis can be performed with either chorionic villus sampling at 10-12 weeks of gestation or by amniocentesis after 15 weeks gestation. The clinical pattern of haemophilia is largely dependent on the severity of the disease. Only patients with <1% factor VIII or IX will have spontaneous bleeds in their muscles and joints. Nowadays, with modern treatment, the clinical picture can be highly changed [11]. With prophylactic therapy the burden of bleeding and arthropathy can be largely prevented and this has changed the attitude of families in making a choice of having a child with severe haemophilia. However, the costs of prophylactic therapy with clotting products is extremely high and most countries can afford it. It is advised that in infants with an inherited congenital bleeding history delivery should be in a hospital. Vaginal delivery is preferable, however invasive methods like subcutaneous electrodes and vacuum extraction are prohibited. Haemophilia is a very well known inherited disease, the inherited patterns is X-linked, therefore boys are affected in 50% of the cases and girls will be carriers in 50% of the children of a known carrier. However, spontaneous cases do occur in up to 50% of the cases with severe haemophilia [12]. Therefore haemophilia can not be excluded with a negative family history.

References

1. Andrew M, Paes B, Milner R, et al. Development of the coagulation system in the full-term infant. Blood 1987;70:165-72.
2. Andrew M, Paes B, Milner R, et al. Development of the coagulation system in the pre-term infant. Blood 1988;80:1998-2005.
3. Goodnight Jr SH, Hathaway WE (eds). Disorders of hemostasis and thrombosis. A clinical guide. Second ed. New York: McGraw-Hill, 2001.

4. Williams MD. Guideline. The investigation and management of neonatal haemostasis and thrombosis. Br J Haematol 2002;119:295-309.
5. Haemostasis and Thrombosis Task Force. Investigation and management of of haemorrhagic disorders in pregnancy. Clin Pathol 1994;47:100-08.
6. Andrew M, Vegh P, Caco C, et al. A randomized controlled trial of platelet transfusions in thrombocytopenic premature infants. J Paediatr 1993;123: 285-91.
7. Oh W, Fanaroff AA, Verter J, et al. Neonatal mortality and morbidity in very low birth weight infants; a seven year trend analysis of the Neonatal Network data. Paediatr Res 1996;39:235A.
8. Cornelissen M, Steegers-Theunissen R, Kollee R, et al. Increased incidence of neonatal vitamin K deficiency resulting form maternal anticonvulsant therapy. Am J Obstetr Gynaecol 1993;168:923-28.
9. Cornelissen M, von Kries R, Loughnan P, Schubiger G. Prevention of vitamin K deficiency bleeding: efficacy of different multiple oral dose schedules of vitamin K. Eur J Paediatr 1997;156:126-30.
10. Ljung R, Tedgard U. Genetic counseling of hemophilia carriers. Semin Thromb Hemostasis 2003;29:31-36.
11. United Kingdom Haemophilia Centre Directors Organisation Executive Committee. Guidelines on therapeutic products to treat haemophilia and other hereditary coagulation disorders. Haemophilia 1997; 3: 63-77.
12. Ljung, R, Sjorin E. Originof mutation in sporadic cases of haemophilia A. Br J Haematol 1999; 106: 870-74.

DISCUSSION

Moderators: C. Dame, A. Brand

M.S. Harvey (Leiden, NL): When children are born only a fraction of them have to have exchange or top up transfusion. But the children are still full of maternal antibody, IgG antibodies outside the blood circulation. So the children go back to another hospital somewhere in the Netherlands and then they are seen as beautiful healthy children. But within six weeks they are anaemic and of course haemolysing there own fresh antigen positive cells. The communication between the obstetricians, the neonatologists and then the neonatologists in the receiving hospital outside our referral hospital is critical. We are phoned up in the laboratory more or less once every two months, by hospitals, somewhere else in the Netherlands, without appropriate information on transfusion history of the child. Something goes wrong in the communication chain.

R.G. Strauss (Iowa City, IA, USA): Much of this foetal monitoring is validated on the basis of D antigen and anti-D. So, when other antigens are involved, is it appropriate to use these tests. How do you actually use them? Is part of the reason for the poor survival with anti-K problems related to undetected Kell positive foetuses?

H.H.H. Kanhai (Leiden, NL): Yes, that's still the problem. The pathophysiology and clinical presentation of Kell immunsation is quite different from D and little c. Therefore the management should be in very experienced hands. Since both ultrasound parameters and bilurubin in amniotic fluid are not reliable for determination of foetal anaemia in Kell immunized foetuses, foetal blood sampling is performed at a lower threshold then we do in the Rhesus D.

A. Brand (Leiden, NL): Related to that question, the false positives and the false negatives in the diamond study, are these particularly in non D cases?

H.H.H. Kanhai: We have excluded the Kells in the study.

H.H.H. Kanhai: Dr. van den Berg, you have a lot of experience with haemophilia. How often have you seen a significant bleeding in relation to the mode of delivery? In relation to the mode of delivery for vaginal, forceps or vacuum, or Caesarean section?

H.M. van den Berg (Utrecht, NL): We don't see it very often, it is in less than 1% of the children born with haemophilia. However, when you perform a vacuum extraction massive cephalic haematoma will occur.

H.H.H. Kanhai: For decades now we are talking about these risks, it must be quantified anyhow. What is the risk if you have an unsuspected haemophilia. What is the risk to have a significant period of bleeding, when you go for a vaginal birth with or without assisted delivery for instance a forceps. Are these data available?

H.M. van den Berg: They are not available. You can look at it just from our cohorts. We have a lot of data on it, but we just started a prospective study in Europe in 20 large haemophilia centres, and this will be one of the aspects we will prospectively investigate.

R. Rinawati (Jakarta, Ind): I have two questions. Because of the limited budget, it is important for us to perform an appropriate laboratory test for DIC. Second, are there any specific clinical symptoms for DIC, especially in the babies, that can guide us to treat this kind of patient.

H.M. van den Berg: The first is difficult for me to answer, because I don't know what kind of laboratory test you have available in Indonesia.

R. Rinawati: Sometimes we have to save the money to buy medicines. So we cannot perform APTT, AT and even fibrinogen. Maybe you can inform us, maybe there is a specific assay.

H.M. van den Berg: Probably the FDP could be most useful, because that test is very fast, if it is increased in comparison with a lower platelet count it gives you a proper diagnosis of DIC. You don't need to do the other tests, because you know that they are decreased When you have a sick child bleeding, you would just have to give them proper therapy. So I don't think you need more tests - do just those two.

R. Suradi (Jakarta, Ind): WHO has suggested to have breast feeding for six months. What do you suggest for vitamin K, how long would you give it and how much? For fully breastfed infants it is now suggested that it should be given for six months. Do you suggest to give vitamin K for as long as that?

H.M. van den Berg: In the Netherlands we give it for the full six months now, when they are totally breastfed, For totally breastfed children. I think you should prolong it after 6 months.

A. Brand: Dr. van den Berg, you mentioned inhibitors. If you look to red cell alloimmunisation, they say that if you transfuse children below the age of one, you have less immunisation for instance in thalassaemia than if you start treatment later. How is it with the inhibitors; is there a relation between the occurrence and starting earlier neonatally?

H.M. van den Berg: We looked at this in our cohort of patients, and recognised that age at first exposure was a very important factor for inhibitor development. It seems to be independent from other factors. Of course we have to realise that in our cohort the children start very early on prophylaxis. So regular treatment is also something that probably even reduces it, because both the Netherlands and Sweden have large experience with prophylactic treatment. They only have around 20% persistent inhibitor patients. That is much lower than in the literature, probably because of very frequent treatment. Of course you have to realise that in children with already massive bleeding they received more subsequent transfusions, or they had surgery at the same time. So we are looking at other confounding factors to see how they have influenced the formation of these inhibitors.

R.G. Strauss: Dr. van den Berg, a question about the non-haemophilia use of activated Factor VII, Factor VIIa. In the infant period, you know it has been used quite a bit for pulmonary haemorrhage and intraventricular haemorrhage. My question is: since the kinetics of VIIa are different, the half live is shorter in infancy; since infant anticoagulant proteins are low; are there special things we ought to be concerned about in terms of risk of thrombosis or altering VIIa dosing? I just wondered what your experience here in the Netherlands was, compared to the US.

H.M. van den Berg: I think the experiences are similar. At the moment we don't use it much, but we really use it in patient where we don't have other possibilities to correct haemostasis, where they still have a very life-threatening bleeding. We give them NovoSeven®. When you give it then you should really give it in a high enough dose, and also very frequently. There has been studies both on continuous infusion and bolus infusion. What I learned from data at the moment, of course all small studies and patient groups that are very difficult to compare, it seems logical to do more in bolus and probably sometimes even every hour. When you control the bleeding, then you can do it at two and three hours and stop. But it is evident, there should be more and better studies on the subject.

R.G. Strauss: The neonate compared to older children, are there any special considerations?

H.M. van den Berg: The thing is that you don't have a real choice at that time. You only do it in case you have a life-threatening bleeding that doesn't respond to all your other measurements, like platelets, FFP and all the other things that you already have done.

R. Rinawati: I have a ten days old infant, with bilirubin level of 20 milligram per decilitre. The baby is fully breastfed and all other causes of jaundice have been excluded. My question is, do you think this baby needs therapy and what bilirubin level do you think is safe to let the baby go home? The last question: what is the long-term prognoses of breast milk jaundice, even though at the moment we know that kernicterus has not been reported for this kind of jaundice.

P.T. Pisciotto (Farmington, CT, USA): That is a very good question. I don't think that we have the answers to all those. The American Academy of Pediatrics (AAP) has come out with guidelines in 1994[1], which are rather specific in terms of healthy infants and when treatment should be done. They do recommend treatment if the bilirubin is at 20 milligrams per decilitre, depending on age in hours. Unfortunately we do not know the long-term outcomes. We do think that more healthy infants can tolerate bilirubins above 20 milligrams per decilitre. But exactly what the cut-off is, is not quite certain.

R. Rinawati: So we can use that guideline from the AAP?

P.T. Pisciotto: I would use the guideline that the American Academy of Pediatrics has recommended.

J.B. Bussel (New York, NY, USA): Dr Urbaniak are you willing to share any information with us about your screening study from Scotland in alloimmune thrombocytopenia?

S.J. Urbaniak (Aberdeen Scotland): We have just completed the analysis of the data, preparing this for publication. There are a lot of numbers, and I'll go slowly through them. We have screened prospectively 26,509 pregnancies, specifically looking for newly identified anti HPA-1a in the at risk population. The women were screened for HPA-1a phenotype, confirmed by genotyping, and were then followed prospectively during pregnancy for the appearance of antibody. We where looking at the natural history of the antibody production and outcome in a first child. There are another four European studies that are either completed or in the process of being completed. Between us we have data on about 100,000 prospectively followed cases. In our particular series we find 1.7% of the Scottish population to be HPA-1a negative, and 8% of these developed newly detected anti-HPA-1a. We excluded all those women with antibodies that we knew from previous history. About a third of the antibody positive cases had a low platelet count, as defined by $<150x10^9$ per Liter, falling within the laboratory definition of NAIT, that is 2.5% of the women all-together.

1. AAP Provisional Committee for Quality Improvement and Subcommittee on Hyperbilirubinemia. Practice parameter: Management of hyperbilirubinemia in the healthy term newborn. Pediatrics 1994;94:558-65.

Twenty percent of the women with antibody developed severe NAIT, sufficient to require treatment. It is of interest that none of the cases in our series had any intracranial haemorrhage or any morbidity associated with the low platelet count. We did not intervene; it was a non-intervention study. I should add though, that we did have HPA matched platelets available for immediate transfusion on delivery, because we knew the status of the mothers' antibodies. We had no adverse outcome and if we combine the results of the 97,000 pregnancies followed throughout Europe in Caucasians, there are only two cases of intracranial haemorrhage that occurred in the prospective studies. One of which occurred antepartum, and one postpartum. The antepartum one was asymptomatic and was identified at follow up by ultrasound scan.

A. Brand: Was that 27,000 HPA negatives or was that 27,000 women and then you select?

S.J. Urbaniak: This was a screening program for women who are randomly presenting to the antenatal clinic, and tested for HPA-1a status: 1.7% in our series and 2.1% in the combined European data all together are HPA negative and form the at-risk population.

A. Brand: What on these figures is the confidence interval for each intracranial haemorrhage?

S.J. Urbaniak: Well, there are already two cases of ICH. I haven't done the mathematics yet, but there were only two cases of ICH from all the combined prospective data on approximately 100,000 women.

A. Brand: You find 8% antibodies. Did you also pre-screen for HLA-DR?

S.J. Urbaniak: No, not prospectively. But when we actually analysed the affected cases, HLA DRB3*01 was also involved. We were specifically looking at anti-HPA-1a identification. So, overall we are only diagnosing a third of those severely affected infants, those that would require immediate HPA matched platelets. If we look at the costs of that, because we did a cost-effectiveness economical analysis, some of the cases had signs like purpura or haematomas which would raise the index of suspicion to make the diagnosis of NAIT in the absence of screening. But two third of the NAIT cases are clinically silent. To identify these cases in a screening program costs 57,000 GB Pounds, € 95,000 or USD 83,000. That would be the costs of screening. Clearly we don't have data to analyse the costs of intervention. But we have to put that into the context of the fact that in all of the prospective series, HPA-matched platelets were immediately available. So I think we have to balance the availability of matched platelets against this low postnatal morbidity.

A. Brand: But that is nothing, 83,000 US dollars?

S.J. Urbaniak: Well that is for the health insurers to debate how that fits into clinical care as a whole. Those are the hard numbers and obviously have to be matched against the benefits.

H.H.H. Kanhai: Have you included in the 97,000 the about 60,000 from the Tromsö study[1]?

S.J. Urbaniak: Yes that is right. Those are from Norway[2]. One case of ICH is from the Cambridge study, and one is from Norway. But the costs I am quoting are the Scottish data, because obviously we were costing within our own context. So that is totally consistent, because we are looking at the additional health care cost. It is obvious these women are being seen and being screened anyway for red cell antibodies, so that is the additional cost of screening for HPA-1a. The message that I have taken from this is that in first-time index pregnancies where the antibodies were detected for the first time, the risks of potential interventions, such as foetal blood sampling to detect whether or not the foetus is going to be at risk is very closely balanced against the potential risks of missing an intracranial haemorrhage, assuming you do something about it. So, we have come to the view that in first-time pregnancies where anti-HPA-1 is detected and the baby is subsequently affected, we would not recommend intervention, such as sticking needles in to confirm the platelet count. In fact, even in a first time case with no history and no previous sibling we would only monitor and have platelets available at delivery.

J.B. Bussel: I think it is extremely valuable. When you consider the costs you need to consider that you at least now know for the next pregnancy who to watch more carefully and you make it pay back in that pregnancy.

S.J. Urbaniak: Yes, personally I am in favour of the introduction of screening, but of course we only got the funding to do it for a fixed period of time. I think there are many tangential benefits, not just simple costs.

M.S. Harvey: Wouldn't it be much cheaper to just screen all neonates for platelet counts?

S.J. Urbaniak: No, this was not the purpose of our particular study, but you know the French group did a study comparing between specific screening for

1. Killie MK, Husebekk A, Skogen B, Olsen J, Kristiansen. Cost-effectveness of antenatal screening for neonatal alloimmune thrombocytopenia (NAITP). Platelets; 2004 (in press).
2. Kjeldsen-Kragh J, Killie MK, Aune B, et al. An intervention program for reducing morbidity and mortalitry associated with neonatal allo-immune thrombocytopenic purpura (NAITP). VIIIth European Congress ISBT, Istanbul 2003. Abstract book:93 (abstract 235).

anti-HPA-1a and screening all neonates. I think they came to the conclusion that targeted screening was more cost effective in their model.

E.F. van Leeuwen: Do you give the mothers with anti-HPA-1A antibodies advice not to use aspirin and to be aware of traumata etc. before the delivery?

S.J. Urbaniak: No, they were just given the normal general advice during pregnancy, because we have no clear epidemiological history of the consequences of first-time antibody detection. Most of the literature is based on cases where there has been a previous infant or sibling affected, and therefore it is largely biased. The point I'm getting at is that in a true first-time index pregnancy the risks are less than the literature suggests. Just one other point is that all but one of the women who developed antibodies in their index pregnancy had been pregnant in the past. So only one was a true primi parous woman. She had no live children, indeed, no previous pregnancies at all. All of the cases that had antibodies had been pregnant in the past, (except one case), even though they didn't have living children. So it looks like you need at least, in most cases, two pregnancies to stimulate the production of antibodies.

H.H.H. Kanhai: One additional short comment to further discourage people who are in favour of invasive management. In the study of July 2003 quoted by Dr. Bussel, the European multicentre study[1] and a previous study from the group of Fisk[2] in 2002, in both studies 6% pregnancy loss was associated with invasive management.

J.F. Harrison (London, UK): Dr. Pisciotto, what is the highest level of bilirubin where you would go for phototherapy and not exchange, and at what point would you decide that phototherapy was not reducing the bilirubin enough and then you would go for exchange?

P.T. Pisciotto: I assume that you are talking about full term infants because the concern has come up in full term infants. I think the bilirubin level at which phototherapy versus exchange transfusion should be used is clearly defined i by the 1994 guidelines, which is essentially what we would follow. The decision whether to stop phototherapy and go to exchange transfusion would probably depend on whether the bilirubin is rising. If we have the infant on photo therapy with rising bilirubin levels, then that would be an indication to switch over to an exchange transfusion. When we put these children on phototherapy, they really

1. Birchall JE, Murphy MF, Kaplan C, Kroll H. European collaborative study of the antenatal management of feto-maternal alloimmune thrombocytopenia. Br J Haematol 2003;122:275-88.
2. Overton TG, Duncan KR, Jolly M, Letsky E, Fisk NM. Serial aggressive platelet transfusion for fetal alloimmune thrombocytopenia: platelet dynamics and perinatal outcome. Am J Obstet Gynecol 2002;186:826-31.

have come down very quickly. I still think that exchange transfusions are being performed very infrequently at this point. But the guidelines from the American Academy of Pediatrics are pretty well set, and those are the guidelines that we would use .

M.S. Harvey: A comment for Dr. Bussel. Maybe I missed it, but I think you missed one piece of the aetiology of neonatal thrombocytopenia. that is of course thrombocytopenia after massive exchange transfusion. It is amazing that this still appears.

The second comment is for Dr. van den Berg. You said, as far as I could understand, 15% of the infants develop persistent inhibitors. Is that correct?

H.M. van den Berg: That is reported. I also think that it is much too high. We saw about 15% for the last 30 years and we did not see any difference in plasma recombinant products.

M.S. Harvey: What about the strategy as far as giving a product? Would you advise changing or stay on the same product? Which would give the best chance of tolerance?

H.M. van den Berg: At the moment it is still advised to stay on the same product. As long as there has been no real evidence that a product is related to inhibitor formation. Of course if that is so, you should stop the product and go to an other product. But for all cases it is better to stay on the same product and get tolerance. So it is not the product that gives you less change to get tolerant. We don't change.

H.L.M. van Straaten (Zwolle, NL): Dr. Pisciotto, once you reach the level of bilirubin at which you decide to start your exchange transfusion, what would you consider to be a reasonable time interval to actually start the exchange transfusion?

P.T. Pisciotto: That's a very good question. Usually what is happening is that the babies are being followed. We are usually warned by the physicians ahead of time, when they feel the baby is not responding. As soon as they feel the baby is not responding they will go ahead and consider doing the exchange transfusion. At that point it is just a matter of preparing the appropriate blood products to release to the nursery. I must say that we rarely do exchange transfusion anymore. I think we probably do one or two a year. So it is very infrequent that infants get to the level of bilirubin at which the physician feels that the exchange transfusion needs to be done. But once they do, then it is just a matter of getting the blood ready and the exchange performed.

A. Brand: Is there anyone in the audience who is willing to tell us what the ultimate length is that you may wait for an exchange transfusion? It is quite actual in the Netherlands, because we have only four divisions. So what is reasonable?

R.G. Strauss: I think I understand the question. Since we collect our own blood at our hospital, it is just a matter of an hour or two between the decision to prepare blood for the exchange and beginning the exchange itself. But I would think that, depending on the rate of bilirubin rise you want to act as quickly as you could – especially, if it is rapidly rising or not responsive with phototherapy.

C. Dame (Berlin, D): I would like to give a short comment. In Germany, the number of exchange transfusions is decreasing more and more. I have the impression that the fellows don't gain the experience to perform the exchange transfusion. We have to consider that a specific training is necessary.

N. Luban (Washington DC, USA): As a tertiary referral centre for neonatology our staff is now performing approximately ten to fifteen exchanges per year. Almost all for G6-PD deficiency and not for Rhesus haemolytic disease. I think that is a very important point. Particularly in areas of the US where there is a large immigrant population, G6-PD deficient hyperbilirubinaemia is much more common. We don't collect a lot of our own blood, so we do depend upon a blood centre, and I would say that no more than three to four hours would be acceptable. In fact in the US, where we have a large amount of litigation and malpractice, anything over four hours would probably end up going to court if there was a bad outcome in the infant.

P.T. Pisciotto: I have to agree with that. Once the decision is made to do exchange transfusion, usually it is the roll of the blood bank to get the blood ready as quickly as possible.

M.S. Harvey: Dr. Brand said that this is a very actual problem in the Netherlands, where 9 regional centres have reduced to four centres. We perform in Leiden, as far as I can remember, about 15 to 20 exchange transfusions a year still. Some of them are of course predictable from the history of the obstetric patient. We used to be able to get an acute transfusion to the ward within two and a half hours. That has now gone up to sometimes 7 hours. I think it is a failure of our new national blood bank organisation.

A. Brand: No comment. I agree indeed with Dr. Dame that the experience with the exchange transfusion should be included in the paediatric education, otherwise you should not be qualified to do it.

E. Ranasinghe (Cambridge, UK): Dr Bussel, our laboratory investigates all suspected cases of neonatal alloimmune thrombocytopenia (NAIT) for the whole of London and the South East of England, so there is a large number of hospitals that we serve. One of the requests that we get is from foetal medicine units. When they scan foetuses and find ventriculomegaly, they always send requests for NAIT investigation regarding these cases to us. Our experience is that out of a large number of these cases we have found only very few real allo-immunisations. In spite of testing for HPA-1, -2, -3, -5 and Gov, which is HPA-15, which forms a considerable workload. It seems that ventriculomegaly could be due to various other causes as well, or are we missing the rare antibodies. My question is: is there a way that the clinicians, the obstetricians could be more selective, so that they can see that this particular ventriculomegaly is due to bleeding and therefore more likely to be due to alloimmunisation. If that is the case then it would help us. Is there a way to check that?

J.B. Bussel: We looked at a series of 21 patients who had had intracranial haemorrhage, not just ventriculomegaly, identified on routine sonography over 15 years, and did not identify any of those as alloimmune thrombocytopenia. Nonetheless there are cases that at least would present with haemorrhage. So if you are talking about ventriculomegaly where no haemorrhage is visible, it might have taken place in the past and resolved and then there is a question of what caused it. I agree with you that makes it less likely, but I think until somebody else comes up with a sufficiently large series to give us some sense of the balance, it would still make sense to work it up, because it would be potentially preventable in the future and at least we would have a cause.

E. Ranasinghe: So you agree that it is justified in doing this anyway at the moment?

J.B. Bussel: I think at the moment it is justified in doing this. I agree with you that the yield is not very high.

C. Dame: Dr. Manno, I would like to ask you about the frequency or the incidence of transplacental transferred anti-phospholipid antibodies. Are there any data available?

C.S. Manno (Philadelphia, PA, USA): What I recall is that several case-reports[1] associated the antibodies with the presence of neonatal arterial cerebral hrombosis, arterial thrombosis and stroke.

C. Dame: Do we know something about the kinetics of the antibodies during the neonatal period? Are they disappearing fast?

1. Golomb MR, MacGregor DL, Domi T, et al. Presumed pre- or perinatal arterial ischemic stroke: risk factors and outcomes. Ann Neurol 2001;50:163-68.

C.S. Manno: They are disappearing over the course of the first two months, in all likelihood.

A. Brand: To make it clear; you really see intracranial thrombosis antenatal due to passive transfer of phospholipid antibodies.

C.S. Manno: It has been reported, yes.

A. Brand: But anti-phospholipid antibodies are very common.

C.S. Manno: Sure. These were the anti-choriolipin antibodies.

A. Brand: Have you any idea of the incidence? Is it really something that you should screen for if you know the mother has these antibodies?

C.S. Manno: So far it is not been associated with something able to be prevented in a very low incidence in the number of mothers who have the phospholipid antibody.

A. Brand: If you say two percent, do you really mean clinical HIT with thrombosis and how is that in the neonate, or do you relate to infants?

C.S. Manno: I think it is a very interesting question about HIT, in the infant or even in the child. I don't know if Dr Bussel has more experience, but for years we said that HIT was just reported in ten to twenty percent of adults treated with heparin and is something not seen in children. This two percent figure to me, before a year ago, would have been a high figure. But I do think that anyone who has being treated with heparin, who develops thrombocytopenia (more than a fifteen percent drop in platelet count) needs to be considered, at least at risk for HIT, because the consequence of heparin induced thrombocytopenia is: 30 percent have a serious thrombosis. It is something that is under-recognised and needs to be considered.

A. Brand: So it should be included in neonatal thrombocytopenia as well? Because all these children will have venous access and receive heparin anyhow.

C.S. Manno: I am not sure that we would see it in the patients who receive heparin to keep their lines open. It is the patient though who has been treated with therapeutic heparin, who developed thrombocytopenia in the absence of another cause of thrombocytopenia. Of course the screening tests that we have for HIT are not very good. The ELISA is specific but not sensitive and the serotonin release is sensitive but not specific. So it is a difficult diagnosis.

C.Th. Smit Sibinga (Groningen, NL): Given the serious consequences of indwelling catheters, either arterial or venous, that may occur in those predisposed patients, wouldn't it be recommendable to have a basic anamnestic screening in place before such invasive technologies are being undertaken?

C.S. Manno: Screening for the thrombophilias?

C.Th. Smit Sibinga: At least have an indication whether there is a risk.

C.S. Manno: I think that the catheters are so important in the therapy of these children that even the detection of for instance Factor V Leiden in the new born would not argue against the use of the catheter. Perhaps the screening of that baby, following of that baby for the development of a thrombus should be closer.

C.Th. Smit Sibinga: I was not mentioning actually or focusing on preventing the use of catheter, because I am well aware of the importance of using them. But trying in a very early stage to prevent thrombosis to occur when inserting an artificial material into a vein or artery. So that was actually the idea.

C.S. Manno: Would you use a treatment to prevent?

C.Th. Smit Sibinga: For instance, yes. Or be extra alert of early symptoms of thrombosis.

C.S. Manno: I think the extra alertness is a very good idea. Although the routine screening of these infants is not yet recommended, certainly it is a very expensive proposition. These work ups are 4000 or 4500 US dollars. Also the results of in particular the genetic testing won't be available for a long time, perhaps after the catheters are removed.

J.B. Bussel: It might or might not be helpful as a screen to do something that is probably totally not done, and that is to take a very careful family history of thrombosis. I mean, I don't think we think that, putting in a catheter in a new born means we should carefully go over the history in the family of heart attacks, strokes, miscarries, etc.. But if we did, it might be interesting to see if you could link that to the risk of thrombosis. In some way that would be a way to triage.

H.M. van den Berg: I think that it is sensible, because what you also demonstrate, it is all exclusively catheters in very young children. So although they have sometimes risk likeness they don't seem to be so very important at that ages, so they should have been multiple risk factored. In those cases you mostly have a positive family history.

J.B. Bussel: Dr Pisciotto, I wondered if you could make a comment on the use of the carbonmonoxide breath test. At least in the US with earlier discharge we are seeing more late hyperbilirubinaemia, after 48 hours. People have wondered if you could use that in stead of doing a direct Coombs test or in stead of a reticulocyte count.

P.T. Pisciotto: Actually using the carbon monoxide breath test is a good indicator of bilirubin production. That's been shown in the literature. It doesn't predict, however, which infants will go on to develop hyperbilirubinaemia. What people look at first is a bilirubin level based on hours, plotted against a nomogram of hours of age-specific serum total bilirubin. It is thought that the combination of looking at the bilirubin level plotted against the nomogram in combination with the end-tidal carbon monoxide may help predict a bit better which infants may develop hyperbilirubinaemia[1]. This approach still needs further evaluation.

1. Prediction of hyperbilirubinemia in near-term and term infants. Pediatrics 2001;108: 31-39.

III. BLOOD TRANSFUSION IN THE NEONATE

NEONATAL THROMBOSIS

L. Raffini, C. Manno[1]

Introduction

Thromboembolic events (TEs) in neonates are becoming more recognized. Infants less than 1 year old account for the largest proportion of paediatric TEs [1]. While still extremely rare in healthy full term infants, premature and ill neonates are at higher risk. The true incidence of TEs in neonates has not been well studied. Estimates from a 1990-1993 Canadian registry demonstrate symptomatic venous thromboembolism (VTE) in 2.4 of 1,000 admissions to neonatal intensive care units [2]. A prospective German study found symptomatic TE in 0.51 of 10,000 live births, with 50% occurring in the venous system and 50% in the arterial [3]. While these numbers may appear relatively small, TEs are not infrequent in major tertiary care centers, and may result in significant acute and chronic morbidity. Improvements in supportive care for critically ill neonates, and increasing awareness of physicians, have likely resulted in more frequent diagnosis of neonatal TEs over the last 10 years.

The developing neonatal haemostatic system and risk factors unique to this age group, pose distinct diagnostic and therapeutic challenges. Despite the fact that neonatal TE's are increasing, in relative terms they are still rare. This has been the major impediment to prospective clinical trials, resulting in a major deficit of evidence-based medicine. Currently, diagnosis and treatment is often extrapolated from adults, though this is unlikely to be the most appropriate approach.

Developmental Haemostasis

Normal haemostasis is achieved through a dynamic balance between thrombin formation, thrombin inhibition, fibrin deposition, and fibrinolysis. The coagulation system in neonates differs from older children and adults. While the basic pathways for coagulation, anticoagulation and fibrinolysis are maintained, the concentrations of many of the factors vary greatly. Reference ranges for coagu-

1. The Children's Hospital of Philadelphia, Division of Hematology, Philadelphia, PA, USA .

lation proteins in healthy term and preterm infants have been established through the significant efforts of the late Maureen Andrew [4-6].

Plasma levels of the vitamin K dependent factors (II, VII, IX and X) are decreased at birth, and are even lower in the preterm infant. They increase rapidly and approach normal levels by 6 months of age. This results in decreased and delayed thrombin generation in newborns, perhaps providing relative protection from thromboembolic events. Levels of the direct thrombin inhibitors, antithrombin (AT) and Heparin Cofactor II (HCII), are also much lower in infants. However, this appears to be compensated for through increased thrombin inhibition via α_2-macroglobulin (α_2-M). This balance helps maintain normal haemostasis. The anticoagulant factors, Protein C and Protein S are also significantly lower in neonates. Protein C levels remain low through much of childhood. Plasminogen and α_1-antiplasmin levels are also decreased, but tissue plasminogen activator levels are higher.

This evolving haemostatic system is largely physiologic, providing relative protection for infants from both bleeding and thrombosis. Ill and premature neonates may be at greater risk for imbalances in these procoagulant and anticoagulant pathways, increasing their risk of thrombosis or bleeding.

Risk Factors

Thrombotic events in neonates, both arterial and venous (excluding stroke), are largely related to catheters, which are often necessary for the care of premature and critically ill neonates. These catheters may damage the endothelial lining and cause blood flow disruption, increasing the risk of thrombosis. Other acquired risk factors for neonatal TEs include prematurity, asphyxia, sepsis, maternal diabetes, transplacental passage of anti-phospholipid antibodies, cardiac disease and dehydration.

There are several congenital abnormalities in coagulation proteins that have been demonstrated to increase the risk of thrombosis in adults. These include deficiencies of Protein C, Protein S and Antithrombin, dysfibrinogenaemias, the Factor V Leiden mutation, and the Prothrombin gene mutation. Other inherited defects that may contribute to thrombophilia included elevated homocysteine and lipoprotein (a). Congenital thrombophilia should be considered in all infants with a clinically significant thrombosis, especially if there is a positive family history. The incidence of congenital prothrombotic disorders in neonates with TE varies widely in the literature. This variability can be accounted for by differences in study design, definition of congenital prothrombotic disorders, small sample sizes, and different patient populations.

Heterozygous deficiencies are unlikely to result in TEs in childhood, unless they are accompanied by additional acquired risk factors. The impact of single gene defects in neonates with catheter related thrombosis is undefined. However, these defects may play a more significant role in infants with non-catheter related abdominal TEs- renal vein, portal vein and hepatic vein [7].

Homozygous or double heterozygous defects, may result in significant symptoms in infancy. The estimated incidence of homozygous Protein C deficiency is 1/250,000-1/500,000 births [8]. There are only a few case reports in the literature of infants with homozygous AT or Protein S deficiency [9]. Neonates with homozygous deficiencies may present with purpura fulminans. This condition is characterized by rapidly spreading skin lesions resulting from thromboses of the small dermal vessels followed by bleeding into the skin [8]. In addition, infants with homozygous deficiencies may also have cerebral thrombosis, ophthalmic thrombosis, DIC and large vessel thrombosis. An infant with purpuric skin lesions of unknown cause should receive initial replacement with FFP. Protein C, Protein S and AT levels should be sent on the infant and both parents. Definitive diagnosis can be difficult in the sick premature neonate who may have undetectable levels of these factors but not have a true genetic deficiency. Protein C and AT concentrates are also available, and have been demonstrated to be effective [10].

Idiopathic VTE are extremely rare in neonates, occurring in less than 1%, most commonly as renal vein thrombosis.

Venous TEs

Central venous lines (CVLs) are associated with up to 90% of neonatal VTE (excluding RVT) [2] . In newborns, umbilical vein catheters (UVCs) are frequently placed through the umbilical vein into the IVC. Portal vein thrombosis may result if the UVC is not placed beyond the ductus venosus, especially when hyperosmolar solutions are infused [11]. IVC obstruction often results in bilateral lower extremity swelling. CVLs may also be placed in the femoral veins or upper extremities, resulting in VTEs in the respective limbs.

Life-threatening complications from VTE include pulmonary embolism, SVC syndrome and clot extension into the heart. The incidence of PE in neonates is not known, and based on autopsy studies, is underestimated due to coexisting respiratory symptoms [11]. Other complications include post-phlebitic syndrome and recurrent thrombosis. One study looking at long term (12 years) follow up of patients with neonatal IVC thrombosis (often accompanied by renal vein thrombosis) found considerable long term morbidity, comprised of extensive internal collaterals, pain, persistent renal disease and arterial hypertension [12].

Arterial TEs

Arterial TEs in neonates are also primarily related to catheters. Umbilical artery catheters (UACs) are frequently used in premature neonates for blood gas analysis and repeated blood sampling. Infants with congenital cardiac defects may require cardiac catheterization. Thrombembolic complications from these lines include mesenteric artery occlusion and necrotising enterocolitis, renal artery thrombosis and renal failure, embolic events to the lower limbs, and embolic events to the CNS via a right to left shunt [11]. There may be impeding loss of limb or organ, requiring immediate attention. Peripheral arterial thromboses may result in a pale, cool, poorly perfused, pulseless extremity [2]. The location of the tip of the UAC (low vs. high) does not seem to influence the risk of TEs [11]. Low dose unfractionated heparin has been demonstrated to maintain UAC patency and prevent symptomatic TEs [11].

Long term complications of arterial TEs include hypertension, abnormal renal function, leg length discrepancies and paraplegia [11].

Renal Vein Thrombosis

Renal vein thrombosis (RVT) is the most common spontaneous TE in neonates. Affected infants may present with haematuria, an abdominal mass and/or thrombocytopenia [2]. Infants of diabetic mothers are at increased risk, although the mechanism for this increased risk is unknown. RVT may be an antenatal event, as the median age of diagnosis is 2 days. Approximately 25% of cases are bilateral [9].

Diagnosis

Though angiography may be considered the gold standard for diagnosis of thrombosis, it is rarely performed in this population. Doppler ultrasound and echocardiography are the most commonly employed imaging studies due to their non-invasiveness, absence of radiation, and ability to be performed at the bedside. However, the sensitivity is not optimal, and Doppler can fail to diagnose both venous and arterial clots. One prospective study compared Doppler echocardiography to contrast venography for the diagnosis of asymptomatic thrombosis associated with UVCs. Thrombi were detected by venogram in 30%. The sensitivity of Doppler echocardiography was poor 21-43% [13]. Other diagnostic imaging options include CT angiography and MR venography, although the sensitivity and specificity of these studies is not known.

Laboratory Testing

When, and if, all neonates with TEs should have comprehensive laboratory testing for known risk factors (Protein C, Protein S, ATIII, Factor V Leiden, Prothrombin gene mutation, homocysteine, lipoprotein (a), anticardiopin antibodies) is controversial.

A causative role of single gene defects is not well documented, although many case series suggest an increased incidence of these risk factors in infants with TE [3, 7]. Evaluation of neonatal coagulation is made complex by the differences in normal ranges that have been established for infants and for older children/adults. Diagnosis of Protein C, Protein S or AT deficiency can be further complicated, as levels may be lower in sick, premature neonates, and because there is variation in the laboratory assays. Low levels must be confirmed when the infant is well, and testing both parents is also recommended before making the diagnosis of a congenital deficiency.

Treatment

Therapeutic options for neonates with thrombosis include observation, anticoagulation, thrombolysis and surgery. The literature is not helpful in guiding management decisions as there are only case reports and small series. Local treatment preferences appear to guide therapy, rather than severity of disease [2, 3].

Observation: For infants with asymptomatic TEs, observation is a reasonable option. If a central catheter is involved, the catheter should be removed. Observation may be necessary in an infant with significant bleeding. Close monitoring is critical, using repeat imaging to ensure the clot has not extended.

Anticoagulation: Neonates with symptomatic TEs are usually treated with anticoagulation to prevent embolisation and clot extension, though the efficacy of this approach has never been documented. In premature and critically ill neonates who may have an increased risk of bleeding, the perceived potential benefit must be weighed against the risk.

Initial anticoagulation options include unfractionated heparin (uFH) and low molecular weight heparin (LMWH). The reduced concentrations of antithrombin in the neonate necessitate higher doses of uFH and LMWH. Because of the ease of dosing need for less monitoring, LMWH is used more and more frequently. Unlike uFH, which is monitored using the aPTT, LMWH is monitored via the anti-Xa activity. The standard starting dose of enoxaparin for infants <2 months is 1.5 mg/kg/dose SQ every 12 hours. A therapeutic anti-Xa level, drawn four hours after the second dose, should be between 0.5-1.0 IU/ml. The dose can be titrated to achieve this range. Once therapeutic, the anti-Xa level should be monitored weekly in a neonate. One disadvantage to LMWH is that it cannot be fully reversed with protamine. The half-life of enoxaparin is 4 hours.
The optimal duration of anticoagulation is not known. Anticoagulation should be continued while the patient has ongoing risk factors, ie. a central catheter. Based on adult data, neonates with a history of a TE are often treated for 3-6 months. Options for outpatient anticoagulation include LMWH, Vitamin K antagonists (coumadin, phenprocoumon), or aspirin. Management of Vitamin K antagonists is difficult in this age group.

Thrombolysis: Thrombolysis should be strongly considered in patients with life or limb threatening thromboses. Numerous small studies have reported their experience of thrombolysis in neonates. There is likely to be a bias in the reported studies favoring lysis, as unsuccessful cases are often not reported. Therapeutic options for thrombolysis include streptokinase, urokinase and recombinant tissue plasminogen activator (rt-PA). Streptokinase is seldom used because of the high incidence of allergic reactions. Urokinase and rt-PA are often used. There is an extremely wide range of doses that have been used and there is no consensus as to the optimal dose. Thrombolysis may be effective, but serious bleeding complications vary from 0-20% [14].

Supplementation of plasminogen using fresh frozen plasma may be necessary because of the low baseline levels in neonates [15].

Surgery: There are multiple case reports of successful surgical thrombectomy in neonates [16, 17]. However, the small size of neonatal vessels, coexisting morbidities, and associated surgical risk, preclude this treatment option in the majority of cases.

Summary

As supportive care for critically ill and premature infants continues to improve, neonatal thromboembolic events are being diagnosed more frequently. The immature haemostatic system may be more susceptible to imbalances. The most important risk factor is the presence of a venous or arterial catheter. The morbidity related to these events can be significant. Well designed, prospective, multiple center studies are necessary to further define the role of genetic risk factors, determine the optimal treatment strategies and understand the long term outcomes.

References:

1. Andrew M, David M, Adams M, et al. Venous thromboembolic complications (VTE) in children: first analyses of the Canadian Registry of VTE. Blood 1994; 83:1251-57.
2. Schmidt B, Andrew M. Neonatal thrombosis: report of a prospective Canadian and international registry. Pediatrics 1995;96:939-43.
3. Nowak-Gottl U, von Kries R, Gobel U. Neonatal symptomatic thromboembolism in Germany: two year survey. Arch Dis Child Fetal Neonatal Ed 1997;76:F163-67.
4. Andrew M, Paes B, Milner R, et al. Development of the human coagulation system in the full-term infant. Blood 1987;70:165-72.
5. Andrew M, Paes B, Milner R, et al. Development of the human coagulation system in the healthy premature infant. Blood 1988;72:1651-57.
6. Andrew M, Vegh P, Johnston M, Bowker J, Ofosu F, Mitchell L. Maturation of the hemostatic system during childhood. Blood 1992;80:1998-2005.
7. Heller C, Schobess R, Kurnik K, et al. Abdominal venous thrombosis in neonates and infants: role of prothrombotic risk factors - a multicentre case-control study. For the Childhood Thrombophilia Study Group. Br J Haematol 2000;111:534-39.
8. Marlar RA, Neumann A. Neonatal purpura fulminans due to homozygous protein C or protein S deficiencies. Semin Thromb Hemost 1990;16:299-309.
9. Chalmers EA. Neonatal thrombosis. J Clin Pathol 2000;53:419-23.
10. Dreyfus M, Masterson M, David M, et al. Replacement therapy with a monoclonal antibody purified protein C concentrate in newborns with se-

vere congenital protein C deficiency. Semin Thromb Hemost 1995;21:371-81.
11. Andrew, M., Monagle P., Brooker L., Thromboembolic Complications during Infancy and Childhood. 2000, Hamilton: B.C. Decker Inc.
12. Hausler M, Duque D, Merz U, Mertens R, Muhler E, Hornchen H. The clinical outcome after inferior vena cava thrombosis in early infancy. Eur J Pediatr 1999;158: 416-20.
13. Roy M, Turner-Gomes S, Gill G, Way C, Mernagh J, Schmidt B. Accuracy of Doppler echocardiography for the diagnosis of thrombosis associated with umbilical venous catheters. J Pediatr 2002;140:131-34.
14. Hartmann J, Hussein A, Trowitzsch E, Becker J, Hennecke KH. Treatment of neonatal thrombus formation with recombinant tissue plasminogen activator: six years experience and review of the literature. Arch Dis Child Fetal Neonatal Ed 2001; 85:F18-22.
15. Schmidt B, Andrew M. Report of Scientific and Standardization Subcommittee on Neonatal Hemostasis Diagnosis and Treatment of Neonatal Thrombosis. Thromb Haemost 1992;67:381-82.
16. Krueger TC, Neblett WW, O'Neill JA, MacDonell RC, Dean RH, Thieme GA. Management of aortic thrombosis secondary to umbilical artery catheters in neonates. J Pediatr Surg 1985;20:328-32.
17. Martin JE, Jr., Moran JF, Cook LS, Goertz KK, Mattioli L. Neonatal aortic thrombosis complicating umbilical artery catheterization: successful treatment with retroperitoneal aortic thrombectomy. Surgery 1989;105:793-96.

CRITERIA FOR SELECTING A RED BLOOD CELL PRODUCT TO TRANSFUSE ANAEMIC INFANTS[1]

R.G. Strauss[2]

Introduction

Many preterm infants, particularly those with birth weight ≤1.0 kg, are given multiple red blood cell (RBC) transfusions during the early weeks of life. Many controversial questions regarding the practice of neonatal RBC transfusion therapy exist, so that practices and policies vary widely – including the clinical indications and physiological basis for RBC transfusions, the choice of RBC product to be transfused, and the need for RBC product modifications such as leukocyte-reduction and gamma-irradiation. This manuscript will critically assess information pertaining to one of these issues – namely, the selection of RBCs stored for up to 42 days after collection in extended-storage preservative solutions for transfusing infants vs the transfusion of fresh RBCs (ie, those stored ≤7 days after donation).

As is true for patients of all ages, efforts have been made to reduce the number of transfusions given to neonates and infants and to limit donor exposures in attempts to minimize the complications of blood transfusion. At the University of Iowa, nearly 100% of extremely preterm infants (birth weight <1.0 kg) require RBC transfusions with 70% of transfusions given during the first month of life [1]. Thus, transfusing aliquots of RBCs, all removed from one unit reserved for the infant (ie, one donor per infant) with the unit stored for up to 42 days, offers a potential means to markedly reduce donor exposure – even when multiple transfusions are given.

The most frequent RBC transfusions given to preterm infants are small-volume transfusions of 10 to 20 mL/kg of body weight of RBCs suspended either in citrate-phosphate-dextrose-adenine solution (CPDA) at haematocrit (HCT) ≅ 70% or in extended storage solutions [AS-1 (Adsol, Baxter Healthcare Corporation, Deerfield, IL), AS-3 (Nutricel, MedSep Corporation, Covina, CA), AS-5 (Optisol, Terumo Medical Corporation, Sumerset, NJ)] at a haematocrit of 60%. To provide a consistent and predictable transfusion response, some centers prefer to centrifuge RBC aliquots before transfusion – regardless of the storage

1. National Institutes of Health Grants P01 HL46925 and RR 00059.

2. Departments of Pathology and Pediatrics, DeGowin Blood Center, University of Iowa College of Medicine, Iowa City, IO, USA.

solution – to prepare a uniform RBC concentrate (haematocrit > 80%) containing relatively small quantities of extracellular fluid [2-4]. However, haemoconcentration is not mandatory because, even in situations where volume overload is a concern, RBC transfusions can be divided into multiple small volume infusions given over several hours.

Most small-volume RBC transfusions are infused slowly over 2 to 4 hours. Because of the small quantity of extracellular fluid (storage or "additive" solution) infused with small-volume transfusions – particularly when the haematocrit is increased by centrifugation – plus the slow rate of transfusion, the type of anticoagulant-preservative solution in which the RBCs are suspended is believed not to pose risks for the majority of premature infants [5]. Accordingly, the traditional use of relatively fresh RBCs (<7 days of storage) has been challenged by several investigators [3,4,6-11] in hopes of diminishing the donor exposure of multitransfused infants by repeated use of a dedicated unit (or part of a unit) of stored RBCs for each infant.

Concerns About and Rationale for Transfusing Stored RBCs

Neonatologists who object to transfusing stored RBCs and insist on fresh RBCs generally raise three major concerns:
- the increase in extracellular (ie, supernatant) potassium (K^+);
- the decrease in RBC 2,3-diphosphoglycerate (2,3-DPG) – both of which occur in RBC units during extended storage; and
- the safety of additives such as mannitol and adenine plus the relatively large amounts of glucose (dextrose) and phosphate present in extended storage preservative solutions.

These concerns are quite legitimate for large volume (≥25 mL/kg) transfusions – especially, when transfused rapidly as in critical care settings or during extracorporeal circulation – but likely do not apply in the small-volume setting, as discussed in the following paragraphs.

Increase in Extracellular Potassium

After 42 days of storage in extended storage media (AS-1, AS-3, AS-5) at a hematocrit of 60%, extracellular K^+ levels in the preservative solution (ie, "plasma") of RBC units approximate 50 mEq/L (0.05 mEq/mL), a concentration that, at first glance, seems alarmingly high. By simple calculations, however, the actual dose of bioavailable K^+ transfused (ie, ionic K^+ in the volume of extracellular fluid infused) during a small volume transfusion is very small. An infant weighing 1 kg, given a 15 mL/kg transfusion of RBCs stored 42 days in extended storage preservative solution and infused at a haematocrit of 60% (ie, drawn directly from of a well-mixed unit) will receive a K^+ dose infused of only 0.3 mEq. The K^+ concentration of RBCs stored in CPDA at haematocrit of 70% will approximate 70 to 80 mEq/L after the 35 days of permitted storage, and the dose of K^+ infused with a 15 mL/kg transfusion to an infant weighing 1 kg is 0.3 to 0.4 mEq. These doses are quite small when compared to the usual daily K^+ requirement of 2 to 3 mEq/kg and, when transfused slowly over 2-4 hours, they have been shown in clinical studies not to cause hyperkalaemia, whether packed RBCs [3,4] or unmodified RBCs [6,7,11] were transfused. However, it must always be remembered that this rationale does not apply to large-volume (>25 mL/kg) transfusions in which larger doses of K^+ may be harmful, especially if infused rapidly (eg, exchange transfusions, extensive surgery, extracorporeal circuits).

Decrease in 2,3-DPG

As for the second concern, 2,3-DPG is totally depleted from RBCs by 21 days of storage, and this is reflected by a P_{50} value that falls from about 27 mmHg in fresh blood to 18 mmHg in stored RBCs at the time of outdate. The 18 mmHg value of older transfused RBCs corresponds to the physiologically low P_{50} value obtained from the blood of many healthy preterm infants at birth, because of the effects of high foetal haemoglobin levels in RBCs of preterm infants. Thus, the low P_{50} of stored transfused RBCs is no worse than that of RBCs produced endogenously by the infant's own bone marrow. Although both the stored blood bank RBCs and those produced by the infant will have a reduced ability to off-load oxygen, the adult RBCs units stored in the blood bank have an advantage over the infant's endogenous RBCs because 2,3-DPG and the P_{50} of transfused adult RBCs (but not endogenous infant RBCs) will increase rapidly after transfusion. In the small-volume (15 mL/kg) transfusion setting, 2,3-DPG levels have been shown to be maintained in infants given stored RBCs [3]. Similarly, fetuses with >80% circulating adult RBCs as a consequence of intrauterine transfusions maintained normal 2,3-DPG levels when sampled by cordocentesis [12]. In the massive exchange transfusion setting, impaired oxygen offloading has been demonstrated in infants given stored RBCs by measurements of 2,3-DPG and P_{50}. Consequently, fresh blood is used frequently in this setting. However, when either stored or fresh RBCs were used for exchange transfusions in one comparative study, the P_{50} in infant blood increased from 17 mmHg two hours after the exchange to 23 mmHg at 24 hours after the exchange with stored RBCs versus an increase to 26 mmHg after the exchange with fresh RBCs – a difference at 24 hours postexchange considered to have neither statistical nor clinical significance [13].

Safety of Additives in Prelervative Solutions

As for the third concern, the quantity of additives present in RBCs stored in extended storage preservative solutions is believed not to be dangerous in small volume (≅15 mL/kg) transfusions [5]. The distinction between small- and large-volume transfusions is important, because the safety of extended-storage solu-

Table 1. Quantity (total mg/kg) of additives infused during a transfusion of 15 mL/kg of AS-1 or AS-3 RBCs at HCT = 60%

Additive	AS-1	AS-3	Toxic dose*
NaCl	42	7.5	137 mg/kg/day
Dextrose	129	23	240 mg/kg/hr
Adenine	0.6	0.6	15 mg/kg/dose
Citrate	9.8	12.6	180 mg/kg/hr
Phosphate	2.0	5.6	> 60 mg/kg/day
Mannitol	33	0	360 mg/kg/day

* Accuracy of toxic dose difficult to predict for transfusions to individual infants because: (1) infusion rates generally are slow, permitting metabolism and distribution of additives from blood into extravascular sites; and (2) dextrose, adenine and phosphate enter RBCs and are somewhat sequestered. Potential toxic doses taken from reference #5.

Table 2. Small-volume transfusions of stored RBCs safely limit donor exposure

Ref	Solution	Storage	Dose	HCT[a]	Trans[b]	Donor[b]
8	CPDA	≤14 days	<60 mL/Tx	NR	13.4	4.2
9	CPDA	≤35 days	NR	NR	3.6	1.5
6	CPDA	≤35 days	15 mL/kg	75%	5.6	2.1
7	CPDA	≤35 days	13 mL/kg	68-75%	6.0	2.0
10	NR	≤35 days	15 mL/kg	NR	5.6	4.9
3	AS-1	≤42 days	15 mL/kg	85%	3.5	1.2
11	AS-2	≤42 days	15 mL/kg	60%	6.7	1.8
4	AS-3	≤42 days	15 mL/kg	85%	3.6	1.3

a. Haematocrit of transfused RBCs; b. mean transfusions and donor exposures per infant.

tion additives has not been convincingly demonstrated in large-volume settings such as exchange transfusions, cardiac bypass or in extracorporeal membrane oxygenation – during the last of which, the additives are circulated repetitively through the infant's body. However, the quantity of additives is quite small in the clinical setting in which an infant receives a single, small-volume RBC transfusion over 2 to 4 hours. Using AS-1 and AS-3 RBCs to illustrate (Table 1), the dose of additives transfused during a typical small volume RBC transfusion is far below levels believed to be toxic [5]. The quantity of additives would be even smaller when packed RBCs (HCT >80%) are transfused. Although multiple transfusions, rather than single, often are given to preterm infants, it is logical to speculate that either single or multiple small-volume transfusions using RBCs from extended storage preservative solutions are safe for neonatal and infant transfusions.

Clinical Experience Transfusing Stored RBCs

To confirm the theoretical calculations discussed in the preceding section with clinical experience, eight reports [3,4,6-11] that documented the successful transfusion of stored, rather than fresh, RBCs for small-volume transfusions are presented by Table 2. In these reports, stored RBCs were transfused safely, without hyperkalaemia or acidosis and, in most instances, with donor exposure decreased compared to that observed with transfusions of fresh RBCs. To illustrate, transfusion studies of AS-1 and AS-3 RBCs stored up to 42 days and given to preterm infants at the University of Iowa Hospitals and Clinics are summarized as follows. The two studies [3,4] were of a two-arm, randomized design in which nursery staff and parents were blinded to the assignment. In one arm, infants with birth weights 0.6 to 1.3 kg received either AS-1 [3] or AS-3 [4] RBCs stored up to 42 days (stored RBCs); in the other study arm, infants received CPDA RBCs stored up to 7 days (fresh RBCs). All transfusions were given uniformly as 15 mL/kg of centrifuged RBCs (haematocrit of 85%) infused over 5 hours. To detect possible clinical transfusion reactions, nurses took seven sets of vital signs and observations during each transfusion – as it began, after

Table 3. Mean changes (delta ± SD) in blood chemistry levels during RBC transfusions*

	CPDA versus AS-1 [3]		**CPDA versus AS-3 [4]**	
	CPDA RBCs	**AS-1 RBCs**	**CPDA RBCs**	**AS-3 RBCs**
Haematocrit (%)	+ 12 ± 4	+ 12 ± 5	+ 12 ± 5	+ 11 ± 4
Glucose (mg/dL)	– 9 ± 32	– 7 ± 25	– 18 ± 40	– 17 ± 24
Lactate (mmol/L)	– 0.3 ± 0.4	– 0.1 ± 0.6	– 0.2 ± 0.3	– 0.5 ± 1.5
pH	0.00 ± 0.05	0.00 ± 0.13	– 0.01 ± 0.09	– 0.03 ± 0.06
Calcium (mg/dL)	– 0.1 ± 0.7	– 0.1 ± 0.5	– 0.1 ± 1.0	+ 0.1 ± 0.6
Sodium (mEq/L)	+ 0.5 ± 4.4	+ 0.5 ± 5.1	– 0.4 ± 5.5	+ 1.9 ± 4.7
Potassium (mEq/L)	+ 0.3 ± 0.9	– 0.2 ± 1.5	+ 0.3 ± 1.2	+ 0.4 ± 0.9
Haematocrit (%)	+ 12 ± 4	+ 12 ± 5	+ 12 ± 5	+ 11 ± 4

* For pre- versus post-transfusion laboratory studies, changes (delta values) observed in infants in one study arm (fresh CPDA RBCs) were compared with infants in the other (stored AS-1 or AS-3 RBCs). Pretransfusion values were subtracted from post-transfusion results, so that a positive delta value indicated an increase of the analyte result after transfusion and a negative value a decrease of the analyte result after transfusion. No statistically significant differences were found using t-test for values with normal distribution and Wilcoxon rank test for values with abnormal distribution.

15 minutes, and hourly thereafter. To detect possible biochemical abnormalities in infant blood, pretransfusion levels of haematocrit, glucose, lactate, pH, ionized calcium, sodium and potassium were measured when RBCs were ordered from the blood bank. Identical posttransfusion studies were performed on infant blood samples drawn shortly after the transfusions were completed.

Complete results were reported in detail elsewhere [3,4], and only the safety aspects of the studies are reported here. None of the CPDA RBCs were stored longer than 7 days, whereas, 47% of AS-1 RBCs and 50% of AS-3 RBCs were stored 15 days or longer before transfusion. No clinical transfusion reactions were observed during 66 AS-1 RBC transfusions given to 19 infants, during 28 AS-3 RBC transfusions given to 11 infants or during 98 CPDA RBC transfusions given to 31 infants [3,4]. No significant differences occurred in the comparative changes between pretransfusion and posttransfusion blood chemistries, whether fresh CPDA RBCs or stored AS-1 or AS-3 RBCs were transfused (Table 3). The hematocrit increased as expected. Changes in levels of glucose, lactate, pH, calcium, sodium, and potassium during transfusion were slight.

After the randomized trials were completed, additional safety data were generated by an open study in which 33 preterm infants (birth weight 0.6 to 1.25 kg) received all RBC transfusions as 15 mL/kg of AS-3 RBCs stored ≤42 days [4]. Of the 120 RBC transfusions given, 78 (65%) were stored 1 through 21 days and 42 (35%) were stored 22 through 42 days. When comparing pretransfusion versus posttransfusion laboratory results of these two groups (ie, <22 days vs ≥22 days), no statistically significant differences were found that could be related to the length of storage (Table 4).

Table 4. Changes in laboratory values* (delta ± SD) of 120 AS-3 RBC transfusions [4]

	Days of storage	
	1 to 21 (N = 78)	**22 to 42 (N = 42)**
Haematocrit (%)	+ 12 ± 5	+ 12 ± 4
Glucose (mg/dL)	– 12 ± 24	– 16 ± 28
Lactate (mmol/L)	– 0. 6 ± 1.1	– 0.2 ± 0.3
pH	0.00 ± 0.08	0.00 ± 0.06
Ca (mg/dL)	– 0.1 ± 0.5	0.0 ± 0. 8
Na (mEq/L)	+ 0.3 ± 4.6	– 0.4 ± 4.7
K (mEq/L)	+ 0.2 ± 0.8	+ 0.2 ± 0.6
Haematocrit (%)	+ 12 ± 5	+ 12 ± 4
Glucose (mg/dL)	– 12 ± 24	– 16 ± 28

* Change = post-transfusion minus pretransfusion values.
Statistical tests used were t-test for pH, Na, K and glucose (normal distribution) and Wilcoxon rank sum test for haematocrit, Ca and lactate (abnormal distribution).
No statistically significant differences were found (p values all > 0.05) comparing 1 to 21 days versus 22 to 42 days of storage.

Conclusions and Recommendations

Thus, RBCs from one donor stored up to 42 days in extended storage preservative solutions such as AS-1, AS-3 or AS-5 can safely provide all RBCs needed by most infants. At the UI DeGowin Blood Center, infants requiring RBC transfusions are assigned to dedicated units of RBCs suspended in extended storage (42-day) preservative solutions. AS-1, AS-3 and AS-5 all have been used. At the time the first transfusion is ordered, one-half of a freshly collected (stored ≤7 days) unit is dedicated to a preterm infant with a birth weight ≤1.0 kg. The remainder of the unit can be assigned to another infant. Thus, one complete unit can serve two very low birth weight infants simultaneously. Larger infants may be assigned, similarly, to a part of a unit, depending on anticipated needs. When RBC transfusions are ordered, aliquots are removed sterilely and issued [2]. Although units are used throughout 42 days of storage, once a unit has been stored 14 days, it has become relatively aged (ie, 14 days of its 42 days have lapsed), and no new infants are assigned to it. When infants assigned to a unit no longer require transfusions, the remainder of the unit is placed in the general inventory for transfusion to older patients. This plan has been shown to be cost-effective [14,15].

References

1. Widness JA, Seward VJ, Kromer IJ, et al. Changing patterns of red blood cell transfusion in very low birthweight infants. J Pediatr 1996;129:680-87.
2. Strauss RG, Villhauer PJ, Cordle DG. A method to collect, store and issue multiple aliquots of packed red blood cells for neonatal transfusions. Vox Sang 1995;68:77–81.
3. Strauss RG, Burmeister LF, Johnson K, et al. AS-1 red blood cells for neonatal transfusions: a randomized trial assessing donor exposure and safety. Transfusion 1996;36:873–78.
4. Strauss RG, Burmeister LF, Johnson K, et al. Feasibility and safety of AS-3 red blood cells for neonatal transfusions. J Pediatr 2000;136:215-19.
5. Luban NLC, Strauss RG, Hume HA. Commentary on the safety of red blood cells preserved in extended storage media for neonatal transfusions. Transfusion 1991;31:229-35.
6. Liu EA, Mannino FL, Lane TA. Prospective, randomized trial of the safety and efficacy of a limited donor exposure transfusion program for premature neonates. J Pediatr 1994;125:92-96.
7. Lee DA, Slagel TA, Jackson TM, Evans CS. Reducing blood donor exposures in low birth weight infants by the use of older, unwashed packed red blood cells. J Pediatr 1995;126:280–86.

Cook S, Gunter J, Wissel M. Effective use of a strategy using assigned red cell units to limit donor exposure for neonatal patients. Transfusion 1993; 33:379-83.

8. Jain R, Jarosz CR, Myers TF. Decreasing blood donor exposure in the neonates by using dedicated donor transfusions. Transfus Sci 1997;18:199-203.
9. Wood A, Wilson N, Skacel P, et al. Reducing donor exposure in preterm infants requiring multiple blood transfusions. Arch Dis Child 1995;72:F29–F33.
10. Jain R, Jarosz C. Safety and efficacy of AS-1 red blood cell use in neonates. Transfus Apher Sci 2001;24:111-15
11. Soothill PW, Lestas AN, Nicolaides KH, et al. 2,3-diphosphoglycerate in normal, anaemic and transfused human fetuses. Clinical Science 1988;74: 527–30.
12. DeLivoria-Papadopoulos M, Morrow G, Oski FA, et al. Exchange transfusion in the newborn infant with fresh and "old" blood: the role of storage on a 2,3-diphosphoglycerate, hemoglobin-oxygen affinity, and oxygen release. J Pediatr 1971;79: 898–903.
13. Hilsenrath P, Nemechek J, Widness JA, et al. Cost-effectiveness of a limited donor blood program for neonatal RBC transfusions. Transfusion 1999;39: 938–43.
14. Wang-Rodriguez J, Mannino FL, Liu E, Lane TA. A novel strategy to limit blood donor exposure and blood waste in multiply transfused premature infants. Transfusion 1996;36:64-70.

HAZARDS OF TRANSFUSION: GvHD

N.L.C. Luban[1]

History

Transfusion-associated graft versus host disease (TA-GvHD), an often fatal immunological complication of blood transfusion, was first reported in the 1960's in individuals with haematological malignancies and infants with congenital immunodeficiencies. In infants, the clinical stigmata was called runting disease [1].

In the past 30 years, we have developed a better understanding of the pathogenesis of TA-GvHD and established preventive strategies, the most successful of which is irradiation of blood and blood components [2-4]. However, many issues still remain. For example, there are no adequate estimates of prevalence or incidence in the U.S., as patients considered to be at risk receive irradiated products. In Japan, the Japanese Red Cross GvHD Study Group and registry estimates 40 cases per year. Homozygosity for one way HLA haplotype sharing in Japan, the use of familial donors and the use of fresh rather than stored red blood cells, may predispose to higher prevalence [5]. In other parts of the world, the prevalence is unknown and systematic reporting systems do not exist. No well established animal or in vitro models of TA-GvHD has been established, making mechanistic studies difficult to perform.

Pathogenesis

In the setting of bone marrow or haematopoietic stem cell transplantation, three prerequisites for the development of GvHD have been proposed: (1) differences in histocompatibility between recipient and donor; (2) presence of immunocompetent cells in the graft; and (3) inability of the host to reject the immunocompetent cells [6]. In TA-GvHD, similar prerequisites occur and are likely causative of the disorder. Most immunocompetent recipients will destroy the donor-derived T cells through lymphocytolysis. However, when an HLA homozygous donor provides blood to an HLA heterozygous recipient who shares one HLA

1. Center for Cancer and Blood Disorders, Chair Laboratory Medicine & Pathology, Director Transfusion Medicine/Donor Center Children's National Medical Center, Washington, DC, USA.

haplotype with the recipient, there may be failure of recognition of the donor cells as being foreign with subsequent engraftment [7,8]. In the case of transplantation and TA-GvHD, the foreign major histocompatibility complex (MHC) antigens and/or minor histocompatibility antigens (minor HA) of the host stimulate clonal T cell expansion and the induction of an inflammatory response with cytokine release. It is this cytokine "storm" that is ultimately responsible for the induction of the process and clinical manifestations of the disorder.

Ferrera et al. have described the Th1/Th2 paradigm, which delineates the cellular origins and differential biologic functions of T-cell-derived cytokines based on murine CD4 differentiation [6]. Th1 CD4 T cells secrete IL-2 as their allostimulator. Th2 CD4 T cells produce IL-4, IL-5, IL-6, IL-10, IL-13 and lesser amounts of TNF-α, while Th1 and 2 both produce IL-3 and granulocyte-macrophage colony stimulating factor. The Type 1 cell is pro-inflammatory and induces cell mediated immunity, while the type-2 cell is considered anti-inflammatory. Differentiation toward type 1 or type 2 is a complicated process which involves early exposure to IL-4 or IL-12, the type of antigen presenting cells, co-stimulating molecules and the presence of macrophages and their unique cytokines. Based on their mouse work, Ferrera et al. propose a three-step process for the development of acute GvHD in the transplant setting which may be comparable to the development of TA-GvHD. In this model, host tissues are damaged through irradiation or chemotherapy, and secrete TNF-α and IL-1 which enhance recognition of host MHC and/or minor HLA antigens by donor T cells. Donor T cell activation results in proliferation of Th1 T cells and secretion of IL-2 and TNF-α, which in turn activate T cells further and induce cytotoxic T lymphocytes (CTL) and natural killer (NK) responses. Subsequently, additional donor and residual host phagocytes are stimulated to produce IL-1 and TNF-α. Stimulated macrophages release the free radical nitric oxide (NO) which has further deleterious effects on host tissues. In addition, NO up-regulates alloreactivity as well as mediates the cytotoxic function of macrophages [9]. A secondary triggering signals lipopolysaccharides (LPS) to stimulate gut-associated macrophages, lymphocytes, keratocytes and dermal fibroblasts and further promotes the inflammatory response and end organ damage that are classical hallmarks of the disorder. Whether the identical pathways are responsible for TA-GvHD is unknown.

The importance of CD4 and CD8 cells in the pathogenesis of TA-GvHD has been studied by Fast et al. in a mouse model [10] and by Nishimura in a patient with TA-GvHD [11] and is further supported by clinical correlation with HIV/AIDS [12]. In the mouse, depletion of CD4+ cells increased the number of donor cells needed to induce TA-GvHD, while depletion of CD8+ and/or NK cells decreased the number of donor cells needed to induce the disorder. In HIV/AIDS, there has been only one report of TA-GvHD [13], despite profound immunosuppression and widespread use of supportive transfusion. Early depletion of CD4 may well protect against establishment of GvHD. Alternatively, activation of CD8+ lymphocytes against HIV infected CD4 T cells may limit the development of the GvHD process [14].

Recently, Kruskal et al. studied infected subjects enrolled in the Viral Activation Transfusion Study. They were unable to demonstrate microchimerism in transfused HIV infected patients, suggesting that such patients are not at risk for TA-GvHD [15].

Clinical Manifestations

Nonspecific findings like fever, anorexia, nausea, vomiting and diarrhoea are seen. Skin manifestations are variable; an erythematous maculopapular eruption may progress to erythroderma with bullae and frank desquamation. Gastrointestinal bleeding is commonly seen, most usually as bloody diarrhoea. Hepatic dysfunction with hyperbilirubinaemia, with a progressively increasing direct fraction, is also seen. In infants, the clinical manifestations are often confused with the signs and symptoms of sepsis or are attributed to other underlying conditions, making diagnosis very difficult. TA-GvHD differs from acute GvHD in the setting of allogeneic transplantation in that the pancytopenia seen is severe and often results in the death of the patient. Diagnosis is often made post mortem and is based on pathognomonic histopathological findings of lymphocyte infiltration in skin, lymph nodes, liver and the gastrointestinal track.

Diagnosis of TA-GvHD

Clinical suspicion may warrant a skin biopsy. Skin biopsy often reveals vacuolization of the epidermal basal cell layer, dermal-epithelial layer separation and formation of bullae; other findings include mononuclear cell migration into the epidermis, hyperkeratosis and dyskeratosis. Liver biopsies may reveal eosinophilic infiltration and degeneration of small bile ducts, peripheral inflammation and lymphocyte infiltration. The bone marrow will demonstrate what is classically described as an "empty marrow" with pancytopenia, fibrosis and some lymphocytic infiltration.

Definitive confirmation is more complicated. Several methods have been utilized to identify lymphocytes of foreign origin in the circulation of a suspected patient or in affected tissue. Serological HLA typing, DNA-based HLA class II typing, karyotype analysis, restriction length polymorphism analysis using probes from both HLA and non HLA regions and genetic fingerprinting using polymorphic microsatellite markers have all been used [16-22]. Fibroblast and buccal mucosal cells of the recipient are often needed as the lymphocytolysis accompanying the disorder prohibits standardized serological HLA typing. Parental or familial specimens may be necessary to deduce a recipient's HLA type [19]. Donor lymphocytes obtained from suspected blood products present in attached remaining blood bag segments often require PCR amplification and sequence specific oligonucleotide probe (SSOP) methodologies to provide confirmation of donor cell origin [23].

Microchimerism and its Relationship to TA-GvHD

In 1996, Busch and Lee demonstrated a thousand fold expansion of donor lymphocytes in the circulation of otherwise healthy recipients 3-5 days following transfusion for elective orthopaedic procedures; within two weeks, the allogeneic cells were cleared [23]. In another study of adult trauma victims, receiving large numbers (4-18 units) of fresh packed red blood cells, 8 of 10 had confirmed microchimerism (MC). Two of the eight still had persistence of MC when studied as long as 1.5 years post transfusion [24]. Kruskall et al. in a study of 93 HIV-infected women who had received blood from male donors, found that five of 47 women randomized to receive non leukocyte reduced RBCs had detectable circulating male donor lymphocytes 1-2 weeks after transfusion and undetectable male donor lymphocytes after 4 weeks. This was in contrast to 46 HIV-infected women who did not have detectable male donor lymphocytes within a month of transfusion [15]. Wang-Rodriquez studied post-transfusion immune modulation in 14 premature infants [25]. Through collaboration with Busch and Lee, she identified two of six female infants, transfused with non leukocyte depleted red blood cells, who developed transient MC detected by Y-chromosome PCR amplification; both cleared these cells by two weeks post transfusion. An additional three infants who received leukocyte depleted red blood cells also had transient MC. Vietor, et al. studied nine surviving recipients of intrauterine trans–fusion whose donors were still available for testing [26]. Using FISH, PCR of Y chromosome specific sequences and assays for the frequencies of cytotoxic T lymphocyte and T helper-lymphocyte precursors, they detected true MC in six out of seven young adults studied twenty years post transfusion. Reed, et al. have developed sequence-specific amplification of DRB1 which permitted identification of minor chimeric populations at the 0.01% level [27]. The establishment of stable MC and identification of its biological consequences is critical for pediatric patients who are expected to live to adulthood, and may well be stable transfusion-induced chimeras, an intriguing and at the same time worrying concept. The persistence of MC may predispose to autoimmune disease [28-30], chronic GvHD, recurrent abortion [31], and may serve as an allogeneic stimulate of latent viral reactivation in the recipient.

Groups at Risk

Patients at risk for TA-GvHD have been described in a number of recent reviews [2-4,7,32]. Additional groups at possible risk continue to be identified. For example, based on two reports of TA-GvHD development in congenital and acquired immunodeficiency in older children [13,22], recommendations have extended the age range patients who might receive of irradiation well past the neonatal age group [34,35]. Given the lack of adequate animal models and definite laboratory tests describing individual TA-GvHD risk, many reports stratify the need for irradiation using such terms as "clearly indicated" or "probably

Table 1. Clinical indications for irradiated products

Foetus/Infant:
– Intrauterine transfusion
– Premature infants
– Congenital immunodeficiency
– Those undergoing exchange transfusion for erythroblastosis
Child/Adult:
– Congenital immunodeficiency
– Haematological malignancy or solid tumor (neuroblastoma, sarcoma,
– Hodgkins disease receiving ablative chemo/radiotherapy)
– Recipient of PBSC, marrow or cord blood
– Recipient of familial blood donation
– Recipient of HLA-matched products
– Lupus or any other condition requiring fludarabine
Potential Indications:
– Term infant
– Recipient and donor pair from a genetically homogeneous population
– Other patients with haematological malignancy or solid tumor receiving immunosuppressive agents

indicated" [2,4,32,33]. In reality, the spectrum of individuals at risk will likely grow as intensive immunomodulatory therapies expand beyond oncological disease and transplantation. (Table 1).

The Irradiation Process

There are several methodologies that can modify the potential for GvHD. These include photoinactivation, PEGylation, ultraviolet light, and irradiation. Of these, only irradiation of whole blood and cellular components is accepted practice by the U.S. FDA. Irradiation of cellular components with ionizing radiation results in the inactivation of T lymphocytes by damaging nuclear DNA either directly or by generating ions and free radicals that have damaging biological actions. This prevents posttransfusion donor T cell proliferation in response to host antigen presenting cells which, in turn, abrogates GvHD [4,36]. Two types of ionizing radiation, γ rays and x-rays, are equivalent in inactivating T lymphocytes in blood components at a given absorbed dose. Gamma rays originate from the radioactive decay process within the atomic nucleus of cesium 137 (^{137}Cs) or cobalt 60 (^{60}Co). Freestanding blood bank gamma irradiators, which are the predominant instruments for blood component irradiation, use either of these two isotopes as an irradiation source. In contrast, X-rays are generated from the interaction of a beam of electrons with a metallic surface.

Linear accelerators that generate X-rays for patient therapy (teletherapy) may serve as an irradiation source for blood and blood components. Recently, the FDA has also approved the use of a free standing X-ray machine (Rad-Source

RS3000, Coral Springs, FL) for irradiation of blood components, which does not require Federal or Nuclear Regulatory Agency licenses.

Instrumentation for Irradiation

The basic operating principles and configurations of a free-standing irradiator with either a Cesium (^{137}Cs) source or a linear accelerator are shown schematically in Figure 1.

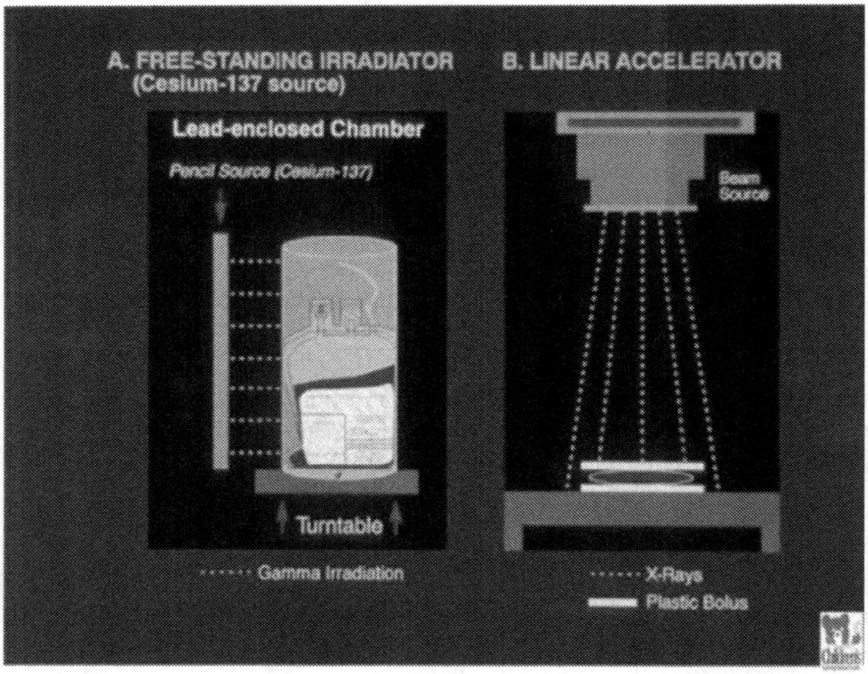

Figure 1.

With a freestanding ^{137}Cs irradiator, blood components are contained within a metal canister that is positioned on a rotating turntable. Continuous rotation allows for the γ rays, originating from one to four closely positioned pencil sources, to penetrate all portions of the blood component. The number of sources and their placement depend on the instrument and model. The speed of rotation of the turntable also depends on the make or model of the instrument. A lead shield encloses the irradiation chamber. Freestanding irradiators employing ^{60}Co as the source of γ rays are comparable except that the canister containing the blood component does not rotate during the irradiation process; rather, tubes of ^{60}Co are placed in a circular array around the entire canister within the lead chamber. When freestanding irradiators are used, the γ rays are attenuated as they pass through air and blood but at different rates [37]. The magnitude of attenuation is greater with ^{137}Cs than with ^{60}Co sources.

Linear accelerators generate a beam of X-rays over a field of given dimension. Routinely, the field is projected on a table-top structure. The blood component is placed (flat) between two sheets of biocompatible plastic several centimeters thick. The plastic on the top of the blood component (i.e., nearer to the radiation source) generates electronic equilibrium of the secondary electrons at the point where they pass through the component container. The plastic sheet on the bottom of the blood component provides for irradiation back-scattering that helps to ensure the homogenous delivery of the x-rays. The blood component is usually left stationary when the entire x-ray dose is being delivered. Alternatively it may be flipped over when one half of the dose has been delivered; this process involves turning off and restarting the linear accelerator during the irradiation procedure. Although it seems as if the practice of flipping is not required, further data are needed.

Components to be Irradiated

The single most important characteristic of a blood component's ability to induce TA-GvHD is the white blood cell content, specifically, lymphocyte content. Based on animal models, and estimates from the bone marrow transplant literature, 5×10^4 to 1×10^5 T cells per kg in an ablated host will induce GvHD [38], while a greater number is likely needed in a non-ablated host. The content of lymphocytes in each blood component differs based on the donor's initial lymphocyte count, the method of collection and any post-collection manipulation and processing. In general, there are likely sufficient lymphocytes present in almost all blood products to induce TA-GvHD in a susceptible recipient (Table 2). During storage, it becomes more difficult to isolate lymphocytes from both red blood cell and platelet concentrates. Detail on the nature of lymphocyte subsets and the molecular changes occurring during storage in different blood products has not been well studied, making risk assessment between a specific class of product and a subcategory of at-risk patients impossible. Of some concern is the fact that there could be a cumulative or synergistic effect from viable T cells present in the multiple transfusions received by a given patient whose own immunological status fluctuates with time from treatment and infectious disease state.

For patients at risk for GvHD, all components that might contain viable T lymphocytes should be irradiated. These components are listed in Table 3. All types of red cells suspended in citrated plasma or in an additive solution, post freezing and thawing [38-41] and filtered products should be irradiated. Although extensive leukocyte reduction through filtration may decrease the potential for GvHD it is not a substitute as there have been reports of TA-GvHD in patients who have received leukocyte depleted (filtered) red cells; however, the extent of leukocyte reduction of the components was not uniformly quantified in such reports [42-45].

Table 2. White blood cell (WBC) content of different blood components

Component	Volume (mL)	Average WBC content
Whole blood	450	$1\text{-}2\times10^9$
Red blood cells	250	$2\text{-}5\times10^9$
Washed red blood cells	Variable	$<5\times10^8$
Deglycerolized red blood cells	250	$\sim10^7$
Platelet concentrate	50-75	4×10^7
Plateletapheresis unit	200-500	3×10^8 *
Cryoprecipitate	25	0
Fresh frozen plasma	125	0
Pediatric frozen plasma	Variable	0
Liquid plasma	125	1.5×10^5
Single-donor plasma	125	0
Granulocyte concentrate	200-500	1×10^{10}

Adapted from Luban NLC. Basics of transfusion medicine. *In* Fuhrman BP, Zimmerman JJ (eds): Pediatric Critical Care. St. Louis: Mosby-Year Book, 1992, pp 829-40.

* Less with new modified chambers.

Table 3. Blood components requiring irradiation for patients at risk of GvHD

All components that might contain viable T lymphocytes (including products collected by apheresis):

- Whole blood
- Cellular components
- Red cells (regardless of anticoagulant or preservative)
- Leukocyte filtered red cells
- Platelet concentrates
- Leukocyte filtered platelet concentrates
- Previously frozen red blood cells
- Non-frozen plasma (fresh plasma)
- Granulocyte concentrates
- Questionable components
    - Fresh frozen plasma
- Frozen plasma
- Unlikely to contain viable T lymphocytes
    - Cryoprecipitate
- PLAS+SD® - Plasma

In addition to the number and specific subtype of T lymphocytes present in a product, patient immunocompetence at the time of transfusion may also influence the development of TA-GvHD. The greater the degree of immunosuppression, the fewer the viable T lymphocytes will be required to produce GvHD in susceptible patients. Some have suggested that cytotoxic T lymphocytes, or interleukin-2 secreting precursors of helper T lymphocytes may be more predictive of GvHD than the number of proliferating T cells alone; until further data are available to confirm adequate removal of these T-cell subtypes by leukocyte reduction, irradiation should be used for blood products destined for patients at risk for GvHD [45].

Blood components given to recipients, whether immunocompromised or immunocompetent, containing lymphocytes that are homozygous for an HLA haplotype that is shared with the recipient, pose a specific risk for TA-GvHD. This circumstance occurs when first and second degree relatives serve as directed donors [7,8,33,35] and when HLA-matched platelet components donated by related or unrelated individuals are transfused [5,7,35,46,47]. Irradiation of blood components must be performed in these situations. Platelet components that have low levels of leukocytes because of their collection through the apheresis process and/or leukocyte filtration should also be irradiated if intended for transfusion to susceptible patients. This is because the minimum number of T lymphocytes that induces TA-GvHD has not yet been delineated.

In contrast, there is controversy over fresh frozen plasma. It is generally accepted that the freezing and thawing processes destroy the T lymphocytes that are present in such plasma. There have been two brief articles suggesting that immunocompetent progenitor cells may be present in frozen-thawed plasma. These authors recommended that frozen-thawed plasma be irradiated [48,49]. Further studies are needed to validate these findings and to assess whether the number of immunocompetent cells, that may be present in thawed fresh frozen plasma, is sufficient to induce GvHD. In rare instances, when non-frozen plasma (termed *fresh Plasma)* is transfused, it should be irradiated because of the presence of a sizable number of viable lymphocytes, approximately 1×10^7 cells, in a component prepared from a unit of whole blood.

Storage of Red Cells and Platelets after Irradiation

Red Cells

Irradiation of red blood cells causes metabolic derangements. The in vivo viability of irradiated red cells, evaluated as the 24-hour recovery, is reduced during storage when compared with non-irradiated red cells [50-53]. This has raised questions concerning the maximum storage time for red cells after irradiation. Davey et al. [50] found that following irradiation with 3000 cGy on day 0, the mean ± SD 24-hour recovery for Adsol-preserved red cells after 42 days of storage was 68.5 ± 8.1 % compared with 78.4 ± 7.1 % for control, non-treated red cells. Subsequent studies employed total storage periods of between 21 and 35 days after day 0 or day 1 irradiation. After storage for 35 days, the mean (± SD) 24-hour recovery for irradiated (3000 cGy) and control Adsol red cells was 78.0 ± 6.8% and 81.8 ± 4.4%, respectively. In studies with a 28-day storage period, the values for irradiated (2500 cGy) and control Adsol red cells were 78.6 ± 5.9% and 84.2 ± 5.1%, respectively [52]. With Nutricel preserved red cells treated with 2000 cGy on day 1, mean 24-hour recovery for control and irradiated red cells were 90.4% and 82.7% after 21 days of storage and 85.0% and 80.7% after 28 days of storage [53]. Moroff et al. [54] evaluated the effect of irradiation on Adsol red cells stored from day 1 to 28 (irradiated day 1, protocol 1), day 14 to 28 (irradiated day 14, protocol 2), day 14 to 42 (irradiated day 14, protocol 3) and day 26 to 28 (irradiated day 26, protocol 4), respectively. In comparison to previous investigations, this study was unique because red cells were studied after being irradiated for various times in storage and then studied after further storage. Protocol 1 mean ± SD recovery was 84.2 ± 5.1% for control RBCs and 78.6 ± 5.9% for irradiated RBCs (n=16; $p < 0.01$). With protocol 3, the recoveries were 76.3 ± 7.0% for control RBCs and 69.5 ± 8.6% for irradiated RBCs (n=16; $p<0.01$). Protocols 2 and 4 demonstrated comparable 24 hour recoveries between control and irradiated RBCs. Long term survival between control and irradiated RBCs were comparable in all protocols confirming previous data that the long term survival of RBCs is minimally influenced by irradiation. Based on multiple linear regression analysis, only the length of storage after irradiation had a significant effect on the 24 hour recovery. No effect was observed with day of irradiation or total storage time. In another study by Moroff et al. [55], in vitro red cell properties such as adenosine triphosphate (ATP) levels and the amount of haemolysis were altered to only a small extent relative to control values with extended storage after irradiation and that potassium leakage from the red cells during storage is substantially enhanced by irradiation. Despite elevated potassium levels, the association between irradiation induced changes in red-cell viability and potassium leakage were not complimentary. Based on analysis of these studies, the Food and Drug Administration (FDA) guidelines call for a 28-day maximum storage period for red cells after irradiation, irrespective of the age of the product when the treatment was performed, with the proviso that the total storage time cannot exceed that for non-irradiated red cells.

Irradiated RBC Transfusion for the Neonate

Irradiated red cells undergo an enhanced efflux of potassium during storage at 1 to 6°C [56,57]. Comparable levels of potassium leakage occur with or without prestorage leukocyte reduction [58]. Washing of units of red cells before transfusion to reduce the supernatant potassium load does not seem to be warranted for most red cell transfusions because post-transfusion dilution prevents increases in plasma potassium [59]. On the other hand, when irradiated red cells are used for neonatal exchange transfusion or the equivalent of a whole blood exchange is anticipated, red cell washing should be considered to prevent the possible adverse cardiotoxicity caused by hyperkalaemia associated with irradiation and storage [60].

Platelets

In contrast to red cells, platelets appear to be unaffected by irradiation. The storage period at 20-24C for irradiated platelet components does not need to be modified. Both in vitro and in vivo platelet properties are not influenced to any extent by irradiation. Many studies have confirmed that platelet properties are retained immediately after conventional levels of irradiation and at the conclusion of a 5-day storage period, whether irradiation is performed prestorage or mid-storage [61-68]. Only one report indicated some differences in selected in vitro parameters between irradiated and control platelets after storage [67].

Granulocytes

Several studies have suggested that irradiation at doses recommended for irradiation of blood components does not affect granulocyte function. Wober et al. [69] found that there was no effect of irradiation doses between 1500 and 2500 cGy on the ability of neutrophils to generate intracellular hydrogen peroxide in the conversion of the non-fluorescent compound 2'-7'-dichlorofluorescen into fluorescent 2'-7'dichlorofluorescein. Wheeler et al. [70] found that buffy coat separated polymorphonuclear leukocytes when treated with 1500 cGy did not demonstrate oxidative or migratory differences in chemiluminescence or chemotaxis under agarose when compared to non-irradiated controls. Patrone et al. [71] found that granulocytes harvested by continuous flow centrifugation using the Aminco Celltrifuge and irradiated at 1500 cGy, demonstrated no differences in chemotaxis compared to granulocytes in precollection venous samples. However, when irradiation doses as high as 10,000 – 40,000 cGy are used, granulocyte motility and bactericidal activity are adversely affected [72].

Selection of Radiation Dose

Early attempts at identifying adequate irradiation dose used mitogen assays [72,73]. LDA measures the clonogenic potential of both CD4+ and CD8+ T cells in a functional assay. It provides a quantification at low T cell numbers. It has been used to determine residual, functional T cells in bone marrows purged of T cells, thus providing a clinical correlate of prevention of GvHD [74]. Assays of T cell proliferation using MLC or mitogens or detection of T cells by flow cytometry can detect up to a two log reduction. PCR techniques are capable of detecting up to 6 log reduction but cannot distinguish viable vs. nonviable cells, and hence are noninformative if cells are inactivated. Studies utilizing a sensitive limiting dilution assay (LDA) indicate that 2500 cGy (measured at the internal midplane of a component) is the most appropriate dose [75,76]. In these experiments, red cell and platelet components were irradiated in their original in plastic containers (blood bags) with increasing doses of radiation. After each irradiation dose, the LDA samples were removed and the clonogenic proliferation of T lymphocytes was measured in the system. With red cell units, 500 cGy had a minimal influence, whereas 1500 cGy inactivated T lymphocyte proliferation by approximately 4 logs; however, some growth was still observed in each experiment. Increasing the dose to 2000 cGy resulted in no T lymphocyte proliferation in all but one experiment. No growth was observed after 2500 cGy [75]. In a subsequent study that used plateletapheresis components with sufficient T lymphocytes to perform the LDA, the influence of 1500 cGy and 2500 cGy was evaluated [76]. With 1500 cGy, substantial inactivation was measured; however, some growth was still observed in all experiments. As noted with the red cell experiments, 2500 cGy resulted in complete abrogation of clonogenic T lymphocyte proliferation. There is a limitation to LDA assays; such assays may fail to detect an as yet undescribed human T cell subset that contributes to GvHD, but despite this limitation it is believed that the current studies provide supportive evidence for the selection of irradiation doses for plateletapheresis and red cell components to abrogate TA-GvHD. Currently, the FDA has recommended that the irradiation process should deliver 2500 cGy to the internal midplane of a freestanding irradiation instrument canister, with a minimum of 1500 cGy at any other point within the canister [77].

Quality Assurance Measures

To assure that the irradiation process is being conducted correctly, specific procedures are recommended for free-standing irradiators and linear accelerators, which are summarized in Table 4 and are detailed in a review [78]. Dose mapping measures the delivery of radiation within a simulated blood component or over an area in which a blood component is placed. This applies to an irradiation field when a linear accelerator is used or to the canister of a free-standing irradiadiator. Dose mapping is the primary means of ensuring that the irradiation process is being conducted correctly. Mapping documents that the intended dose of irradiation is being delivered at a specific location (such as the central midplane. of a canister), and how the delivered irradiation dose varies within a simulated component or over a given area. This permits extrapolation of the maximum and minimum doses being delivered [79]. Dose mapping should be performed with sensitive dosimetry techniques. A number of commercially available systems have been developed in recent years. Other quality assurance measures that need to be done include the routine confirmation that the turntable is operating correctly (for ^{137}Cs irradiators), measurements to ensure that the timing device is accurate, and the periodic lengthening of the irradiation time to correct for source decay. With linear accelerators, it is necessary to measure the characteristics of the x-ray beam to ensure consistency of delivery. Confirming that a blood component has, in actuality, been irradiated is also an important part of a quality assurance program. Several indicator labels are available for this purpose.

Confirming that Irradiation Occurred

It is important to have positive confirmation that the irradiation process has taken place in the case of operator failure and/or instrumentation malfunction. Several commercial products are available including a radiation-sensitive indicator label developed specifically for this purpose (International Specialty Prod-

Table 4. Quality assurance guidelines for irradiating blood components

Dose:
2500 cGy to the central midplane of a canister (free-standing irradiator) or to the centre of an irradiation field (linear accelerator) with a minimum of 1500 cGy.
Dose mapping (free-standing irradiators):
Routinely, once a year (^{137}Cs) or twice a year (^{60}Co) and after major repairs; using a fully filled canister (water/plastic) with a dosimetry system to map the distribution of the absorbed dose.
Dose mapping (Linear accelerators):
Recommend yearly dose mapping with an ionization chamber and a water phantom. More frequent evaluation of instrument conditions to ensure consistency of x-rays.
Correction for radioisotopic decay:
– With ^{137}Cs as the source, annually
– With ^{60}Co as the source, quarterly
Turntable rotation (free-standing ^{137}Cs irradiators)
Daily verification:
Storage time for red cells after irradiation.
For up to 28 days; total storage time cannot exceed maximum storage time for unirradiated red cells.
Storage time for platelets after irradiation.
No change due to irradiation procedure.

Adapted from Reference 78.

ucts, Wayne, NJ). This label contains a radiation sensitive film strip placed on the external surface of the blood component. Irradiation causes visually distinct changes and results in an appearance change from clear red to opaque with obliteration of the word "NOT." When the label is placed on a blood component, there is a visual record that the irradiation process took place. The reliability of this type of indicator has been documented in a multi-site study [80].

Two versions of the indicator label have been manufactured. The difference is the range of radiation needed to cause a change in the radiation-sensitive film. The ratings for these indicators are 1500 cGy or 2500 cGy. The ratings serve as an approximate guideline for the amount of absorbed radiation that will be needed to completely change the window from reddish to opaque with complete obliteration of the word "NOT". Because the indicator labels are designed for and are used to confirm that the irradiation process has occurred, our laboratory utilizes the 1500 cGy label as the most appropriate tool to perform this quality control measure. This is based on the routinely observed pattern of dose distribution to a blood component in a canister of a free-standing irradiator. Despite a targeted central dose of 2500 cGy, there will be spots at which the dose will be less [81]. If the theoretical dose map presented in Figure 2 is used as an example, there will be a spot that will receive only 1800 cGy. If the 2500 cGy-rated label were to be located on the external surface of a component, there may be

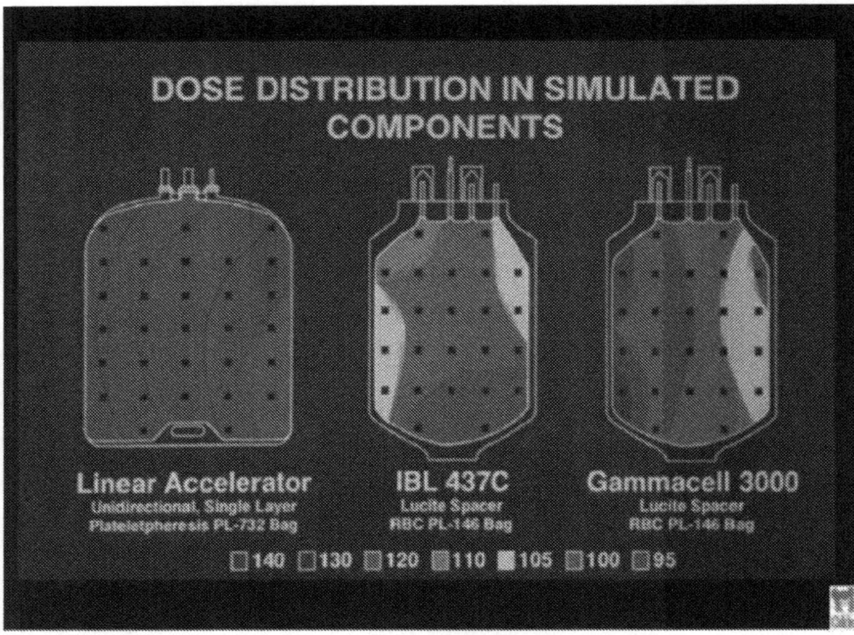

Figure 2.

minimal changes in the appearance of the radiation-sensitive film window. This would result in a judgment that the blood component was not irradiated, when in actuality it was treated satisfactorily.

New Methods in the Prevention of TA-GvHD

In the future, photochemical treatment (PCT) using psoralens and long wavelength ultraviolet irradiation (UVA) that have been developed to reduce the risk of bacterial and viral contaminants of platelet transfusions as well as other agents that disrupt or modify DNA replication of microorganisms may be used in the inactivation of leukocytes in blood products. Psoralens bind reversibly to nucleic acids by intercolation and, after UVA illumination, from covalent monoadducts and cross links with RNA and DNA. Among a broad group of compounds, the psoralen S-59 has been shown to be particularly effective in inactivating bacteria and viruses, without adversely affecting in vitro and in vivo platelet function [82].

Recently, S-59 and PCT has been studied for its possible inactivation of leukocytes in platelet concentrates [82,83]. PCT inactivation of T cells was evaluated utilizing four assay systems. These assay systems included T cell quantitation, inhibition of cytokine synthesis, modification of leukocyte genomic DNA by quantification of psoralen-DNA adducts and inhibition replication of T cells using PCR amplification of genomic DNA sequences. These studies demonstrated significantly reduced or absent cytokine generation and greater DNA strand break induction in platelet concentrates treated with PCT as compared to those treated with irradiation [82,83]. Furthermore, LDA was used to confirm inactivation of T cells in the platelet concentrates. To further support the efficacy of S-59 and PCT, a murine F1 hybrid-transfusion-induced GvHD model was tested [84]. No GvHD was noted in mice receiving splenocytes treated with either 2500 cGy or 150 µmol/LS-59 and 2.1 J/cm^2 UVA. In another set of experiments, PCT to prevent GvHD in an immunocompromised mouse model was studied [85]. These studies taken together suggest that PCT may well be an alternative to irradiation and further, provide a mechanism to prevent increase in cytokine concentration in platelet concentrates. The limitation of PCT methodology is the need for UVA penetration, which is not currently possible with red blood cell products. Several strategies are currently being studied in an attempt to overcome this limitation. Other agents such as PEN110, a low-molecular weight electrophilic compound, have been shown to chemically modify DNA and result in inhibition of DNA replication. Such compounds do not require an activation step and have been demonstrated to inactivate mononuclear cells present in RBC units [86]. Another method of inactivating WBC uses ultraviolet B irradiation to induce immune tolerance in donor leukocytes [87]. Further research in the safety of such approaches is warranted.

Treatment of TA-GvHD

Despite the mortality (80-90%) associated with TA-GvHD, effective treatment remains elusive [4]. Immunosuppressive therapy, the mainstay of treatment of transplantation associated GvHD is of unproven value in TA-GvHD and immunosuppressive agents such as steroids, methotrexate, anti-thymocyte globulin, cyclosporin and OKT3 have been associated with disappointing results. A recent report described the early detection and successful treatment of TA-GvHD using solumedrol, cyclosporin A, followed by high dose Cytoxan and anti-thymocyte globulin and autologous peripheral blood stem cell infusion [88]. Such cases are the exception and the best treatment for TA-GvHD remains prevention.

References

1. von Fliedner V, Higby DJ, Kim U. Graft-versus-host reaction following blood product transfusion. Am J Med 1972;72:951.
2. Anderson KC, Weinstein HJ: Transfusion-associated graft-versus-host disease. New Eng J Med 1990; 323:315-21.
3. Webb IJ, Anderson KC. Transfusion-associated graft-versus-host disease in Anderson KC, Ness PM, (eds.) Scientific Basis of Transfusion Medicine. Philadelphia, PA. WB Saunders, 2000, pp. 420-25.
4. Linden JV, Pisciotto PT: Transfusion-associated graft-versus-host disease and blood irradiation. Transfus Med Rev 1992; 6:116-23.

5. Ohto H, Anderson KC: Survey of transfusion-associated graft-versus-host disease in immunocompetent recipients. Transfus Med Rev 1996;10:31-43.
6. Ferrera JM, Krenger W. Graft-versus-host disease. The influence of type 1 and type 2 T cell cytokines. Transfus Med Rev 1998;12:1-17.
7. McMilan KD. Johnson RL: HLA-homozygosity and the risk of related-donor transfusion-associated graft-versus-host disease. Transfus Med Rev 1993; 7:37-41.
8. Petz LD, Calhoun L, Yam P, et al: Transfusion-associated graft-versus-host disease in Immunocompetent patients: Report of a fatal case associated with transfusion of blood from a second-degree relative, and a survey of predisposing factors. Transfusion 1993;33:742-50.
9. Worrall NK, Lazenby WD, Misko TP, et al. Modulation of in vivo alloreactivity by inhibition of inducible nitric oxide synthetase. J Exp Med. 1995; 181:63-70
10. Fast LD, Valeri CR, Crowley JP. Immune responses to major histocompatibility complex homozygous lymphoid cells in murine F1 hybrid recipients: implications for transfusion-associated graft-versus-host disease. Blood 1995;86:3090.
11. Nishimura M, Uchida S, Mitsunaga S, et al. Characterization of T-cell clones derived from peripheral blood lymphocytes of a patient with transfusion-associated graft-versus-host disease: Fas-mediated killing by CD4+ and CD8+ cytotoxic T-cell clones and tumor necrosis factor beta production by CD4+ T-cell clones. Blood 1997;89:1440.
12. Ammann AJ. Hypothesis: absence of graft-versus-host disease in AIDS is a consequence of HIV-1 infection of CD4+ T cells. J Acquir Immune Defic Syndr 1993; 6:1224.
13. Klein C, Fraitag S, Foulon E, Raffoux C, Bodener C, Blanche S. Moderate and t transient transfusion-associated cutaneous graft versus host disease in a child infected by human immunodeficiency virus. Am J Med 1996;101: 445-6.
14. Brubaker DB. Immunopathogenic mechanisms of post-transfusion graft versus host disease. Proc Soc Exp Biol Med 1993;202:122-47.
15. Kruskall MS, Lee TH, Assmann SF et al. Survival of transfused donor white blood cells in HIV-infected recipients. Blood 2001;98:272-9.
16. Blundell, EL, Pamphilon DH, Anderson NA et al. Transfusion-associated graft- versus-host disease, monoclonal gammopathy and PCR. Br J Haematol 1992;82: 622-23.
17. Capon SM, DePond WD, Tyan DB et al. Transfusion associated graft-versus-host disease in an immunocompetent patient. Ann Intern Med 1991;114: 1025-26.
18. Drobyski W, Thibodeau S, Truitt RL, et al. Third-party-mediated graft rejection and graft-versus-host disease after T-cell-depleted bone marrow transplantation, as demonstrated by hypervariable DNA probes and HLA-DR polymorphism. Blood 1989;74:2285-94.

19. Kunstmann E, Bocker T, Roewer L, Sauer H, Mempel W, Epplen JT. Diagnosis of transfusion-associated graft versus-host disease by genetic fingerprinting and polymerase chain reaction. Transfusion 1992;32:766-770.
20. Depalma L, Bahrami KR, Kapur S, et al. Amplified fragment length polymorphism analysis in the evaluation of post-transfusion graft versus host disease. J Thoracic Cardiovasc Surg 1994;108:182-84.
21. Wang L, Juji T, Tokunaga K, et al. Polymorphic microsatellite markers for the diagnosis of graft-versus-host disease. N Engl J Med 1994;330:398-401.
22. Friedman DF, Kwittken P, Cizman B, et al. Dan-based HLA typing of nonhematopoeitic tissue used to select the marrow transplant donor for successful treatment of transfusion-associated graft-versus-host disease. Clin Diagn Lab Immunol 1994;1: 590-96.
23. Lee TH, Donegan E, Slichter S, Busch MP. Transient increase in circulating donor leukocytes after allogeneic transfusions in immunocompetent recipients compatible with donor cell proliferation. Blood 1996;85:1207-14.
24. Lee TH, Paglieroni T, Ohto H, Holland PV, Busch MP. Survival of donor leukocyte subpopulations in immunocompetent transfusion recipients: frequent long term microchimerism in severe trauma patients. Blood 1999;93: 3127-39.
25. Wang-Rodriguez J, Fry E, Fiebig E, et al. Immune response to blood transfusion in very-low-birthweight infants. Transfusion 2000;40:25-34.
26. Vietor HE, Hallensleben E, van Bree SP, et al. Survival of donor cells 25 years after intrauterine transfusion. Blood 2000;95:2709-14.
27. Reed WF, Lee TH, Trachlenberg E, Vinson M, Busch MP. Detection of microchimerism by PCR as a function of amplification strategy. Transfusion 2001; 41:39-44.
28. Nelson J, Furst D, Maloney S, et al. Microchimerism and HLA compatible relationships of pregnancy in scleroderma. Lancet 1998;351:559-62.
29. Arlett CM, Smith JB, Jimenez SA. Identification of fetal DNA and cells in skin lesions from women with systemic sclerosis. N Engl J Med 1998; 333:1186-91.
30. vans PC, Lambert N, Maloney S, Furst D, Moore J, Nelson J. Long-term fetal microchimerism in peripheral blood mononuclear cell subsets in healthy women and women with scleroderma. Blood 1999;93:2033-37.
31. Daya S, Gunby J, Clark DA. Intravenous immunoglobulin therapy for recurrent spontaneous abortion: a meta-analysis. Am J Reprod Immunol 1998;39: 69-76.
32. Williamson LM, Warwick RM: Transfusion-associated graft-versus-host disease and its prevention. Blood Reviews 1995; 9:251-61.
33. Kanter MH: Transfusion-associated graft-versus-host disease: Do transfusions from second-degree relatives pose a greater risk than those from first-degree relatives? Transfusion 1992; 32:323-27.
34. Luban NL, DePalma L. Transfusion-associated graft-versus-host disease in the neonate-expanding the spectrum of disease. Transfusion 1996; 36:101-03 (editorial).

35. Ohto H, Anderson KC. Post-transfusion graft-versus-host disease in Japanese newborns. Transfusion 1996; 36:117-23.
36. Shlomchik WD, Couzens MS, Tang CB, et al. Prevention of graft versus host disease by inactivation of host antigen-presenting cells. Science 1999; 285:412- 15.
37. Fearon TC, Luban NLC: Practical dosimetric aspects of blood and blood product irradiation. Transfusion 1986; 26:457-59.
38. Davey RJ: The effect of irradiation on blood components, in Baldwin ML and Jefferies LC (eds): Irradiation of Blood Components. Bethesda, MD. American Association of Blood Banks 1992; pp. 51-62.
39. Suda BA, Leitman SF, Davey RJ: Characteristics of red cells irradiated and subsequently frozen for long term storage. Transfusion 1993;33:389-92.
40. Miraglia CC, Anderson G, Mintz PD: Effect of freezing on the in vivo recovery of irradiated red cells. Transfusion 1994;34:775-78.
41. Crowley JP, Skrabut EM, Valeri CR: lmmunocompetent lymphocytes in previously frozen washed red cells. Vox Sang 1974; 26:513-17.
42. Akahoshi M. Takanashi M, Masuda M, et al: A case of transfusion-associated graft-versus-host disease not prevented by white cell-reduction filters. Transfusion 1992; 32:169-72.
43. Heim MU, Munker R, Sauer H, et al. Graft-versus-host Krankheit(GVH mit letalem ausgang nach der gabe von gefilterten erythrozytenkonzentraten (Ek). Infusionstherapie 1991; 18:8-9.
44. Hayashi H, Nishiuchi T, Tamura H, et al. Transfusion associated graft-versus-host disease caused by leukocyte filtered stored blood. Anesthesiology 1993; 79:1419-21.
45. Anderson KC: Leukodepleted cellular blood components for prevention of transfusion-associated graft-versus-host disease. Transfus Sc. 1995; 16:265-68.
46. Benson K, Marks AR, Marshall MJ, et al: Fatal graft-versus-host disease associated with transfusions of HLA-matched, HLA-homozygous platelets from unrelated donors. Transfusion 1994;34:432-37.
47. Grishaber JE, Birney SM, Strauss RG: Potential for host transfusion-associated graft-versus-host disease due to apheresis platelets matched for HLA class I antigens. Transfusion 1993; 33:910-14.
48. Wielding JU, Vehmeyer K, Dittman J, et al: Contamination of fresh-frozen plasma with viable white cells and proliferable stem cells. Transfusion 1994; 34:185-86. (letter)
49. Bernvill SS, Abdulatiff M, Al-Sedairy S, et al: Fresh frozen plasma contains viable progenitor cells-should we irradiate. Vox Sang 1994; 67:405. (letter)
50. Davey RJ, McCoy NC, Yu M, et al: The effect of pre-storage irradiation on post- transfusion red cell survival. Transfusion 1992; 32:525-28.
51. Mintz PD, Anderson G: Effect of gamma irradiation on the in vivo recovery of stored red blood cells. Ann Clin Lab Sci 1993; 23:216-20.

52. Moroff G, Holme S, Heaton A, et al: Effect of gamma irradiation on viability of AS-3.h WC, Cimino DF: The effect of pre-storage gamma irradiation on post-transfusion red blood cell recovery. Transfusion 1991;31:50S, (abstr).

53. Moroff G, Holme S, AuBuchon JP, et al: Viability and in vitro properties of AS-1 red cells after gamma irradiation. Transfusion 1999; 39:128-34.
54. Moroff G, George VM, Siegl AM, et al: The influence of irradiation on stored platelets. Transfusion 1986; 26:453-56.
55. Ramirez AM, Woodfield DG, Scott R, et al: High potassium levels in stored irradiated blood. Transfusion 1987; 27:444-45.
56. Rivet C, Baxter A, Rock G: Potassium levels in irradiated blood. Transfusion 1989; 29:185.
57. Swann ID, Williamson LM: Potassium loss from leukodepleted red cells following γ-irradiation. Vox Sang 1996; 70:117-18.
58. Strauss RG: Routine washing of irradiated red cells before transfusion seems unwarranted. Transfusion 1990; 30:675-77.
59. Luban NLC, Strauss RG, Hume HA: Commentary on the safety of red cells preserved in extended-storage media for neonatal transfusion. Transfusion 1991; 31:229-35.
60. Espersen GT, Ernst E, Christiansen OB. et al: Irradiated blood platelet concentrates stored for five days-evaluation by in vitro tests. Vox Sang 1988; 55:218-21.
61. Duguid JK, Carr R, Jenkins JA, et al: Clinical evaluation of the effects of storage time and irradiation on transfused platelets. Vox Sang 1991; 60:151-54.
62. Read EJ, Kodis C, Carter CS, et al: Viability of platelets following storage in the irradiated state. A paired-controlled study. Transfusion 1988; 28:446-50.
63. Rock G, Adams GA, Labow RS: The effects of irradiation on platelet function. Transfusion 1988;28:451-55.
64. Sweeney JD, Holme S, Moroff G: Storage of apheresis platelets after gamma irradiation. Transfusion 1994; 34:779-83.
65. Seghatchian MJ, Stivala JFA: Effect of 25 Gy gamma irradiation on storage stability of three types of platelet concentrates: a comparative analysis with paired controls and random preparation. Transfus Sci 1995; 16:121-29.
66. Bessos H, Atkinson A, Murphy WG, et al: A comparison of in vitro storage markers between gamma-irradiated and non-irradiated apheresis platelet concentrates. Transfus Sci 1995; 16:131-34.
67. Anderson KC, Goodnough LT, Sayers M, et al: Variation in blood component irradiation practice: Implications for prevention of transfusion-associated graft- versus-host disease. Blood 1991; 77:2096-102.
68. Wolber RA, Duque RE, Robinson JP, Oberman HA. Oxidative product formation in irradiated neutrophils. A flow cytometric analysis. Transfusion 1987; 27:167-70.

69. Wheeler JG, Abramson JS, Ekstrand K. Function of irradiated polymorphonuclear leukocytes obtained by buffy-coat centrifugation. Transfusion 1984;24:238-39.
70. Patrone F, Dallegri F, Brema F, Sacchetti C. Effects of irradiation and storage on granulocytes harvested by continuous-flow centrifugation. Exp Hematol 1979;7: 131-36.
71. Valerius HN, Johansen KS, Nielsen OS, Platz P, Rosenkvist J. Sorensen H. Effect of in vitro X-irradiation on lymphocyte and granulocoyte function. Scand J Haematol 1981;27:9-18.
72. Rosen NR, Weidner JG, Bold HD, et al: Prevention of transfusion-associated graft-versus-host disease: selection of an adequate dose of gamma irradiation. Transfusion 1993; 33:125-27.
73. Quinones RR, Gutierrez RH, Dinndorf PA, et al. Extended cycle elutriation to adjust T-cell content in HLA-disparate bone marrow transplantation. Blood 1993;82:307-17.
74. Pelszynski MM, Moroff G, Luban NLC, et al: Effect of gammą irradiation of red blood cell units on T-cell inactivation as assessed by limiting dilution analysis: implications for preventing transfusion-associated graft-versus-host disease. Blood 1994; 83: 1683-89.
75. Luban NLC, Drothler D, Moroff G, et al: Irradiation of platelet components: inhibition of lymphocyte proliferation assessed by limiting dilution analysis. Transfusion 2000; 40:348-52.
76. Center for Biologics Evaluation and Research, Food and Drug Administration: Recommendations regarding license amendments and procedures for gamma irradiation of blood products. Department of Health and Human Services, July 22, 1993.
77. Moroff G, Luban NL. The irradiation of blood and blood components to prevent graft-versus-host disease: technical issues and guidelines. Transfus Med Rev 1997; 11:15-26.
78. Masterson ME, Febo R: Pre-transfusion blood irradiation: Clinical rationale and dosimetric considerations. Med Phys 1992; 19:649-57.
79. Leitman SF, Silberstein L, Fairman RM, et al: Use of a radiation-sensitive film label in the quality control of irradiated blood components. Transfusion 1992; 32:4S (abstr).
80. Luban NLC, Fearon T, Leitman SF, et al: Absorption of gamma irradiation in simulated blood components using cesium irradiators. Transfusion 1995; 35:63S, (abstr).
81. Lin L, Cook DN, Wiesehahn GP, et al. Photochemical inactivation of viruses and bacteria in human platelet concentrates using a novel psoralen and long wavelength UV light. Transfusion 1997;37:423.
82. Hei DJ, Grass J, Lin L, Corash L, Cimino G. Elimination of cytokine production in stored platelet concentrate aliquots by photochemical treatment with psoralen plus ultraviolet A light. Transfusion 1999;39:239-48.
83. Grass JA, Hei DJ, Metchette K, et al. Inactivation of leukocytes in platelet concentrates by psoralen plus UVA. Blood 1998;91:2180-88.

84. Grass JA, Wafa T, Reames A, et al. Prevention of transfusion-associated graft-versus-host disease by photochemical treatment. Blood 1999;93: 3140-47.
85. Fast LD, DiLeone G, Edson CM, Purmal A. PEN110 treatment functionally inactivates the PBMNCs present in RBC units: comparison to the effects of exposure to gamma irradiation. Transfusion 2002;42:1318-25.
86. del Rosario ML, Zuclai JR, Kao KJ. Prevention of graft-versus-host disease by induciton of immune tolerance with ultraviolet B-irradiated leukocytes in H-2 diparate bone marrow donor. Blood 1999;15:3558-64.
87. Hutchinson K, Kopko PM, Muto KN, et al. Early diagnosis and successful treatment of a patient with transfusion-associated GVHD with autologous peripheral blood progenitor cell transplantation. Transfusion 2003;42: 1567-72.

NON-IMMUNE, NON-INFECTIOUS COMPLICATIONS OF TRANSFUSION

P.T. Pisciotto[1]

Introduction

Some of the more frequent adverse effects of transfusion that are seen in older children and adults, such as immunologically mediated febrile or allergic reactions, are rarely reported in the newborn. Neonates, however, are more vulnerable to metabolic complications and susceptible to potential toxic effects of various compounds as a result of the immature nature of their organ systems. Transfusion practices for neonates are continually changing as medical advances are made in the care of these critically ill newborns. Recent data shows that there is a decrease in overall administration of neonatal transfusions with most red blood cell (RBC) transfusions being given to infants who are less than 1000 g or extremely low birth weight (ELBW) infants [1,2]. These ELBW infants often have major clinical problems as a result of their prematurity. Even though the use of surfactant has reduced the mortality from respiratory failure, the vast majority of infants will need some form of assisted ventilation requiring clinical monitoring [3]. A high percentage of infants will have cardiovascular problems in the form of a patent ductus arteriosus (PDA) that may require either medical or surgical treatment and careful fluid balance [4]. Fluid and electrolyte management is a challenge in these ELBW infants. As a result of the large surface area to body weight ratio and an underdeveloped epidermis evaporative losses can be significant. The immature kidney has limited concentrating ability providing a large amount of dilute urine. These infants therefore are vulnerable to dehydration and hyperosmolality, which may increase the risk for intraventricular hemorrhage (IVH) [4]. Electrolyte abnormalities such as hypernatraemia, hyponatraemia and hyperkalaemia are frequently seen, the latter occurring even in the absence of oliguria and potassium intake [5]. Acid and base imbalance will also vary depending on the degree of renal maturity. Glucose homeostasis is a problem as a result of poor glycogen stores and the immaturity of the adaptive mechanism of the endocrine system to control glucose levels. Because of the slow metabolic adaptation, rapid and significant changes in glucose intake are usually avoided. Calcium homeostasis is also altered as a result of renal imma-

1. Department of Laboratory Medicine, University of Connecticut Health Center, Farmington, CT, USA.

turity and parathyroid dysfunction [4]. The other groups of infants who regularly receive transfusions are those requiring exchange transfusions, extra–corporeal membrane oxygenation (ECMO) and cardiopulmonary bypass. Each of these procedures, which often involve either preterm or full term infants, require a massive transfusion since it involves exchange of the infant's blood volume multiple times. These procedures, in combination with organ immaturity of the infant will potentiate the metabolic complications that are associated with massive transfusion.

Extended Storage/Additive Solutions

CPDA-1 has been the preferred anticoagulant/red cell storage solution for neonatal transfusion for some time [6]. As a result of concern regarding donor exposure in the neonatal period strategies to limit donor exposure have been explored. Feasibility studies looking at the safety of using extended storage of red cells were first performed using CPDA-1 RBCs. Lui et al. [7], in a prospective randomized study in very low birth weight infants (VLBW) less than 1500 g looked at the efficacy and safety of using fresh CPDA-1 RBCs (less than 5 days) versus CPDA-1 RBCs stored for an extended period. The study found that donor exposure was decreased without incidence of hyperkalaemia or acidosis. A similar finding was observed when extended storage CPDA-1 RBCs were used versus washed RBCs [8]. In both of these studies relatively few units were stored beyond 20 days and additive solution (AS) red cell units were not evaluated. The introduction of additive solutions for use as anticoagulant-preservatives has several advantages including storage for 42 days, increased plasma extraction and better flow characteristics since the final haematocrit is

Table 1. Formulation of anticoagulant-preservative

Constituent	CPD	CP2D	CPDA-1	AS-1	AS-3	AS-5
Volume (mL)	63	63	63	100	100	100
Final Hct (%)	70-75	70-75	70-75	55-60	55-60	55-60
Sodium chloride (mg)	None	None	None	900	410	877
Dextrose (mg)	1610	3220	2010	2200	1100	900
Adenine (mg)	None	None	17.3	27	30	30
Mannitol (mg)	None	None	None	750	None	525
Trisodium citrate (mg)	1660	1660	1660	None	588	None
Citric acid (mg)	188	188	188	None	42	None
Sodium phosphate (mg)	140	140	140	None	276	None
Final Hct RBC Unit (%)	70-75	70-75	70-75	55-60	55-60	55-60
Storage Time (days)	21	21	35	42	42	42

approximately 60%. Improvement over CPDA-1 is ascribed to increased levels of dextrose and adenine for intracellular metabolism and in some additive solutions also mannitol, which diminishes red cell lysis (Table 1). Concerns, how ever, have been raised over the safety of transfusing additive solutions into neonates, particularly when units may be fresh or transfusion volumes are large. Metabolites of adenine are known to be nephrotoxic in animal studies. Approximately 5% of adenine that is infused is converted to 2,8-dioxyadenine (DOA) in vivo, which is insoluble and precipitates in kidney tubules [9]. Renal toxicity is also a concern with mannitol infusion, as well as the potential for a diuretic effect, which may cause unacceptable fluctuations in cerebral blood flow in infants that are already at risk for IVH. The ability to handle glucose and citrate loads has also been questioned. A theoretical model, looking at the amount of additive solution transfused in a small volume transfusion of AS-1 RBCs at a Hct of either 80% or 60% versus toxic levels suggests that there should be no substantial risk with small volume transfusions [10]. The metabolic and physiologic safety of AS-1 RBCs has also been demonstrated in ELBW infants through controlled, randomized studies. Sixteen premature infants (mean birth weight 863 g) were randomized to receive either CPDA-1 or ADSOL (AS-1) RBCs less than 5 days old at a dose of 17 mL/kg in a randomized double blind crossover study. AS-1 RBC units were utilized unmanipulated with a hct of approximately 60% versus CPDA-1 RBC units with a Hct of approximately 75%. All blood was irradiated, filtered and infused over 3 hours, with all other non-essential intravenous (I.V.) fluids discontinued. Glucose homeostasis was better preserved with AS-1 RBCs than observed with CPDA-1 RBC [11]. In terms of mannitol or adenine effects there was no difference in urine output or osmolality measured in a 24 hour urine pre and post transfusion and there was no difference in serum creatinine or BUN measured out to 4 hours post transfusion. There was a persistent increase (measured out to 4 hours post transfusion) in ammonia levels over baseline with both types of components used, but the concentrations remained below clinically significant levels. It was postulated that this might have represented an excessive load of ammonia for the immature infant to metabolize. The post transfusion hemoglobin was lower, reflecting the lower Hct of the aliquot transfused. A follow-up study of AS-1 red cells used out to 21 days showed similar results [12]. Additional studies looking at transfusing AS-1 and AS-3 RBC units to outdate versus fresh CPDA-1 RBC units (< 7days) showed no evidence of transfusion reactions, no metabolic changes and decreased donor exposure [13,14]. In these studies infants were transfused with 15 mL/kg over 5 hours. Red blood cells were packed to a hct of approximately 85% removing a large proportion of the additive solution and the blood was gamma-irradiated just prior to transfusion. Twenty to 30% of units transfused were older than 22 days. Renal and hepatic chemistry tests as well as 2,3-DPG levels were measured weekly in infants receiving fresh CPDA-1 units versus stored AS-1 units and there was no clinically significant difference detected [13]. These studies support the calculated model predicting that the use of additive solution red cells, even without additional processing, poses no substantial risk when used for small volume transfusions in the premature infant.

Clinical studies comparing the relative safety of using AS red cells in the setting of a large volume transfusion (either in the form of exchange transfusion, massive blood loss or ECMO) have not been performed. Performance of exchange transfusion for hyperbilirubinaemia using either AS-1 RBCs or red cells collected in saline adenine glucose mannitol (SAGM) unmodified has been associated with the development of hypoproteinaemia/hypoabluminaemia post transfusion, returning to near baseline levels within one day [15,16]. Decreased availability of albumin in the setting of increased bilirubin levels can potentially increase the risk for bilirubin toxicity. Based on theoretical mathematical calculation the use of reconstituted whole blood using AS-1 RBC and CPD plasma in the exchange transfusion setting could pose problems with glucose and citrate doses infused [10] (Table 2). This will be discussed further in the respective metabolic sections. The amount of adenine and mannitol infused in this particular setting is relatively small since a large proportion of these additives are removed during the preparation of the reconstituted component. As a result of the continuous infusion of blood and components in the setting of ECMO or cardiac bypass surgery it is difficult, even on a theoretical basis, to determine the amount of these constituents that may be present at any time period. Due to the uncertainty however, it has been suggested that removal of additive solution through centrifugation or washing and resuspension in appropriate fluid should be considered [10].

Table 2. Quantity of additives infused during exchange transfusion with reconstituted wholeblood* in a 3 kg infant

Additive	Reconstituted Whole Blood (mg/mL)	Total Transfused (mg)	Transfusion (mg/kg)	Potential Toxic Dose (mg/kg)
Dextrose	5.60	1075.0	358.0	240/hour
Sodium	1.00	192.0	64.0	137/day
Citrate	2.70	518.0	173.0	180/hour
Phosphate	0.16	31.0	10.0	>60/day
Adenine	0.04	7.7	2.6	15/dose
Mannitol	0.22	42.0	14.0	360/day

* One unit of reconstituted whole blood using AS-1 RBCs and CPD plasma - calculated for a one volume exchange (80 mL/kg) total volume of 240 mL with 192 mL retention. Modified from Luban et al. [10

Metabolic Complications

Hypoglycaemia/Hyperglycaemia – Impaired glucose homeostasis is a major concern in the premature infant. Glucose turnover relates to the production of glucose by the liver in relationship to use by the brain and other tissues. Turnover in neonates (4-8 mg/dL) greatly exceeds that of adults and is greatest in premature infants due in part to the ratio of brain to body mass, emphasizing the importance of glucose as fuel for the brain. Unfortunately there is no definitive data as to the exact level of glucose at which hypoglycaemic-induced neurodevelopmental sequelae may occur. Since infants who are hypoglycaemic are often asymptomatic, or when symptoms are present they tend to be non-specific and variable, monitoring of infants using chemical analysis is usually performed. The chemical definition of hypoglycaemia is a plasma glucose level of <40 mg/dL in the first 24 hours or <45 mg/dL subsequently [17]. The incidence of hypoglycaemia occurring in premature infants has been reported to be 1.5% to 5.5%. Concern that hypoglycemia during routine transfusions may go unrecognized was first raised in 1985 [18]. This was based on a report of 14 episodes of severe hypoglycemia (<2 μmol/L [<40 mg/dL]) in 6 infants (BW 650 to 1530 g) receiving CPDA-1 blood or FFP whose blood glucose was otherwise stable. During the transfusions all other I.V. fluids were discontinued. Glucose homeostasis was monitored in 16 premature infants with a mean BW of 863 g and gestational age of 26 weeks who received transfusions with either CPDA-1 or AS-1 RBCs at 17 ml/kg over 3 hours [11]. All other non-essential I.V. fluids were discontinued. Glucose levels were monitored before transfusion and then every 30 to 60 minutes using glucose oxidase strips. Glucose was administered if levels fell <40 mg/dL or there were clinical symptoms. One hour into the infusion the glucose levels dropped by 42% ± 11 with AS-1 RBCs and 54% ± 13 with CPDA-1 RBCs and continued to drop throughout the transfusion. Supplemental glucose was required within 2 hours of the transfusion in 64% of the infants transfused with CPDA-1 RBCs and 15% of the infants transfused with AS-1 RBCs. A higher percentage of the infants remained euglycaemic with AS-1 RBCs as a result of the higher glucose concentration in this component. A similar incidence (16%) of transfusion-associated hypoglycaemia was observed with older units of AS-1 RBCs (out to 21 days), despite decreasing glucose concentrations in stored units [12]. Based on calculated amounts of additive solutions in CPDA1 and AS-1 RBCs [10] the infusion of 17 ml/kg over 3 hours as in the study above, without any additional I.V., would drop the glucose infusion to approximately 0.4 mg/kg/min and 0.8 mg/kg/min respectively. This is well below the glucose infusion necessary to maintain euglycaemia.

Hypoglycaemia has also been reported to occur in association with exchange transfusion. A retrospective review of adverse effects of exchange transfusion spanning a 15-year time period (1980-1995) reported that 106 neonates out of 15,000 neonatal admissions (0.7%) underwent 140 exchange transfusions [19]. Two infants developed hypoglycaemia (1.4% of exchange transfusion) described as mild and asymptomatic. (Jackson) ABO-compatible Whole Blood collected in CPDA-1 or group O CPDA-1 RBCs resuspended in compatible plasma were used for the exchange. Hypoglycemia occurring in this scenario is the result of high glucose loads that stimulate endogenous insulin secretion and rebound hypoglycaemia [20]. The intermittent infusion of glucose from the donor blood masks the hypoglycemia effect of increased insulin secretion that occurs during the exchange. Therefore the glucose levels usually reach a nadir at approximately 2 hours after the exchange transfusion. Infants who are hypoglycaemic before the exchange are more prone to this effect.

Neonatal hyperglycemia is a concern in the premature infant since it has been postulated that the change in osmolality that may occur (each 18 mg/dL of blood glucose adds 1 mOsm/dL) could result in rapid fluid shifts in the brain, which in turn may increase the risk of intraventricular haemorrhage [17]. Hyperglycemia in the premature infant is usually defined as a glucose level of greater than 150 mg/dL. There are several factors that have been attributed to the hyperglycemia that is observed in very premature infants including decreased insulin production, peripheral insulin resistance, decreased or abnormal insulin receptors and stress, which results in mobilization of glycogen stores [21]. The reported incidence of hyperglycemia in premature infants has ranged from 20% to 72% [21]. The increased glucose loads that are associated with a large volume transfusion may not be well tolerated in an ELBW infant, particularly in clinical situations (i.e. sepsis) where the infant may already be at increased risk for hyperglycemia. This may be of particular concern in infants who may require transfusion during surgical procedures under general anesthesia, since this has been associated with the development of hyperglycemia [22].

Hypocalcaemia – As with hypoglycaemia, neonatal hypocalcaemia may also be asymptomatic. Total calcium levels < 7 mg/dL in premature infants or ionized calcium levels below 3.0mg/dL are abnormal. Low levels of ionized calcium are associated with a prolongation of the QT interval, indicating a measurable effect on cellular excitability, even though the heart rate remains stable [23]. Decreased ionized calcium has been reported to occur in both full term and premature infants in association with exchange transfusion. Sodium citrate used as an anticoagulant binds ionized calcium and the citrate load infused during exchange transfusion can reach extremely high levels (Table 2). Citrate levels in the bloodstream will depend on several factors including the rate and duration of administration, the recipient's blood volume, and the recipient's ability to metabolize and excrete the compound. Citrate is metabolized to bicarbonate by the liver, kidney and skeletal muscle and usually does not cause a problem until the rate of infusion exceeds the rate of metabolism and excretion. Exchange transfusions are usually performed at a rate that is no faster than 5 mL/kg BW/3 minutes. In a 3 kg infant this would calculate to a citrate load of approximately 3-4 mg/kg/minute infused into a plasma compartment of less than 150 mL. The kidney and liver, which are the main sites of citrate metabolism, are not fully functional in the neonate and muscle mass is small. Conditions such as hypothermia and acidosis will reduce the clearance of citrate from the kidney and liver [24]. The decrease in ionized calcium associated with exchange transfusion in the neonate tends to follow a pattern. There is a significant and rapid decrease in calcium within the first 100 to 200 mL with a slower decrease thereafter and return to normal within the first hour post exchange [25]. Symptomatic hypocalcaemia was one of the more serious morbidities in a retrospective review of 106 infants who underwent exchange transfusion [19]. Four (5%) of 81 healthy infants had transient symptomatic hypocalcaemia associated with electrocardiogram changes, irritability and jitteriness and 28 (34.6%) additional infants had asymptomatic hypocalcaemia. Two of 25 ill infants (8%) developed symptomatic hypocalcaemia with one experiencing a cardiac arrest. Ten additional infants (40%) developed asymptomatic hypocalcaemia. These were all double volume exchange transfusions performed using either ABO-compatible whole blood anticoagulated with CPDA-1 or group O CPDA-1 RBCs resuspended in compatible plasma. All blood was less than 5 days old and the exchange was completed within 2 hours.

Hyperkalaemia – Hyperkalaemia is one of the most life threatening electrolyte disturbances in the newborn. Plasma potassium levels in the premature infant rise over the first few days even in the absence of exogenous potassium intake. This increase is the result of several factors including immaturity of the renal distal tubules, a relative hyopaldosteronism and a potassium shift from the intracellular to the extracellular compartment [26]. The development of hyperkalaemia in the premature infant has been associated with cardiac arrhythmias [27]. Hyperkalaemia in the newborn can also occur as a result of excessive iatrogenic administration and has been reported following massive transfusion [28,29]. Plasma potassium increases progressively in Whole Blood and RBCs with storage, as a result of leakage of intracellular potassium, reaching concentrations of 75-100 mEq/L in CPDA-1 RBCs by 35 days and approximately 50 mEq/L in AS RBCs by 42 days. Irradiation of red cells prior to storage potentiates the storage lesion of red cells with increased plasma potassium concentration from what is normally observed occurring within 48 hours of irradiation [30]. Total potassium concentration infused is relative to the amount of plasma present in the component. The morbidity of transfusion-associated hyperkaalemia depends on the quantity of blood transfused, the extracellular potassium concentration, rate of transfusion, site of infusion, the intracellular versus extracellular distribution of potassium in the recipient and the clinical condition of the recipient. There are several clinical conditions that can alter potassium distribution influencing the risk of hyperkalaemia including acid-base status, previous potassium load, renal function and medication. Evidence based medicine has shown that small volume transfusions (i.e.15 mL/kg) of stored red cells out to expiration administered slowly over 3 to 4 hours usually does not pose a problem in relatively healthy infants [31]. If one calculates the amount of potassium infused in this scenario it does not come near the infant's daily requirement. However, in situations where there is rapid blood transfusion, particularly in conjunction with low cardiac output and the use of a central venous access, there usually is not sufficient time for an appreciable amount of potassium to be redistributed between extracellular and intracellular compartments resulting in hyperkalaemia and potential cardiac arrest. Cardiac arrest reported in a 14 day old infant was associated with the infusion of 60 mL of 32 day old blood, with a plasma concentration of approximately 60 mEq/L, over 10 to 15 minutes into a CVP line during cardiac surgery [29]. It has been determined that the ratio of transfusion rate to venous return, defined as the cardiac output plus the transfusion rate, is important in terms of potassium concentration and development of hyperkalaemia [32]. When the ratio was <0.1 clinically dangerous levels of potassium were not identified, but if the rate were >0.7 the transfusion of even potassium poor plasma (10 mEq/L) could result in hyperkalaemia and when plasma potassium levels in transfused blood were in the range of 20 mEq/L rates of <0.3 could result in dangerous levels of serum potassium. Therefore in the setting of massive transfusion the freshest component available or processing of the unit (i.e. washing or centrifugation with removal of supernatant) to minimize plasma supernatant and therefore potassium concentration should be considered if time permits.

While iatrogenic hyperkalaemia associated with transfusion is recognize to occur with stored RBCs other conditions may alter the integrity of transfused red cells resulting in release of potassium. There are numerous non-immuno–logic causes of haemolysis including excessive infusion pressure, freezing or overheating blood, or addition of incompatible I.V. fluids or medications to blood units. Inherited abnormalities of transfused red cells such as red cells deficient in glucose-6-phosphate dehydrogenase (G-6PD) or red cells from donors with sickle cell trait have been reported to cause hemolysis in the neonate and is of particular concern in those infants who may be severely stressed or hypoxic [34,35]. An increase in potassium as a result of hemolysis would most likely be associated with other indications of red cell damage such as hyperbilirubinaemia and possibly haemoglobinuria. Once immunologic causes of haemolysis have been ruled out it is important to investigate other reasons for red cell destruction.

Potential Toxicities of Transfusion

Plasticizer – Polyvinyl chloride plastics (PVC) are used in a wide array of medical devices including feeding tubes, umbilical catheters, ECMO circuits, endotracheal tubes, blood bags and intravenous tubing. Plasticizer is added to PVC in order to impart flexibility and durability. One of the most common in use is di-2-ethylhexyl phthalate (DEHP), which is a lyphophilic compound. Medical devices have been reported to contain on average 30% to 40% DEHP by weight [35]. Since DEHP is not chemically bound to the plastic matrix it, has been shown to leach into biological fluids containing lipid, such as all blood components. The concentration present in a blood bag depends on the temperature, duration of storage and composition or lipid content of the component [38]. DEHP is metabolized to its toxic metabolite mon-(2-ethylhexyl)-phthalate (MEHP) and, in the healthy individual, is rapidly excreted by the kidneys as conjugated (glucuronide) oxidation products of MEHP. Premature and full term infants do not have mature glucoronidation and therefore MEHP may have a longer half-life in the body. Toxicological studies in animals, and in vitro, have linked exposure to DEHP and metabolites to adverse effects of the liver, kidneys, heart, lung, reproductive system as well fetal effects [35,36]. The developing testis may be more susceptible to the testicular toxicity of DEHP with the Sertoli cells being the likely target. While high levels of DEHP have been observed in infants undergoing exchange transfusion and ECMO, no evidence of acute toxicity has been reported to date [37,38]. There have been no studies evaluating the effect of DEHP exposure on testicular function in humans. The extraction of DEHP has been found to directly correlate with the duration of exposure, which is higher for infants on ECMO then those undergoing exchange transfusion or cardiopulmonary bypass. Little release of DEHP has been observed with the use of heparin-coated tubing [38]. Further research would be necessary to determine which toxic effects seen in animals may also be present in humans. The Centers for Devices and Radiological Health of The Food and Drug Administration (FDA) have recommended that procedures should not be avoided but that substitute devices should be used if possible and if not, attempts should be made to minimize exposure by using the freshest blood component stored at the lowest temperature and heparin-coated tubing should be used in circuits [39].

Lead Exposure – Lead is known to be toxic to the nervous system, but there is no well-defined threshold level at which lead-associated deficits will develop. There has been an association established between the exposure of low to moderate levels of lead in early childhood and modest declines in psychometric intelligence [40]. The Centers for Diseases Control and Prevention (CDC) and the World Health Organization (WHO) have set a blood lead concentration of 10 μg/dL or higher as a level of concern [41,42]. A recent report indicates that blood lead concentrations even below 10 μg/dL have been found to be inversely associated with children's IQ scores at three and five years of age [43].

The lifetime average blood lead concentration, which was determined by computing the area under the blood lead curve from 6 though 36 months or 6 through 60 months of age and dividing by the corresponding age span, was found to best reflect chronic exposure. There are several environmental sources of lead exposure. Data has shown that blood transfusions represent a source of lead exposure for premature infants [44]. Concentration of lead in blood units has been reported to range from 0 to 19 μg/L (median 2.5 μg/L). A lead concentration in packed RBCs that was $\geq$ 5 mg/dL did result in an elevated post-transfusion blood lead in some infants [44]. A dose response relationship between the amount of lead in the transfused blood and the increase in lead concentration was determined and for every μg of lead transfused over a dose of 1.5 μg/kg there was a linear increase in post transfusion lead. However, there was no significant effect of lead dose on lead concentration in the infants by 4 weeks of age, and therefore no evidence of long-term elevation [44]. Further investigation would be necessary before definitive recommendations for routine screening of blood for lead levels could be determined.

References

1. Wildness JA, Seward VJ, Kromer IJ, Burmeister LF, Bell EF, Strauss RJ. Changing patterns of red blood cell transfusion in very low birth weight infants. J Pediatr 1996;129:680-87.
2. Maier RF, Sonntag J, Walka MM, Liu G, Metze BC, Obladen M. Changing practices of red blood cell transfusions in infants with birth weights less than 1000 g. J Pediatr 2000;136:220-24.
3. Corbet A, Bucciarelli R, Goldman S, Mammel M, Wold D, Long W. Decreased mortality rate among small premature infants treated at birth with a single dose of synthetic surfactant: A multicenter controlled trial. J Pediatr 1991;118:277-84.
4. Papageorgiou A, Bardin CL. The extremely-low-birth-weight infant. In; Avery GB, Fletcher MA, MacDonald MG, eds. Neonatal pathophysiology and management of the newborn. Philadelphia: Lippincott, Williams & Wilkens, 1999:445-72.
5. Sato K, Tsutomu K, Iwao H, Ueda K. Internal potassium shift in premature infants: cause of nonoliguric hyperkalemia. J Pediatr 1995;126:109-13.
6. Levy GJ, Strauss RG, Hume H et al. National survey of neonatal transfusion practices: I. Red blood cell therapy. Pediatrics 1993;91:523-29.
7. Liu EA, Mannino FL, Lane TA. Prospective, randomized trial of the safety and efficacy of a limited donor exposure transfusion program for premature neonates. J Pediatr 1994;125:92-96.
8. Lee DA, Slagle TA, Jackson TM, Evans CS. Reducing blood donor exposure in low birth weight infants by the use of older, unwashed packed red blood cells. J Pediatr 1995; 126:280-86.
9. Simon ER. Adenine in blood banking. Transfusion 1977;17:317-25.
10. Luban NLC, Strauss RG, Hume HA. Commentary on the safety of red cells preserved in extended-storage media for neonatal transfusions. Transfusion 1991;31: 229-35.
11. Goodstein MEL, Locke RG, Wlodarczyk D, Goldsmith LS, Rubenstein SD, Herman JH. A comparison of two preservation solutions for erythrocyte transfusions in newborn infants. J Pediatr 1993;123:783-88.
12. Goodstein MH, Herman JH, Smith JF, Rubenstein SD. Metabolic consequences in very low birth weight infants transfused with older AS-1 preserved erythrocytes. Pediatr Pathol Lab Med 1999;18:173-85.
13. Strauss RG, Burmeister LF, Johnson K, et al. AS-1 red cells for neonatal transfusions: a randomized trial assessing donor exposure and safety. Transfusion 1996;36: 873-78.
14. Strauss RG, Burmeister LF, Johnson K, Cress G, Cordle D. Feasibility and safety of AS-3 red blood cells for neonatal transfusions. J Pediatr 2000; 136:215-19.
15. Tuchschmid P, Mieth D, Burger R, Duc G. Potential hazard of hypoalbuminemia in newborn babies after exchange transfusions with ADSOL red blood cell concentration (letter). Pediatrics 1990;85:234-35.

16. Ryan SW, Bhadura B, Harran MJ. Concern over safety of SAGM blood. (letter) Arch Dis Child 1988;63:104.
17. McGowen JE, Hagedorn ML, Price WR, Hay WW. Glucose homeostasis. In: Merenstein GB, Gardner SL, eds. Handbook of neonatal intensive care. St Louis: Mosby Year Book, 1993:169-83.
18. MacMahon P, Jones ST, Kovar IZ. Hypoglycemia and blood transfusion in the newborn (letter). Lancet 1985;2:388.
19. Jackson JC. Adverse events associated with exchange transfusion in healthy and ill newborns. Pediatrics 1997;99:E7.
20. Schiff D, Arabda JV, Colle E, Stern L. Metabolic effects of exchange transfusion. II. Delayed hypoglycemia following exchange transfusion with citrated blood. J Pediatr 1971;79:589-93.
21. Pildes RS. Neonatal hyperglycemia. J Pediatr 1986;109:905-7.
22. Srinivasin G, Jain RS, Kannan CR. Glucose homeostasis during anesthesia and surgery in infants. J Pediatr Surg 1986;21:718-21.
23. Colletti RB, Pan MW, Smith EWP, Genell M. Detection of hypocalcemia in susceptible neonates: The Q-oTc interval. N Engl J Med 1974;290:931-35.
24. Dzik WH, Kirkley SA. Citrate toxicity during massive blood tansfusion. Transfus Med Rev 1988;2:7a6-94.
25. Gershanik JJ, Levkoff AH, Duncan R. Serum ionized calcium values in relation to exchange transfusion. J Pediatr 1973;82:847-50.
26. Lorenz JM, Kleinmman LI, Markarian K. Potassium metabolism in extremely low birth weight infants in the first week of life. J Pediatr 1997;131: 81-86.
27. Shortland D, Trounce JQ, Levene MI. Hyperkalemia, cardiac arrhythmias, and cerebral lesions in high-risk infants. Arch Dis Child 1987;62:1139-42.
28. Scanlon JW, Krakaur R. Hyperkalemia following exchange transfusion. J Pediatr 1980;96:108-10.
29. Hall TL, Barnes A, Miller JR et al Neonatal mortality following transfusion of red cells with high potassium levels. Transfusion 1993;33:616-19.
30. Hillyer CD, Tiegerman KO, Berkman EM. Evaluation of the red cell storage lesion after irradiation in filtered packed red cell units. Transfusion 1991;31:497-99.
31. Strauss RG. Data-driven blood banking practices for neonatal RBC transfusions. Transfusion 2000;40:1528-40.
32. Brown KA, Bissonnette B, McIntyre B. Hyperkalemia during rapid blood transfusion and hypovolemic cardiac arrest in children. Can J Anaesth 1990; 37:747-54.
33. Minmouni F, Shohat S, Reisdner SH. G6PD deficient donor blood as a cause of haemolysis in two premature infants. Isr J Med Sci 1986;22:120-22.
34. Murphy RJC, Malhotra C, Sweet AY. Death following as exchange transfusion with hemoglobin SC blood. J Pediatr 1980;96:110-12.

35. Tickner JA, Schettler T, Guidotti T, McCally M, Rossi M. Health risks posed by use of di-2 ethyle phthalate (DEHP) in PVC medical devices: a critical review. Am J Ind Med 2001;39:100-11.
36. Latini G. Potential hazards of exposure to di-(2-ethylhexyl)-phthalate in babies. Biol Neonate 2000;78:269-76.
37. Shea KM. Pediatric exposure and potential toxicity of phthalate plasticizers. Pediatrics 2003;111:1467-74.
38. Karle VA, Short BL, Martin GR, et al. Extracorporeal membrane oxygenation exposis infants to the plasticizer, di(2-ethylhexyl)phthalate. Crit Care Med 1997;25: 696-703.
39. US Food and Drug Administration, Center for Devices and Radiological Health Safety assessment of di(2-ethylhexyl)phthalate (DEHP) released from PVC medical devices. Rockville, MD: Center for Devices and Radio–logic Health;2001. Available at: http://www.fda.gov/cdrh/ost/dehp-pvc.pdf.
40. Needleman H, Schell A, Bellinger D, Leviton A, Allred EN. The long term effects of exposure to low doses of lead in childhood: an 11-year follow-up report. N Engl J Med 1990;322:83-88.
41. Preventing lead poisoning in young children: a statement by the Centers for Disease Control, October 1991.
42. International Programme on Chemical Safety. Inorganic lead. Environmental health criteria 165. Geneva: World Health Organization, 1995.
43. Canfield RL, Henderson CR, Cory-Slechta DA, Cox C, Jusko TA, Lanphear BP. Intellectual impairment in children with blood lead concentrations below 10 µg per deciliter. N Engl J Med 2003;348:1517-26.
44. Bearer CF, O'Riordan MA, Powers, R. Lead exposure from blood transfusion to premature infants. J Pediatr 2000;137:549-54.

EXTRACORPOREAL MEMBRANE OXYGENATION IN THE NEONATE WITH RESPIRATORY FAILURE

N.L.C. Luban[1], B.L. Short[2]

Introduction

In 1944, Kolff and Berk observed that blood became oxygenated as it passed through cellophane chambers of an artificial kidney membrane [1]. This historic observation led to the recognition that blood could be oxygenated through a semipermeable membrane lung [2]. In 1956, the development of the first membrane lung, which used an ethylcellulose membrane [3], opened the door for the study of prolonged cardiopulmonary bypass and the potential application of extracorporeal membrane oxygenation (ECMO) as an artificial lung. The concept of an artificial placenta capable of continuing *ex utero* the gas-exchange functions of the placenta developed in parallel with that of an artificial lung. In 1961, Callaghan and colleagues began using animal models of respiratory distress syndrome (RDS) of the newborn to test the efficacy of an extracorporeal oxygenation circuit as an artificial placenta [3], which was later expanded to premature infants [4-6]. This was an extremely important period for the development and refinement of the mechanical and surgical techniques that laid the foundation for the subsequent success of ECMO. The full potential of ECMO for infants in severe respiratory failure was not realized until it was used on term infants. In 1976, Bartlett et al., reported the first neonatal ECMO survivor, a term infant with severe meconium aspiration syndrome (MAS) [7]. During the subsequent 10 years, neonatal ECMO was used to treat 99 term infants with respiratory failure in three centres in the United States with an overall survival rate of 65%. Since 1986, and more than 18,000 infants have been treated in more than 90 ECMO programs with an overall survival rate of 77% (Figure 1) [8]. ECMO is also being used to support the cardiac patient post-operatively and

1. Interim Executive Director, Center for Cancer and Blood Disorders, Chair Lab Med & Pathol, Director, Transfusion Medicine/The Edward J. Miller Donor Center Children's National Medical Center, Vice Chair for Academic Affairs, Dept of Pediatrics, Professor of Pediatrics and Pathology, The George Washington Univ School of Medicine, Washington, DC.
2. Chief, Div of Neonatology, Children's National Medical Center, Professor of Pediatrics, The George Washington Univ School of Medicine Washington, DC.

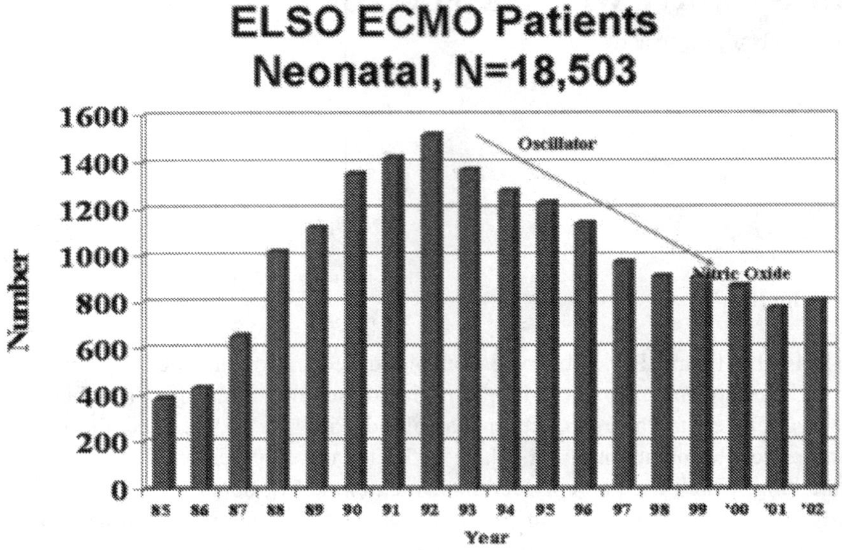

Figure 1. ECMO patients reported to the ELSO Registry.

the older child and adult in respiratory failure. This chapter will only address the use of ECMO in the neonatal patient with respiratory failure.

The most common use for ECMO is in the term or near-term infant in respiratory failure due to MAS, idiopathic persistent pulmonary hypertension (PPHN), congenital diaphragmatic hernia (CDH), sepsis and pneumonia, or hyaline membrane disease (HMD). Although overall survival is 77% nationally, the best results are for the MAS (94%) and PPHN (79%) groups. In some institutions, the survival rate for the MAS patient may be as high as 100%, PPHN 94%, and sepsis/pneumonia 100%. New therapies such as inhaled nitric oxide (iNO) and high frequency ventilation (HFV) have been added to the armamentarium of therapy, and some concerns have been raised that these may be delaying the initiation of ECMO. Survival does not seem to be adversely effected [9]. With the initiation of these additional therapies pre-ECMO, however, length of time an ECMO has increased from 5 to 9 days. Surfactant therapy and HFV have decreased the number of infants requiring ECMO. The survival rate for the CDH population requiring ECMO has not increased over time and remains between 50-60% nationally, perhaps because of the heterogeneity of this group of infants, with varying degrees of pulmonary hypoplasia and pulmonary hypertension [10,11]. Only 30% to 40% of the CDH population requires ECMO therapy, with a survival rate close to 100%. With ECMO therapy, the overall survival rate for the CDH population is over 70% with some centres reporting rates of 80% [12,13]. Most centres are now repairing the diaphragmatic defect in the critical CDH while the infants is on ECMO or immediately post ECMO [10].

The potential risks associated with ECMO therapy include those associated with ligation of the carotid artery (in venoarterial ECMO) and jugular vein, prolonged exposure to systemic heparinization, alterations in pulsatile blood flow patterns, exposure to potential toxins such as phthalate esters (i.e., plasticizer) from the circuit, and others yet to be determined [14,15]. With its long-term outcome still unknown, use of ECMO is presently limited to the term or near-term infant with a 20% or less chance of survival predicted with conventional therapy.

ECMO Criteria

Several important inclusion criteria for neonatal ECMO are based on known complications of the procedure and include:

1 – Age and weight limitations

The requirement for systemic heparinization of the ECMO patient places significant limitations on the population that can be treated. Use of ECMO in premature infants weighing less than 2,000 g or younger than 34 weeks gestation resulted in significant mortality from intracranial haemorrhage (ICH) [16-18]. This increased risk was likely the result of systemic heparinization combined with a direct effect of ECMO on the brain [19,20]. Once the pathophysiology of intracranial bleeds in ECMO are understood, therapies may alter the risk and thus permit lower application of their technique at a gestational age [19,20].

2 – Haematologic limitations

Systemic heparinization is required for the procedure which places the infant with a pre-existing coagulopathy or with bleeding complications at extreme risk. All attempts should be made to correct any coagulopathy before instituting ECMO. The septic infant is of particular concern because of the commonly associated coagulopathy. Correction of coagulopathy and meticulous heparin management has resulted in successful treatment of some septic infants [21]. The necessity for heparinization during ECMO precludes the treatment of infants with major ICH. Infants with grade I to II ICH or small parenchymal haemorrhages can be treated if heparin management is monitored closely and activated clotting times (ACTs) are kept low (e.g., 160 to 180 seconds).

3 – Prior mechanical ventilation

ECMO therapy is not initiated if the infant has been on assisted ventilation for 10-14 days; this is because of the probable development of chronic lung disease after aggressive assisted ventilation of this duration. ECMO cannot reverse this disease process within a safe period. After 3 weeks of ECMO, the risks for complications related to the ECMO procedure itself, such as clot formation, nosocomial infections (e.g., neck wound infections), and mechanical failures (e.g., tubing rupture), increase. The maximal time that a neonatal patient can be kept on ECMO is unknown, but in view of the increasing risk of complications and lack of response beyond 3 weeks, most centres limit time on the circuit to that period. Infants chronic lung disease, who do not improve in a short period, should not be considered for ECMO unless a life-threatening underlying disease state, like acute pulmonary hypertension or sepsis/pneumonia, known to be rapidly reversed by ECMO.

4 – Cardiopulmonary disease

Candidates for ECMO must have reversible lung disease and significant cardiac disease must be ruled out. However, infants with severe reversible lung disease superimposed on congenital heart disease may be candidates for ECMO support before cardiac surgery. Infants with congenital diaphragmatic hernia are excellent candidates for ECMO but intra-operative bleeding must be carefully controlled [22,23].

Pre-ECMO Procedures

Before transfer of a patient to an ECMO centre, studies should include an echocardiogram to rule out congenital heart disease; cranial ultrasound scan to rule out significant ICH; coagulation studies, including a partial thromboplastin time, prothrombin time, fibrinogen level, fibrin degradation products, and platelet count; calcium and electrolyte levels; leukocyte count with a differential; haemoglobin and haematocrit levels. These studies help the team at the ECMO centre determine whether the patient should be considered for ECMO and prepare the infant for transport with appropriate fluids. Blood group and antibody screen should be called to the referring hospital to provide the ECMO centre with the ability to assess inventory and be prepared for the infant's arrival.

On admission to the ECMO centre, the appropriateness of the patient as an ECMO candidate is assessed. The ultrasound examination of the central nervous system (CNS) is repeated to ensure that ICH did not occur during transport. If there is any question about the possibility of cardiac disease, the ECHO is repeated. Doppler flow techniques are used to document the severity of pulmonary hypertension, valuable data in the event that infant does not wean from ECMO. Serum electrolyte and calcium levels, haemoglobin and haematocrit, clotting studies including fibrinogen level, fibrin degradation products, partial thromboplastin and prothrombin times, platelet count, and a baseline ACT are obtained to detect abnormalities that require correction before initiation of ECMO.

The ECMO Procedure

Venoarterial Method

Venoarterial (VA) ECMO is the gold standard and involves the use of two catheters: venous outflow catheter is placed in the right internal jugular vein with with the tip in the right atrium and the arterial return catheter is placed in the

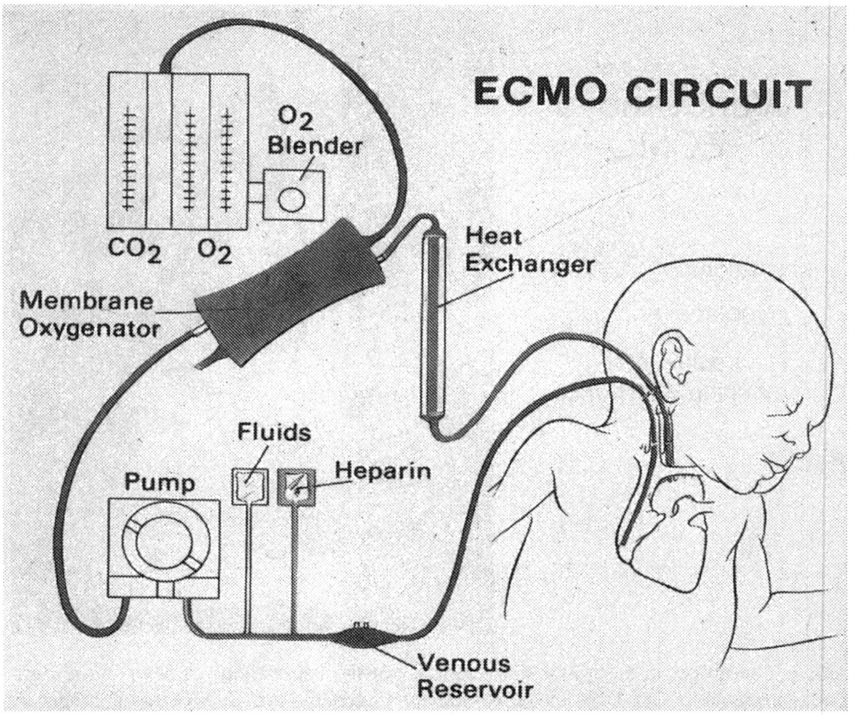

Figure 2. Components of the venoarterial extracorporeal membrane oxygenation circuit. (From Short BL. Physiology of extracorporeal membrane oxygenation (ECMO). In Polin RA, Fox WW, eds. Fetal and neonatal physiology. Philadelphia: WB Saunders, 1992:932.).

right carotid artery with the tip at the junction with the aortic arch. Blood is removed through the jugular catheter by means of gravity drainage into a venous reservoir (Figure 2). Blood is pulled out of the reservoir by a roller occlusion pump and pumped through the membrane lung, where gas exchange occurs. Gases transfer across the silicone membrane lung into the blood because of pressure gradients while increasing the oxygen level and removing carbon dioxide. Blood is then pumped into the heat exchanger, where it is warmed to body temperature and returned to the infant through the arterial catheter. This form of bypass provides both pulmonary and cardiac support. Oxygenation is achieved by allowing the pump to support as much of the cardiac output as is needed to oxygenate the infant, usually at 120 to 150 mL/kg/min in the first few days.

However, ligation of the carotid artery, alteration of pulsatile arterial blood flow patterns, and the possibility that particulate matter or air may enter the cerebral or coronary circulation remain as major concerns.

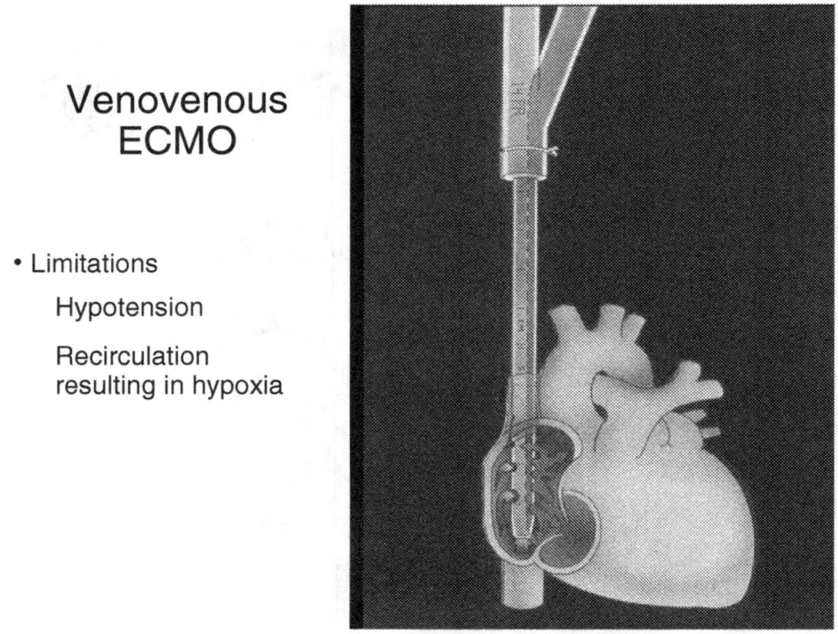

Figure 3. The inflow and outflow characteristics of the venovenous catheter in the right atrium. (From Short BL, O'Brien A, Poindexter C, eds. CNMC ECMO training manual. Washington, DC: CNMC, 1993.)

Venovenous Method

Venovenous (VV) techniques for ECMO have been developed to obviate the need for carotid ligation. In VV ECMO, a single double-lumen catheter is placed through the internal jugular vein into the right atrium (Figure 3) [24,25]. This catheter has inflow and outflow ports that attach to the circuit. Blood return and outflow occur in the right atrium so that recirculation occurs resulting in less oxygenation. Because the heart serves as the pump for VV ECMO, the use of this methodology depends on intact cardiac function. The advantages of this technique include no ligation of the carotid artery, maintenance of normal pulsatile blood flow, and the theoretical advantage that particulate matter entering the circuit enters through the lungs rather than the cerebral or coronary circulation. Disadvantages are the lack of cardiac support and limited oxygenation.

Equipment and Systems

ECMO equipment is essentially modified cardiopulmonary bypass circuitry designed for short-term use (Figure 4). The limitations of each element of the circuit must be understood and considered to ensure safe and effective use. Each ECMO centre designs an ECMO circuit using equipment evaluated and designed

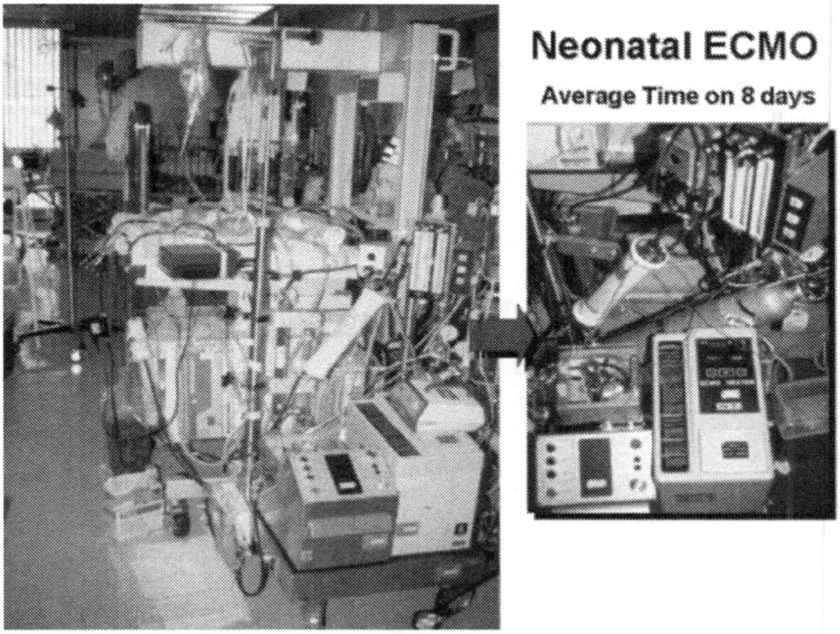

Figure 4. The extracorporeal membrane oxygenation system used at the Children's National Medical Center has a modular design.

to meet space and other unique requirements of their centre. Bioengineering experts and cardiopulmonary perfusionists are consulted in the design and evaluation of the ECMO circuit. The only membrane lung approved for long-term ECMO use in the United States is the silicone membrane lung made by Medtronics. The $0.8m^2$ membrane is most commonly used for neonates, and can support oxygenation up to a Q of 1 L/min. Carbon dioxide transfer is so efficient with this membrane that CO_2 must be added to the gases flowing into the membrane.

Patient Management

A team approach to the management of the ECMO patient is critical. Each member of the team, the bedside nurse, respiratory therapist, and ECMO specialist, should have a clearly delineated set of responsibilities to ensure efficient and effective care [26]. Since the major complications while on ECMO are related to bleeding and/or coagulation issues, a key member of the team should be a paediatric haematologist and/or the blood bank specialist. This relationship is critical for programs treating post-operative cardiac patients.

CNMC Blood Bank Protocol for Neonatal ECMO

Product	Age	Attribute	Purpose
PRBC	< 7 d	CPDA 1 or Adsol packed if time permits	Prime
PRBC	< 10 d	CPDA 1 or Adsol by syringe or transfer bag	Top-up tx Hct 35–40%
PRBC	< 10 d	CPDA 1 or Adsol min. 175 mL in cooler	Decannulate
PLT	–	Random unit or pheresis aliquot; volume reduced for renal failure	Clinical bleeding, PLT > 100–200K
FFP – pedipacks	–	10–20 mL/kg	Hepatic failure, clinical bleeding with adequate PLT count
Cryo	–	1 bag/3 kg	Hypofibrinoginaemia clinical bleeding
All units prestorage leukocyte reduced; RBCs are sickle cell negative. Irradiation based on 1° dx / familial donation.			

Figure 5. Blood/blood component specifications.

Daily Medical Management (Figure 5)

Most neonatal patients, with the exception of those with CDH, are maintained on ECMO for 7-8 days. During this period, reversal of disease occurs and the infant can be slowly weaned off ECMO to minimal ventilator settings and extubated within 24 to 48 hours after coming off the ECMO circuit. The rapidity of recovery is remarkable, given the severity of the illness of these infants. Many physiologic changes occur rapidly in ECMO infants making daily care a fine art. All infants are systemically heparinized, so tasks such as suctioning of the airway must be done with caution. The membrane lung consumes platelets, resulting in a fairly high platelet transfusion rate in these patients. Platelet counts are maintained at a specific level, depending on the risk for bleeding. Patients with a low risk for bleeding usually have their platelet counts maintained >100,000 per mm^2, while those with acute bleeding complications require platelet counts at >150,000 to 200,000. Fibrinogen level are usually maintained >150 mg/dL.

After stabilization, the infant is placed on lung-rest settings on the ventilator. It is typical for the lungs to appear opaque on chest radiographs during the first 1 to 3 days of ECMO [27-29]. This radiologic finding is caused by the acute decrease in ventilatory settings, capillary leak, activation of complement as a result of interaction of blood products with the artificial surfaces in the circuit, and surfactant deficiency secondary to lung injury [30,31].

Heparin is administered continuously into the ECMO circuit to prevent clotting [26], but management will vary, depending on events before and during

ECMO. Heparin management is optimised when there is a decrease in the risk for fibrin and clot formation in the circuit while minimizing the risk for bleeding complications in the patient. Because heparinization must be evaluated rapidly at the bedside, most centres use the ACT [32] with appropriate quality control. The ACT is determined in a system that uses activators, such as glass beads, to initiate the clotting cascade. The specimen is warmed to accelerate the clotting process. This test gives values of 80 to 120 seconds in a nonheparinised infant, compared with standard non-activated bleeding time values longer than 5 minutes [32].

The primary cause of death in the ECMO population is ICH [16,17,33]. The risk factors associated with the development of an ICH include significant hypoxic or ischaemic cerebral insult before ECMO, sepsis with coagulopathy, or gestational age less than 37 weeks. Initial heparin management is based on pretreatment risk factors.

Fibrin formation is related to flow rate; if there are low *Q*s in the circuit, the heparin dose is increased to decrease the risk for clot formation. At the beginning of an ECMO run, blood flow rates are high, and the ACTs can be maintained in a lower range. At the end of a run, the ACTs are increased, especially when the idling phase (i.e., 60 to 80 mL/min) is reached. When *Q* in the circuit is below 150 mL/min, ACTs are increased to 200 to 220 seconds.

Clinical factors that affect the ACT values are renal function (heparin excretion is directly proportional to urine output), transfusion of unheparinised blood products or platelets, and a significant patent ductus arteriosus with a left-to-right shunt that may decrease renal blood flow.

As the arterial blood gases and venous saturations improve, weaning can occur. Idling flows, (defined as flows at 10% of the cardiac output, i.e., 60 to 80 mL/min) are continued for 6 to 8 hours, and if blood gases normalize during this period, most infants are taken off ECMO. In our institution, the average time to extubation post ECMO is 23 hours. The CDH patient is an exception; these patients require slower weaning to ensure that pulmonary hypertension does not recur. Haemoglobin, haematocrit, calcium, and electrolyte measurements should be obtained 6 to 8 hours after ECMO. These can then be monitored every 24 hours or as clinically indicated. The platelet count should be followed closely (i.e., values every 12 hours for 24 hours) because rebound thrombocytopenia may occur. After extubation, the infant usually requires oxygen therapy for another 5 to 7 days. Most ECMO infants feed poorly and require feeding by gavage for a few days.

Because not all intracranial abnormalities are detected by ultrasound, a computed tomographic or magnetic resonance scan is recommended before discharge [33]. A baseline hearing screen and a neurologic assessment are also recommended before discharge. All infants should be followed in a neonatal high-risk follow-up program.

Outcome Data

Most centres report that 60% to 70% of ECMO survivors are normal at 1 to 2 years of age [34-36]. Poor outcome is associated with severe abnormality on neuro-imaging, chronic lung disease, prematurity, and beta streptococcal sepsis [34,37-39]. Glass, et al. found 37% of infants were at risk for school failure [40] at 5 years of age. Rais-Bahrami, et.al, found a similar risk in the population of "near-miss" ECMO patients, defined as those referred for ECMO, but who improved without ECMO [41]. Wagner, et. al., followed the ECMO population studied in the Glass study into school and found a high percentage (37%) had academic problems [42]. Therefore, a neuropsychological evaluation prior to starting grade school identify those children who may benefit from special education programs.

The need for carotid artery ligation for VA ECMO has caused concern that right-sided CNS lesions may result; most studies have not shown this to be true [27,32,33,39]. Analysis of the first 360 patients treated at Children's National Medical Center did not reveal lateralising hemorrhagic or non-haemorrhagic abnormalities, but there was a high incidence of posterior fossa haemorrhage, raising the concern that jugular venous ligation might increase venous back pressure and the risk of haemorrhage [43]. Data published by Taylor and Walker showed that decreased sagittal sinus blood flow velocity is associated with ICH (70%) in the ECMO population [44]. Whether this is cause or effect has yet to be determined. Also noted in this study was a marked decrease in sagittal sinus blood flow when the infants head was turned to the left, obstructing the left internal jugular vein when the right was ligated, resulting in obstruction of venous flow. The association of this with cerebral haemorrhage could not be determine because of the small number of patients, but supports the need to keep the infants head midline during the ECMO run. Many ECMO centres now place jugular bulb catheters in the right internal jugular vein, advanced up to the jugular bulb area, to drain the venous outflow from the brain into the venous side of the circuit, and thus reduce the potential obstruction caused by the venous catheter and ligation of the jugular vein.

The infant with CDH may have unique long-term problems, including significant gastroesophageal reflux and chronic lung disease [10,23]. These infants require close follow-up in a multidisciplinary clinic to prevent problems such as failure to thrive and respiratory compromise.

Little is known regarding clinical factors associated with increased blood utilization in neonates on ECMO. Clinical experience suggests that neonates with increased mortality on ECMO have higher blood utilization rates. We sought to confirm this by conducting a retrospective analysis of 640 neonates on ECMO from 1984 to 2001. Medical and transfusion records were reviewed for primary diagnosis, age, weight, gender, ethnicity, 1 min and 5 minute APGAR scores, presence of intracranial haemorrhage (ICH) or non-ICH, performance of exchange transfusion, volume of component blood use, and days on ECMO. Blood utilization rate (BUR) expressed as mL/kg/days (on ECMO) was calculated for each patient.

Of the 640 patients, there were 255 (39.8%) with meconium aspiration syndrome (MAS), 141 (22.0%) with persistent pulmonary hypertension of the newborn (PPHN), 70 (10.9%) with left congenital diaphragmatic hernia (L-CDH), 44 (6.9%) with Group B Streptococcus sepsis (GBSS), 33 (5.2%) who were septic (non-GBSS), 28 (4.4%) with respiratory distress syndrome (RDS), 22 (3.4%) with right congenital diaphragmatic hernia (R-CDH), 17 (2.7%) with hyaline membrane disease (HMD), and 30 (4.7%) with other diagnoses. The mortality rate for each diagnosis was 5.5, 13.5, 48.6, 20.4, 12.1, 17.9, 38.4, 11.8, and 40.0 percent respectively. Overall mortality rate was 17 percent. A significantly higher blood utilization rate was seen with deceased versus surviving patients [45]. Factors associated with significantly higher blood utilization rates, included lower gestation age, use of exchange transfusions, cryoprecipitate transfusion, having both ICH and non-ICH vs either alone, and longer duration on ECMO. Factors not associated with increased blood utilization included 1 and 5 minute APGAR scores and ethnicity. These findings are consistent with that of Goodman et al who saw an increase in mortality in transfused versus non-transfused paediatric intensive care patients, and Herbert et al who illustrated that there was a decrease in mortality of patients who were on restrictive transfusion regimens and received fewer blood transfusions [46,47]. With ECMO, restrictive transfusion regimens may prove to be impossible unless haemodilution and other blood conservation techniques can be utilized.

Summary

Care of the ECMO patient requires highly trained nurses, respiratory therapists, perfusionists, ECMO trained physicians, and participation of paediatric haematologists and/or paediatric blood banking experts. The team must continually evaluate the treatment modalities and use the information to improve techniques and to define the indications for ECMO therapy.

References

1. Kolff WJ, Berk HT. Artificial kidney: a dialyzer with a great area. Acta Med Scand 1944;17:121.
2. Clowes GHA Jr, Hopkins AL, Neville WE. An artificial lung dependent upon diffusion of oxygen and carbon dioxide through plastic membranes. J Thorac Surg 1956;32:630.
3. Callaghan JC, delos Angeles J. Long-term extracorporeal circulation in the development of an artificial placenta for respiratory distress syndrome of the newborn. Surg Forum 1961;12:215.
4. Rashkind WJ, Freeman A, Klein D, Toft RW. Evolution of a disposable plastic low volume, pumpless oxygenator as a lung substitute. J Pediatr 1965; 66:94.

5. White JJ, Andrews HG, Risemberg H, et al. Prolonged respiratory support in newborn infants with a membrane oxygenator. Surgery 1971;70:288.
6. Dorson WJ, Baker E, Cohen ML, et al. A perfusion system for infants. Trans Am Soc Artif Intern Organs 1969;15:155.
7. Bartlett RH, Gazzaniga AB, Jefferies MR, et al. Extracorporeal membrane oxygenation (ECMO) cardiopulmonary support in infancy. Trans Am Soc Artif Intern Organs 1976;22:80.
8. Data from the Extracoporeal Life Support Organization quarterly report, July 2003.
9. Gill BS, Neville HL, Khan AM, Cox CS Jr., Lally KP. Delayed institution of extracorporeal membrane oxygenation is associated with increased mortality rate and prolonged hospital stay. J Pediatr Surg 2002;37(1):7.
10. Van Meurs K and Short BL. State-of-the-Art management of congenital diaphragmatic hernia: a neonatologist's perspective. Pediatrics in Review, 20:e79-e87, 1999.
11. Sanchez LS, O'Brien A, Anderson KD, et al. Best postductal PO_2 and PCO_2 do not predict outcome of CDH infants in extremis, stabilized with ECMO prior to surgical repair. Pediatr Res 1992;31:221A.
12. Boloker J, Bateman DA, Wung JT, Stolar CJ. Congenital diaphragmatic hernia in 120 infants treated consecutively with permissive hyper-apnea/ spontaneous respiration/elective repair. J Pediatr Surg 2002;37:357.
13. Kays DW, Langham MR, Ledbetter DJ, Talbert JL. Detrimental effects of standard medical therapy in congenital diaphragmatic hernia. Ann of Surg 1999;230:340.
14. Karle VA, Short BL, Martin GR, et al. Extracorporeal membrane oxygenation exposes infants to the plasticizer, di(2-ethylhexyl)phthalate. Crit Care Med 1997;25: 696.
15. Schneider B, Schena J, Troug R, et al. Exposure to di(2-ethylhexyl)phthalate in infants receiving extracorporeal membrane oxygenation. N Engl J Med 1989;320: 1563.
16. Cilley RE, Zwischenferger JB, Andrews AF, et al. Intracranial hemorrhage during extracorporeal membrane oxygenation in neonates. Pediatrics 1986; 78:699.
17. Revenis ME, Glass P, Short B. Mortality and morbidity among lower birth weight (2–2.5 kg) infants treated with extracorporeal membrane oxygenation (ECMO). J Pediatr 1992;121:452.
18. Toomasian JM, Snedecor SM, Cornell RG, et al. National experience with xtracorporeal membrane oxygenation for newborn respiratory failure. Trans Am Soc Artif Intern Organs 1988;34:140.
19. Short BL, Walker LK, Bendu KS, Traystman RJ. Impairment of cerebral autoregulation during extracorporeal membrane oxygenation. Pediatr Res 1993;33:289.
20. Short BL, Walker LK, Gleason CA, et al. Effects of extracorporeal membrane oxygenation on cerebral blood flow and cerebral oxygen metabolism in newborn sheep. Pediatr Res 1990;28:50.

21. McCune S, Short BL, Miller MK, et al. Extracorporeal membrane oxygenation therapy in neonates with septic shock. J Pediatr Surg 1990;25:479.
22. Newman KD, Van Meurs KP, Short BL, Anderson KD. Extracorporeal membrane oxygenation and congenital diaphragmatic hernia – should any infant be excluded? J Pediatr Surg 1990;25:1048.
23. Van Meurs KP, Newman KD, Anderson KD, Short BL. Effect of extracorporeal membrane oxygenation on survival of infants with congenital diaphragmatic hernia. J Pediatr 1990;117:954.
24. Anderson HL, Otsu T, Chapman RA, Bartlett RH. Venovenous extracorporeal life support in neonates using a double lumen catheter. Trans Am Soc Artif Intern Organs 1989;35:650.
25. Rais-Bahrami K, Walton DM, Sell JR, Rivera O, Mikesell GT, Short BL. Improved oxygenation with reduced recirculation during venovenous ECMO: comparison of two catheters. Perfusion 2002;17:415.
26. Short BL. Clinical management of the neonatal ECMO patient. In Arensman RM, Cornish D, eds. Extracorporeal life support. Cambridge, MA: Blackwell Scientific, 1993.
27. Taylor GA, Short BL, Kreismer P. Extracorporeal membrane oxygenation: radiographic appearance of the neonatal chest. Am J Radiol 1986;146:1257.
28. Lotze A, Short BL, Taylor GA. The use of lung compliance as a parameter for improvement in lung function in newborns with respiratory failure requiring extracorporeal membrane oxygenation. Crit Care Med 1987;15:226.
29. Keszler M, Subramanian KN, Smith YA, et al. Pulmonary management during extracorporeal membrane oxygenation. Crit Care Med 1989;17:495-500.
30. Lotze A, Whitsett JA, Kammerman L, et al. Surfactant protein A concentrations in tracheal aspirate fluid from infants requiring extracorporeal membrane oxygenation. J Pediatr 1990;116:435.
31. Anderson JM, Kottke-Marchant K. Platelet interactions with biomaterials and artificial devices. In Williams DF, ed. Blood compatibility, vol I. Boca Raton: CRC Press, 1987:127.
32. Hattersley P. Activated coagulation time of whole blood. JAMA 1966;196:436.
33. Taylor GA, Short BL, Fitz CR. Imaging of cerebrovascular injury in infants treated with extracorporeal membrane oxygenation. J Pediatr 1989;114:635.
34. Bulas DI, Taylor GA, O'Donnell, Short BL, Fitz CR, Vezina G. Intracranial abnormalities in infants treated with extracorporeal membrane oxygenation: update on sonographic and CT findings. Am J Neuroradiol 1996;17:287.
35. Glass P, Miller M, Short B. Morbidity for survivors of extracorporeal membrane oxygenation: neurodevelopmental outcome at 1 year of age. Pediatrics 1989;83:72.
36. Schumacher RE, Palmer TW, Roloff DW, et al. Follow-up of infants treated with extracorporeal membrane oxygenation for newborn respiratory failure. Pediatrics 1991;87:451.

37. Towne BH, Lott IT, Hicks DA, Healey T. Long-term follow-up of infants and children treated with extracorporeal membrane oxygenation (ECMO): a preliminary report. J Pediatr Surg 1985;20:410.
38. Glass P, Bulas DI, Wagner AE, et al. Severity of brain injury following neonatal ECMO and outcome at age 5. Dev Med Child Neurol 1997;39: 441-48.
39. Schumacher RE, Barks JDE, Johnston MV, et al. Right-sided brain lesions in infants following extracorporeal membrane oxygenation. Pediatrics 1988; 82:155.
40. Bulas DI, Glass P, O'Donnell RM, Taylor GA, Short BL, Vezina GL. Neonates treated with ECMO: Predictive value of early CT and US neuroimaging findings on short-term neurodevelopmental outcome. Radiology 1995; 195:407.
41. Glass P, Wagner AE, Papero PH, et al. Neurodevelopmental status at age five years of neonates treated with extracorporeal membrane oxygenation. J Pediatr 1995;127(3):447.
42. Rais-Bahrami K, Wagner AE, Coffman C, Galss P, Short BL. Neurodevelopmental outcome in ECMO vs near-miss ECMO patients at 5 years of age. Clinical Pediatr 2000;39:145.
43. Wagner AE, Coffman CE, Short BL, Glass P. Neuropsychological outcome and educational adjustment to first grade of ECMO-treated neonates. Pediatr Res 39; Suppl 2;283.
44. Bulas DI, Taylor GA, Fitz CR, et al. Posterior fossa intracranial hemorrhage in infants treated with extracorporeal membrane oxygenation: sonographic findings. Am J Roentgenol 1991;156:571.
45. Taylor GA, Walker LK. Doppler US evaluation of the intracranial venous system following ligation of the right jugular vein in infants treated with extracorporeal membrane oxygenation. Radiology 1992;183:453.
46. Wong ECC, Baxter C, Huang Z, Rais-Bahrami K, Luban NLC, Short B. Increased mortality is associated with increased blood utilization in neonates undergoing extracorporeal membrane oxygenation (ECMO). Pediatric Research 2003;53:50A.
47. Goodman AM, Pollack MM, Patel KM, Luban NLC. Pediatric Red Blood Cell Transfusions Increase Resource Use. J Pediatr 2003;142:123-7.
48. Hebert PC, Wells G, Blajchman MA, et al. A multicenter, randomized, controlled clinical trial of transfusion requirements in critical care. N Engl J Med 1999;340:409-17.

DISCUSSION

Moderators: R.G. Strauss and E.F. van Leeuwen

G. Walther-Wenke (Munster, D): What is a premature infant? Can you give us a clear definition of the risk group?

N. Luban (Washington DC, USA): Prematurity is classically described as less than 34 weeks. We tend to use an arbitrary cut off not of weeks gestation, but rather of birth weight. The weight cut off that we use is 1500 grams.

G. Walther-Wenke: So there is no clear definition, because in Germany we use 37 weeks.

N. Luban: Let me tell you exactly where we came up with the gram weight. That was actually based on a review of serial autopsies of infants, looking for the development of T cells. Perhaps Dr Dame would like to speak to that point. We came up to that not on the basis of gestation age, but rather on the basis of – presumed on autopsy – clear T cell deficiency. One could certainly argue, but that was how we came up with that.

R.G. Strauss (Iowa City, IA, USA): Maybe I could comment on why one decides to use gamma irradiation or not. A part of it is related to science. The article that Dr. Luban referred to[1], looking at all the cases of transfusion-related Graft versus Host Disease under 1 year of age, that with rare exception, they all occurred in recognised high-risk groups. There were only 5 instances where there were no recognised high-risk groups. Three of those infants were very small preterm babies under 1500 grams, some under 1 kilo birth weight. The other two were surgical patients who received multiple blood products. So they got multiple transfusions, and they were probably immunosuppressed from their illness. On a purely scientific basis, we probably really don't have to gamma irradiate, except for high-risk groups. Perhaps very small preterm infants, who are critically ill might warrant it. Would preterm babies need gamma irradiated blood? Scientifically, I would say no. For example, an uncomplicated term infant going to cardiac surgery, assuming they don't have the Di George syndrome or an immuno-

1. Strauss RG. Data-driven blood banking practices for neonatal RBC transfusions. Transfusion 2000;40:1528-40.

deficiency state. Scientifically, I think you can make a case for saying, you don't have to give gamma irradiated blood except for high-risk disorders. On the other hand, what is the standard of practice. In the United States, it is estimated that between 70 and 90 percent – it is a little hard to come up with the exact numbers – of University centres give gamma irradiated blood to all infants in the NICU[1]. Community hospitals are down to about 50 percent or so, who gamma irradiate. So, if you have an infant that develops transfusion related Graft versus Host Disease and you did not give gamma irradiated blood, somebody will say, "Well, over 90 percent of all University centres, where there are all these smart people who know everything, irradiate. How can you violate that standard of practice? Thus, you can see, we are forced in the United States to give gamma irradiated blood. As a final point, what are the down sides of giving gamma irradiated blood? Well, relatively few. Certainly, potassium rises quickly in the extracellular fluid, if you irradiate blood. You have to worry about potassium dose in a surgical setting when you are giving large amounts of blood rapidly. On the other hand, for small volume transfusions given slowly, it is really not much of a problem. The slightly shorter post-transfusion RBC survival is not really a striking problem.

Thus, scientifically, it is very hard to justify gamma irradiation for all infants. At a practical level it is almost always done. So I think you are at risk both legally and ethically, if you fail to gamma irradiate blood in the US. We are gamma irradiating blood for all infants up to one year of age because it is very hard for us in the blood centre to know who is a high-risk infant and who isn't. At Johns Hopkins, they irradiate up to the age of six years, which I think is excessively long. But Dr. Paul Ness, Medical Director, feels it is the appropriate thing to do. As a point already made, there are hundreds of thousands of babies over the last 30 years or so, that have not received gamma irradiated blood, and there are only very few case reports of transfusion-related Graft versus Host Disease. Thus, we probably do much more irradiation than necessary.

G. Walther-Wenke: Sorry, but I am not really pleased with these answers, because I think we need clear guidelines for this important question. Another thing is what about exchange transfusion. In Germany guidelines[1,2] say we should irradiate all the blood. Should we or should we not?

R.G. Strauss: Exchange transfusion by itself is one of the high-risk indications.

E.F. van Leeuwen (Amsterdam, NL): For all children?

---

1. Wissenschaftlicher Beirat der Bundesärztekammer und Paul-Ehrlich-Institut (2000). Richtlinien zur Gewinnung von Blut und Blutbestandteilen und zur Anwendung von Blutprodukten (Hämotherapie). Dtsch Ärzteverlag, Köln. http://www.baek.de.
2. Vorstand und Wissenschaftlicher Beirat der Bundärztekammer (2001). Leitlinien zur Therapie mit Blutkomponenten und Plasmaderivaten. Dtsch Ärzteverlag, Köln. http: //www.baek.de.

R.G. Strauss: For all children under one year of age. Although the data are limited, there were several infants reported with exchange transfusion only and fatal Graft versus Host Disease.

E.F. van Leeuwen: And what was the product? Was it fresh whole blood?

R.G. Strauss: It was either fresh blood or blood reconstituted, I don't recall every instance.

E.F. van Leeuwen: Because we use reconstituted blood, leukocyte depleted by buffy coat removal and filtration, etc. Of course you have a large volume.

R.G. Strauss: I agree with all that you say. All I can say is that the reports are that it does occur. If we are spending billions of dollars to try to prevent one instance of transfusion related HIV, it is hard to imagine not doing a little gamma irradiation to try to prevent a much more frequent occurrence, which is Graft versus Host Disease, following exchange transfusion. For me to not do it, is very hard in a moral and legal sense.

E.F. van Leeuwen: Then you have a very defensive way of treating children and all the case histories are based on old case histories treated with former products. The same as the preterm children.

N. Luban: That is true. There are no incidence figures. The only registry that exist that I am aware of is the Japanese registry[1]. This Japanese registry gives us valuable information, but it is a very different population, very narrow HLA phenotypes and they exclusively use fresh whole blood. So can one extrapolate from that registry information to other areas of the world? I doubt it. But that is the only information that we have to work on. Yes, in the US we do practice defensive medicine, there is no question about that.

M.S. Harvey (Leiden, NL): About guidelines: We do irradiate for all immunodeficiencies acquired or natural, intrauterine transfusions, below 32 weeks or below 1500 grams, and we do irradiate all the exchange transfusions. But I agree with Dr. van Leeuwen, it is not really necessary, but it is practical.

CMV – the article of Nichols in Blood[2], do you think there is really an indication for CMV seronegative donor units in intrauterine transfusions, haploidentical stem cell transplantations and so on.

---

1. Asai T, Inaba S, Ohto H, et al. Guidelines for irradiation of blast and blood component to prevent graft versus host disease in Japan. Transfus Med 2000;10:315-20.
2. Nichols WG, Price TH, Gooley T, Corey L, Boeckh M. Transfusion-transmitted cytomegalovirus infection after receipt of leukoreduced blood products. Blood 2003; 101:4195-200.

R.G. Strauss: To answer your question, I think in all these instances you mention, you have to give blood that is safe for CMV. Whether it is leukocyte reduced or seronegative or some combination. The paper by G. Nichols was from the Fred Hutchinson Centre in Seattle, WA. They use, for their transplant patients, whatever CMV safe blood they can get. Combinations of CMV seronegative, leukocyte reduced largely by filtration, leukocyte reduced platelets by apheresis techniques. They observed a certain historical rate of CMV infection in their patients. I don't remember the precise number. Because they were switching to apheresis products, they felt that, perhaps, leukocyte reduction would not be as good. Also, their patients were receiving more red cell transfusions. They were worried, since none of the ways of preventing CMV – leukocyte reduction or serology testing of donors – is perfect. They thought that they might see an increase in CMV. When they did surveillance and found CMV antigen, they increased Gancyclovir and IVIG, and other means of treating CMV. Thus, they really never saw any clinical evidence of CMV infection, they just saw changes in antigen, which they treated. When they looked at patients studied recently, who developed CMV antigenaemia, more often than historically, they noted that recent patient received more blood transfusions. Their practices remain the same, as they prescribe CMV seronegative, leukocyte-reduced and all sorts of mixtures. So their conclusion was that we should try to do better to prevent CMV. They did not say that CMV seronegative was better than leukocyte reduction. They never looked at the study in this particular way. My way of interpreting is, when you have a process that does not prevent something 100 percent of the time – and I think we all agree that leukocyte reduction probably prevents CMV somewhere between 98 and 99 percent, there is still 1 percent chance of break-through infection despite leukocyte reduction. When you use blood from seronegative donors, the rates are about the same, one to three percent of people who get blood from seronegative donors will develop CMV. Whenever you have two things that don't work perfectly, of course, there are going to be break-through infections – especially, if you are transfusing people more and more. Whether you can improve the safety by using seronegative blood instead of leukocyte reduced, or in our centre leukocyte reduced instead of seronegative, or whether you want to combine them together, you still have two methods that are not perfect. When putting them together, maybe they work better. Logic will tell you that they probably would. However CMV is such an infrequent infection, I don't think there are ever going to be data to show that combining the two, leukocyte reduction and blood from seronegatives, is going to be better. But if logic is the way you want to go, and if you have plenty of money at your institution and a lot of availability of seronegative blood, you can do both things or you can pick and chose one or the other for different patient groups. To me that doesn't make much sense. I think prestorage leukocyte reduction, done in the blood centre where there is careful quality control, is the best way to go. But if people would rather use both, it is hard to argue, there just are no data.

M.S. Harvey: I just checked with the blood centre last week and I understand they still have the same policy: do both in very specific indications. The last question – is there indication for giving Parvo B19 safe blood to neonates?

N. Luban: I spend two and a half days discussing that with the FDA and the American Red Cross. My conclusion is, there is only one indication and that would be intrauterine transfusion to an infant of an either CMV seronegative or Parvo PCR negative mother. Other than that I think is a lot about nothing, but that is my personal opinion.

J.F. Harrison (London, UK): Dr Strauss, is there any evidence that we should not use red cells in optimal additives less than five days old, for either exchange transfusion or for large volume transfusions in children less than six months. What is the evidence that we shouldn't use this?

R.G. Strauss: To my knowledge, there are no data to show in large volume transfusions, like exchange transfusion or priming of ECMO circuits, that that is necessarily wrong. Several years ago Dr. Luban, Dr. Hume and I published an intellectual exercise looking at the potential toxic doses of these additives[1]. If you gave a large volume transfusion, would you exceed the toxic dose and so theoretically could there be a problem? The conclusion was that there, theoretically, could be a problem – especially in extracorporeal circuits where the blood is being washed through the babies body over and over again. Potentially, there would be the possibility, especially in a procedure of several hours, where all of the body compartments could be saturated with this additives. Do we really have any clinical data to show that anything bad happened to these babies? No, not that I know of. People, anecdotally have told me, "we use Adsol in extracorporeal bypass for cardiac surgery all the time, and we haven't seen any problems." But my answer always is, "Well how did you look for a problem?" There are some data in baby cats that in cardiac bypass, if one uses AS1, because of the high glucose concentration, extreme hyperglycaemia in the brain can occur with CNS problems. Following cardiac bypass surgery, central nervous system dysfunction is fairly common. Thus, how would you distinguish whether CNS dysfunction in an infant might be related to hyperglycaemia or just the bypass itself. So, we are just very cautious if it is going to be a large volume transfusion, especially in an extracorporeal circuit and we wash out the additives and resuspend the RBCs in whatever fluid is going to be used in a circuit, crystalloid or plasma. We are trying to be conservative and try to do what seems to be the safest.

N. Luban: For open heart procedures and extracorporeal membrane oxygenation we try to use CPD, CPD A1 if we are sure. But because of blood group or gen-

1. Luban NLC, Strauss RG, Hume HA. Commentary on the safety of red cells preserved in extended-storage media for neonatal transfusions. Transfusion 1991;31:229-35.

eral shortages we will use additive solutions, but we will pack off the additive and then we will add back crystalloid plasma if it is going to be used in the bypass.

*C.S. Manno (*Philadelphia*, PA, USA)*: If we don't have red cells and CPD we use additive solution red cells, two units to prime pump and then we use fresh whole blood at the end of bypasses, which is an entirely different discussion.

R.G. Strauss: Do you remove the additive?

C.S. Manno: We don't.

R.G. Strauss: So it is a difference of practice.

J.F. Harrison: Dr. Luban, we use a lot of homozygous class I HLA platelet donors. They are homozygous for common haplotypes like A1B8. A lot of the platelets which are not HLA matched, then go to patients who are immonosuppressed, and we know they are from donors homozygous to common tissue types. I wonder whether we should be irradiating them all. We irradiate them when they are HLA matched, but not if they are issued as 'random' platelets. But they could by chance be HLA matched.

N. Luban: Certainly that is one of the reasons that many University hospitals in the US that have oncology and transplant units, will irradiate all products for those recipients. That is the practice both at the Children's Hospital of Philadelphia, in Washington DC and also in Iowa City. Again a very different international perspective because of access to the equipment and the necessity of maintaining the quality control, but it is for exactly that reason that we would encourage it.

M.S. Harvey: I have an answer to Dr. Piciotto's question about intrauterine transfusions. We stipulate to our local blood bank, that we want intrauterine transfusions made up of not more than five days old erythrocytes that have been pre-storage filtered, from CMV seronegative donors and of course compatible with the mother. They are stored in Saline Adenine Glucose Mannitol. This is removed and replaced within four hours before transfusion by physiological saline without added protein, to an Hct of about 80 percent. The units are irradiated also directly after being made up and we try to get them out to the clinic as I said, within two hours. So we never give out old intrauterine transfusion units.

Second: I would suggest that if you are worried about potassium levels you can do two simple things. One is, never transfuse from a normal, maybe aged erythrocyte unit, more than 80 millilitres per kilogram, and the second is of course never transfuse erythrocytes that have been irradiated more than 24 hours before giving out to the clinic. And the last question of course, if you are worried about hypocalcaemia and so on after exchange transfusion, why don't we go back to heparin exchange transfusions.

P.T. Pisciotto: I think in the US it would be very hard to go back to heparin. I don't know, perhaps someone else would like to make a comment on that?

R.G. Strauss: If one collects blood in heparin, it doesn't store very well. So how would one go about doing infectious disease testing and all those other things, and still have blood that is worth anything when all of that is finished. That is my problem.

M.S. Harvey: I don't know what you do for HLA compatible platelets, but they come to us within 24 hours after collection, granulocytes would be on the ward within 12 hours after apheresis. So I think the blood bank should and could do acute testing.

R.G. Strauss: For products like granulocytes and HLA matched platelets, it is fairly common for blood centres to select a donor who has been tested recently, at our place within the last 10 days, who is in the regular pool and has been tested multiple times to suggest that they are biologically safe. Granulocytes of course have to be given before donation testing is done, so donor testing is waived. I suppose, if you have testing laboratories that turn things around very quickly including nucleic amplification tests, then you can await test results.

E.F. van Leeuwen: But in case of heparin plasma, you are also able to freeze it and store it that way. But, there is also another side effect of heparin plasma. You heparinise the child deeply in a period that you have a lot of pressure differences and so on. So you have also the bleeding problem in heparinisation, and of course glucose.

M.S. Harvey: Our exchange units are made up from erythrocytes from one donor, and of course fresh frozen AB plasma hopefully from a non pregnant donor, which is defrosted and made up to a Hct of about 40 to 50 percent.

R.G. Strauss: The question I was going to ask is if you wash red cells with saline, how soon do you demand that these be transfused?

M.S. Harvey: As soon as possible of course.

R.G. Strauss: Do you have a limit?

M.S. Harvey: We try to restrict to four hours. But unfortunately it is out of control, because sometimes the procedure itself takes quite a long time.

R.G. Strauss: The comment is – if one washes red cells and then serially samples them for supernatant potassium, within about four hours potassium is already starting to rise. Within 12 hours, it is approaching 12 to 15 milli-equivalents per litre. So if you are washing cells to lower the potassium, they really can not be kept very long. This rise occurs whether you try to put albumin in the wash "to protect" or whether you are just using saline, or saline with a pH that has been adjusted to 7.4. So we "shoot ourself in the foot" if we wash to "clean" RBCs and, then do not insist on them being transfused very quickly.

A. Brand (Leiden, NL): Dr. Luban showed that if you use stored irradiated blood, I could see in three of the four controlled randomized trials there was at least ten percent difference in 24 hours recovery. So there is a difference, and you should realize that you cannot simply exchange non-irradiated blood for irradiated blood. The second point is – has any of you looked carefully into for instance scavenger potentials of red cells stored in particular in storage solution and in relation to irradiation. Of course all these metabolic parameters are important, but there are other parameters that maybe important for instance for brain damage such as free ion. So what is the scavenger potential? All these parameters have not been measured in a systematic way as far as I know.

N. Luban: There are two articles in the literature[1, 2] out of the Massachusetts General Hospital. Dr. Dzik has looked at free ion radical generation in irradiated blood. In one of the two studies he attempted to modify that by putting in some sort of a quenching solution. But all of this was done in an in vitro system; subsequent animal work has not been done. So that is an area that has not been very well explored at all. There are a few abstracts in the literature and one of them actually we presented – this was a fellow's work and she never managed to get it to publication phase – where the donors of the blood were encouraged for one month prior to donation to take vitamin E and vitamin C and donate a unit. The unit was irradiated at three different levels, and we looked at in vitro parameters. We were unable to get this into a biosurvival study, but that would have been a logical next step. Individuals who take 400 IU of vitamin E and 500 milligrams of vitamin C clearly have a protective effect on particularly potassium and LDH leakage from irradiated blood. So those are the only three evaluations that I am aware of.

A. Brand: I agree with you that it is limited what is available, but we should be careful not to leave the audience with the idea that nothing is happening in the combination of storage and irradiation. That is all that I want to say. There was also this year (2003) one publication in Transfusion Medicine[3] on 5 days old blood, 120 millilitres given two days after irradiation in cardiac surgery and

1. Anand AJ, Dzik WH, Iman A, Sadrzadeh SM. Radiation-induced red cell damage: role of reactive oxygen species. Transfusion 1997;37:160-65.
2. Sharifi S, Dzik WH, Sadrzadeh SM. Human plasma and tirilazad inesylate protect stored human erythrocytes against the oxidative damage of gamma-irradiation. Transfusion Med 2000;10:125-30.
3. Baz EMK, Kanazi GE, Mahfouz RAR, Obied MY. An unusual case of hyperkalaemia-induced cardiac arrest in a paediatric patient during transfusion of a "fresh" 6-day-old blood unit. Transfusion Med 2002;12:383-86.

there was a fatal cardiac arrest. It still happens, so we should be careful and not say, well if you're in doubt irradiate.

R.G. Strauss: That is a good point. I think one has to weigh all of the points: what is the purpose you are doing it for, what are the other situations involved with the patient and what is the situation with irradiation at your own centre. We have our own irradiator. Many of you perhaps have an irradiator in your blood bank, many don't. But if you have your own irradiator, so that you irradiate RBCs and transfuse promptly, these down-sides are minimised. The shortened survival that has been reported were at the limits of storage. So when you irradiate and transfuse promptly, there is no demonstrable shortening of survival or damage to the red cells that can be detected at a clinical level. If you are at a centre who has to get blood irradiated from a regional centre, you may store it for several days or weeks or so. Then problems may arise, and I think you should be a little more cautious in what you irradiate for.

The other point is the potassium. When you irradiate and the extracellular potassium goes up, it rises very promptly over three to five days, but it actually stabilises at maximum at about 70 millimoles per litre if you are using standard storage medium. If you are using CPDA, it goes up to a hundred or more because of the smaller amount of plasma. So you can actually calculate how much potassium is going to be given and the rate at which it is going to be infused. Then, you can either infuse it slowly, or you can wash it, or you can get fresher blood. I agree totally, I think you have to look at each transfusion, each patient and balance all of those things, and then decide which you are going to do.

A. Brand: That reminds me of what Dr. Pisciotto said about the case in intrauterine transfusion who developed a bradycardia. I think bradycardiac is a complication – Dr Bussel may confirm – in intrauterine transfusion. You also see it in platelets transfusions, in which you do not have those potassium problems. In fact you should not be so very afraid. We had a really major problem 3 years ago in which the intrauterine red cells were not resolved in 0.9 percent saline, but in 9 percent saline. The red cells looked awful, they had spikes and were completely sticky. There where four patients transfused, and two children died. We can't prove of course that it is not related to the transfusion. However, two of them stayed alive. We started to calculate before intrauterine and after intrauterine transfusion and found that the buffering capacity of the foetal placental unit is so extremely large that even this huge amount of potassium was removed almost immediately, 15 minutes after transfusion. So even during the transfusion you have already an equilibrium.

E. Ranasinghe (Cambridge, UK): We in the UK adhere to BCSH guidelines on irradiation, which do not recommend irradiation of all units for transfusion. At the moment it is recommended for babies at risk only. However, what I want to mention is that in view of the fact that congenital immunodeficiency can not be diagnosed with confidence at the time of birth and it might take even up to four months or six months to diagnose this condition, don't you think it is after all a good idea to irradiate all neonatal cellular transfusion products.

R.G. Strauss: That is precisely what we do, until the age of one year for that reason, and why the people at the Johns Hopkins irradiate up to six years of age. I believe Dr Manno irradiates up to 14 years. The calculations we did in Iowa with our population is at congenital immunodeficiency disease of a T cell variety, severe enough that you would suspect Graft versus Host Disease might occur. We thought this came about 1 in 100,000 births. I think Dr. Manno was mentioning another calculation at Hopkins as 1 in 50,000 birth. So it is very uncommon, but nonetheless in a referral hospital you may see it at a higher rate. If you are in a community hospital where you give relatively few red cell transfusions, mostly for surgery, a lot of the high risk babies are referred to elsewhere, and the risk of Graft versus Host Disease would probably be much smaller. And if you didn't have your own irradiator, which you probably would not, you may not irradiate blood very often at all in that situation. I think we are all well intended, we just have to examine what our needs are, and try to do what is best for the babies in our own setting. It is important to have a written protocol, so that you can follow things in a consistent fashion at your own hospital. That is probably the first and major step.

N. Luban: I think your British Society of Haematology guidelines were usually reviewed at 3 to 5 year intervals. What I would recommend is making sure that you have a thorough review of literature, and evaluate that literature a propos of the patient populations that you are dealing with, because there isn't any right or wrong answer necessarily. As we were discussing, there are no incidence figures and there are no prevalence figures. You are working backwards from an old literature and you will not see a new literature, because no one will publish case reports on Graft versus Host Disease now, unless there is some miraculous therapeutic intervention that has worked to improve the mortality rate. You will begin to see a few articles in the literature on, for example, the use of bone marrow transplantation for transfusion associated Graft versus Host Disease. It gets to the tip of the iceberg phenomenon. You only know of a few, you can only define a limited group of patients of risk. Then do you intervene for the bottom of the iceberg, or do just stick to those specific groups. At Hopkins one of the reasons why they have the programme that they established and can use it so easily, is that it is a 1700 bed mixed paediatric and adult hospital. So when they irradiate units they can distribute them to the adult patients and always have only the freshest, just irradiated units to distribute and to give out to the neonatal intensive care unit and their paediatric floors. In other institutions that becomes very difficult, if not impossible. So inventory control has to be an important part of the decision making.

E. Ranasinghe: In England the responsibility for irradiation lies with the blood transfusion service actually. Where ever the patient is, in a small hospital or a referral hospital, the national blood service is responsible for issuing the blood after irradiation. That is the problem.

E.F. van Leeuwen: But this supports the importance of a good registration of all side effects of blood transfusion. We should not make our rules out of case publications, but out of registries.

J.B. Bussel (New York, NY, USA): Dr Brand reminded me that not everybody in the audience would know that when you give a red cell transfusion to small babies – five ml per kilo per hour, but when you are giving it to a foetus that is usually 5 ml per kilo per minute. So there are differences potentially for potassium that would be important. While the placenta is a wonderful capacitance vessel for taking out red cells, intact or damaged, I don't know what it would do with plasma. We had done a study[1] trying to look at slightly larger transfusions to see if we could decrease the interval of IUTs. We could decrease the interval, but we did get a little more bradycardia. We attributed it to the volume, but it may or may not have been something else.

C.S. Manno: Dr Luban, when your ECMO team calls you that they want to put a baby on, and you have hard packed additive storage red cells, and then they decide not to put that baby on, what do you do with the hard packed additive solution cells?

N. Luban: Usually give it to a sickle cell patient.

C.S. Manno: So you can quickly re-circulate that?

N. Luban: Yes.

C.S. Manno: What if it happens at 6 o'clock at night and your patients are not coming in until ten o'clock the next day for their transfusion. You feel good about storing that for 18 hours?

N. Luban: What we would do is to just quarantine and dump the unit.

C.S. Manno: So if you can use it right away, you will.

N. Luban: We will.

---

1. Inglis, SR, Lysikiewicz, A, Sonnenblick, AL, Bussel, J, Chervenak, FA. Advantages of larger volume, less frequent intrauterine red blood cell transfusions for maternal red cell alloimmunization. Am J Perinatol 1996;13:27-33.

C.S. Manno: For emergency ECMO, if somebody decides to end and they want blood at the bedside for stopping, do you have a system for using O negative cells or do you always give them type specific?

N. Luban: We try to give them type specific whenever possible, to decrease overuse of O's. That pretty much has worked out successfully. When we initially began, and I am not sure exactly where this came from, it could well have come from Michigan, which is where the whole concept of ECMO began with Dr Bartlett, who by the way is a paediatric surgeon, not a neonatologist, there would be a request for O. Many of these kids would then be supported through an 8, 12, 15 or 22 day process on O only, never reverting back to group and type specific. When we began in the seventies we did follow that process, but switched relatively rapidly to group and type specific. Also important for emergency procedures is, to have a well established system for transport of a unit with temperature control to the bedside and a system to get the unit back in case it is not used.

R.G. Strauss: At our place we have a unit at the bedside for emergencies. We keep the packed unit for up to one week. If it is not used, we throw it out without really knowing how well the red cells are preserved in the packed stage. How do you do this, do you have a red cell at the bedside for a blowing circuit, and what is it?

N. Luban: We are lucky in that we are not an astronomically large hospital. So someone can run down and pick up a unit from us. We do not keep a unit at the bedside, but we have an emergency shelf. Obviously these children do not have repetitive cross matches. I didn't mention that, but you have exceeded their blood volume multiple times, so one does not do repeated cross matching with these units. It is essentially an emergency release of an O unit.

P.T. Pisciotto: How often do you see this occurring? How often do you have to go to this emergency type?

N. Luban: I would say that the one blown circuit that I showed, I will vividly remember until the day I die. That is the only blown circuit that we have ever had. The decanulation of course occurs every time. But luckily the unit which we send up in a cooler, most often comes back, not entered, never used, goes back on the shelf and gets used for someone else.

C.S. Manno: We have a refrigerator, called ECMO-refrigerator, which is distant from the blood bank, monitored by the blood bank twice a day. It holds two O negative units. We have one in the cardiac unit as well for pulling the lines out at the end of the long post-operative period of two days to about six days. So because of that size of our hospital, there is more distance and a little more trust between us and the people who use the blood in the refrigerators.

R.G. Strauss: And are they packed?

C.S. Manno: They are just O negative additive solution units. They are not packed. Because of this question, I don't know what happens to the red cells that are packed.

R.G. Strauss: For those of you who haven't read the original paper on the development of this, it is quite interesting. It used an interesting statistical design called 'play the winner' or something like that. Efficacy was decided on a study involving fewer than ten patients.

E.F. van Leeuwen: Dr. Pisciotto concerning the letter in the Lancet[1] about the lead intoxication: do we have to test all donors for repetitive transfusion in the newborn, and dedicate one unit to one newborn and in large volume transfusions do we have to screen the donors for high lead levels in their blood? Is there any reason for it?

P.T Pisciotto: At this point this is still under investigation. In the United States there has been a report out of California[2] where there were high levels of lead observed in premature infants after blood transfusion. This is the only area where this has been studied. They were seeing high lead levels in some of their blood products. But we really don't know what the long term effects of that will be. I think that there will be more investigation before there will be recommendation for universal screening.

---

1. Bearer CE, Linsalata N, Yomtovian R et al. Blood transfusions: a hidden source of lead exposure. Lancet 2003;362: 332.
2. Bearer CE, O'Riordan MA, Power R. Lead exposure from blood transfusion to premature infants. J Pediatr 2000;137:549-54.

IV. CELLULAR THERAPIES IN NEONATOLOGY

GENETIC ENGINEERING FOR THE FOETUS AND NEONATE

K..M. Axsom, C.S. Manno[1]

In Utero Haematopoietic Stem Cell Transplantation

Technological advances allow for prenatal diagnosis of many genetic abnormalities and may provide the opportunity for treatment early in gestation or neonatal life. Stem cells provide a unique opportunity to treat genetic diseases because they are multi-potent and demonstrate life-long self-renewal. Two approaches for treatment of genetic disease early in life are *in utero* haematopoietic stem cell transplantation (IUHSCTx) and neonatal haematopoietic stem cell directed gene therapy. Target diseases for these therapies are listed in Table 1.

Table 1. Target diseases for IUHSCTx or neonatal haematopoietic stem cell directed gene therapy

Class of disorder	**Disease**
Haemoglobinopathies and other erythrocyte defects	– ß-Thalassaemia, Sickle cell disease
	– Fanconi's anaemia
	– G6PD deficiency
	– Cytoskeletal defects
Immune-deficiency syndromes	– SCID
	– Wiskott-Aldrich syndrome
	– CD40 ligand deficiency
	– Agammaglobulinanaemia
Leukocyte defects	– Chronic granulomatous disease
	– Leukocyte adhesion defect
Lysosomal storage disease	– Gaucher disease
	– Hurler's syndrome
Leukodystrophies	– X-adrenoleukodystrophy
	– Metachromatic leukodystrophy

The ability to diagnose disease early in gestation, by weeks 10 to 12, provides the opportunity to administer prenatal genetic therapies to prevent or aid

1. The Children's Hospital of Philadelphia, Division of Hematology, Philadelphia, PA, USA.

future treatment of the anticipated postnatal disease. Stem cells administered during foetal life can be used to deliver a normal gene, replace an abnormal or deficient stem cell (e.g. haemoglobinopathies), or to induce prenatal tolerance to donor cells in preparation for postnatal solid organ or stem cell transplant without immune suppression or graft rejection. Stem cells demonstrate plasticity and, in the foetus, have the potential for migration to numerous tissues. Haematopoietic stem cells (HSCs) are of particular interest because they demonstrate self-renewal and differentiation are well understood, relatively simple to obtain, and express HLA antigens that are useful in establishing immune tolerance. The foetus is an attractive target for stem cell transplantation because the immune system is immature and tolerance to donor antigens can be achieved. Finally, because the foetus is very small, administering a high dose of HSCs is relatively easy.

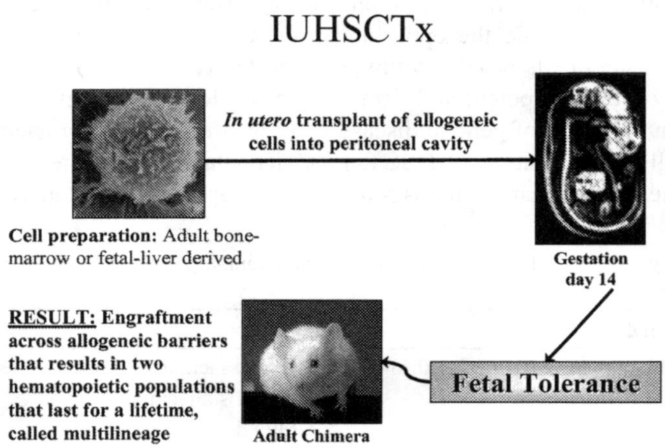

Figure 1. Schematic for murine chimera development.

Arguably the most important feature of IUHSCTx is the foetus's immature immune system and ability to become tolerant to donor cells. The foetal immune system matures around gestational week 14 in a two-step process, a positive selection process of self-antigens followed by a deletion process based on high-affinity for self-antigens. This two-step process results in a repertoire of lymphocytes that react against foreign antigens. Introduction of allogeneic or xenogeneic HSCs before immune maturation, theoretically, allows positive selection and prenatal tolerance to donor cells. The result is a chimeric individual who maintains both native and transplanted HSCs, which ultimately cure disease, improve functioning, or enable postnatal donor stem cell or organ transplantation.

In utero haematopoietic stem cell transplantation (IUHSCTx) has been examined as an approach to the treatment of many diseases, particularly the haemoglobinopathies. In animal models, IUHSCTx is performed by injecting adult haematopoietic stem cells or foetal liver stem cells into the foetal peritoneal cavity prior to immune system maturation. As the immune system matures the foetus is tolerised to the donor cells and will, theoretically, exist as an adult chimera (see Figure 1). IUHSCTx alone may be beneficial for some diseases as the donor cells will have a selective advantage or minimal donor cell engraftment is required to achieve a therapeutic response. Other diseases may benefit from IUHSCTx and postnatal therapies, such as stem cell or organ transplant. These diseases require a higher level of mixed haematopoietic chimerism than that achieved with IUHSCTx alone (see Table 2). These diseases are targeted for IUHSCTx because of the theoretical therapeutic response of a mixed chimerism.

Table 2. Target diseases for IUHSCTx

Diseases that may benefit from IUHSCTx alone	**Diseases that would benefit from a combination of IUHSCTx and postnatal strategies**
Selective advantage for donor cells: – *SCID:* X-linked, ADA-deficiency, ZAP 70, Jac 3 – Wiskott Aldrich – *Chromosomal breakage:* Fanconi anaemia, Bloom syndrome	Potential treatment with mixed chimerism: – *Haemoglobinopathies:* β-Thalassaemia, α-Thalassaemia, sickle cell disease
Minimal engraftment required to be therapeutic: – Hyper IgM syndrome – CGD	Postnatal therapy requiring prenatal tolerance induction because lack of matched sibling donor: – Diseases that can be diagnosed early in gestation and successfully treated by postnatal stem cell transplant

Animal IUHSCTx studies have, so far, shown engraftment levels that are well below what would be considered therapeutic for most target diseases. For β-thalassaemia and sickle cell disease clinical improvement would be characterized as a chimera having as little as 15-20% engraftment. One study compared the use of adult haematopoietic stem cells to foetal liver cells in murine models for β-thalassaemia and sickle cell disease. Higher levels of engraftment were seen with transplanted foetal liver cells. While allogeneic mixed chimerism was sustained in approximately 50% of mice that lived, interestingly, haematologic parameter improvement was not sustained despite donor erythropoiesis having a selective advantage [1].

Human IUHSCTx Clinical Trials

In 1999, 26 human cases of IUHSCTx were reported. Targeted diseases for IUHSCTx included Rh-disease, bare lymphocyte syndrome, SCID, α and ß-thal-

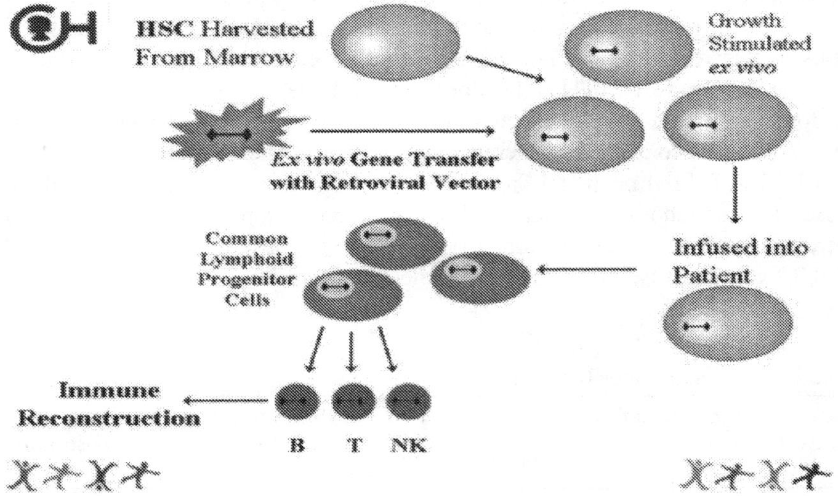

Figure 2. Schematic for an X-linked SCID trial. From: Hacein-Bey-Abina, S. et al. NEJM. 2002.

assaemias, Nieman-Pick type A CGD, Chediak-Higashi, Hurler's disease, sickle cell disease, and globoid leukodystrophy. Fourteen of the 26 survived the procedure. Twelve were performed at greater than 14 weeks gestation, after immune system maturation. Nine of 26 had stem cell engraftment. Three of the nine died, three had original disease, and two were reported as clinically normal. Interestingly, three of the nine who had stem cell engraftment were treated after gestational week 14 (including the 2 clinically normal children).

The key questions of this new treatment approach are: Is there space in the foetal haematopoietic compartment for donor cells? Does space need to be made through myeloablation? Can donor cells effectively compete with host cells to achieve significant postnatal expression? Is the early gestational foetus able to become tolerant to the foreign antigen?

Gene Therapy for X-Linked Severe Combined Immune Deficiency

Severe combined immune deficiency (SCID) is characterized by abnormalities in lymphocyte development and function. If untreated, most children with SCID will die within the first two years of life due to overwhelming infection. Current treatment for SCID is bone marrow transplantation (BMT) from an HLA matched sibling donor with resultant survival rates approaching 90% or haploidentical BMT from a parent or HLA-matched BMT from a non-related donor have a survival rate between 50-70% [2]. The most frequently encountered SCID is the X-linked variant, which is characterized by a defect in the *gamma c* chain, an essential component of five cytokine receptors a necessary for T cells and natural killer cell development.

Gene therapy for SCID has been investigated and tested in humans. Infused genetically altered cells have selective advantage over endogenous cells and are able to colonize the lymphoid system. Human clinical trials for ADA-deficient SCID [3] and X-linked SCID [4] have shown promising results; however, recent serious adverse events related to study procedures in the X-linked SCID trial have puzzled the scientific community. A schematic for the X-linked SCID trial is shown in Figure 2.

SCID Clinical Trials and Leukaemia

The report on first five subjects in the X-linked SCID trial [4] revealed that transplant of the retroviral treated cells in four of five subjects resulted in development of a functional immune system two to three months after receiving the gene therapy, as shown by protective T-cell immunity and partial restoration of B-cell and natural killer (NK) cell populations. The immune system repair was incomplete; the treatment still provided protective immunity. To date, 11 subjects have been enrolled in this trial. Ten of 11 subjects have sustained correction of the T-cell deficiency. The one subject who did not undergo HSC engraftment was ill at the time of the procedure.

In September 2002, a subject presented with hepatosplenomegaly and WBC of 300,000/mm3 and was subsequently diagnosed with T-cell leukaemia. In January 2003, a second subject was diagnosed with T-cell leukaemia. These cases of leukaemia following gene therapy are unique, in that no leukaemia or other cancers were observed in animal studies, only one case of murine tumor formation has been reported in retroviral transduction of HSCs1, other human trials with similar vector and methodology have not seen oncogenesis, and insertional mutagenesis thought an unlikely risk with this vector.

There are obvious similarities in these children. Both cases detected around 2.5 years following stem cell engraftment, the children are the youngest treated in this trial, the T-cell clone is detectible in both patients' serum taken one year post-treatment, and the gene integration site was near the known oncogene LMO2.

There are many unanswered questions remaining:

1. Is retroviral integration causally linked to leukaemogenesis? Tumor formation can occur if a normally silenced oncogene is activated. Retrovirus is used to uncover novel oncogenes through insertion-induced mutagenesis. However, there is no other report of gene therapy vector insertion-induced mutagenesis using a retroviral vector
2. Is integration near LMO2 site a frequent event or one that occurs in select patients? Analysis of leukaemic cells showed that the therapeutic gene integrated near the known oncogene LMO2, which encodes a LIM domain protein that binds DNA transcription factors.
3. Is the gamma c gene expression different when the gene is derived from a recombinant retroviral vector under control of the vector's LTR? The latency that preceded leukaemia development suggests that LMO2 expression con-

fers only a small increase in proliferation or that secondary transforming events are required to cause proliferation of the leukaemic T-cell. The gamma c gene may provide proliferative or anti-apoptotic effect in combination with insertional activation of LMO2.

4. Are there other genetic co-factors that cooperate with LMO2 to promote leukaemia development? It is known that tumours that persist in immunodeficient mice are rejected in normal mice. All subjects in this gene transfer trial had subnormal NK-cell numbers, which may have placed these subjects at an increased risk for tumour development.

Future Directions

Scientists are establishing IUHSCTx methods that will improve stem cell engraftment and looking to develop Phase I clinical trials in the future. Currently, the human retroviral gene transfer studies remain on hold until the big questions are answered and risk factors for leukaemia development are identified. Physicians, scientists, and families will have to carefully weigh the risks and benefits of the X-linked SCID trial before moving on to the next phase.

References

1. Hayashi S, Abdulmalik O, Peranteau WH, et al. Mixed chimerism following in utero hematopoietic stem cell transplantation in murine models of hemoglobinopathy. Exp Hematol 2003;31:176-84.
2. Antoine C, Muller S, Cant A, et al. Long-term survival and transplantation of haemopoietic stem cells for immunodeficiencies: report of the European experience 1968-99. Lancet 2003;361:553-60.
3. Aiuti A, Slavin S, Aker M, et al. Correction of ADA-SCID by stem cell gene therapy combined with nonmyeloablative conditioning. Science 2002; 296:2410-13.
4. Hacein-Bey-Abina S, Le Deist F, Carlier F, et al. Sustained correction of X-linked severe combined immunodeficiency by ex vivo gene therapy. N Engl J Med 2002; 346:1185-93.

META-ANALYSIS AND EVIDENCE-BASED DECISION MAKING IN NEONATAL CARE[1]

R.G. Strauss[2]

Introduction

Therapies are prescribed for neonates and infants with the intent that they will be beneficial, that the benefits are likely to outweigh any risks and, hopefully, that the therapies will be judged to be cost effective and provide years of quality life at an acceptable price. All agree that therapeutic decisions should follow the principles of "evidenced-based medicine" whenever possible. Briefly stated, these principles are to avoid therapies for which efficacy has not been proven and to prescribe efficacious therapies only when indicated. Consequently, risks of adverse effects are taken only when benefits are likely, and healthcare resources are used optimally.

Efficacy is most convincingly established – and the most frequently encountered toxicities often identified – by prospective clinical trials in which comparable subjects are randomly allocated either to receive the investigational therapy being evaluated ("Treatment Arm") or to be treated in the usual way (i.e., standard care) without receiving the investigational therapy ("Control Arm"). Whenever possible, everyone involved (i.e., patient, patient's family and investigators) are unaware of the assignment (i.e., "blinded" as in a placebo-controlled study). If blinding is impossible, observations and endpoints should be as objective as possible (i.e., avoid subjectivity), and/or the observations should be analyzed and interpreted by "blinded" or impartial assessors to avoid bias. Before initiation, trials must be designed so that sufficient numbers of subjects are enrolled to answer the question posed (i.e., to test the hypothesis) with rigorous statistical significance/confidence, and plans made to ensure complete and accurate collection of data for analysis, interpretation and reporting.

Because of the heterogeneity of critically-ill patients, honest differences of medical/scientific opinion pertaining to administration of either the investigational and/or the standard therapies being studied, and variations/flaws in experimental design, the results and/or interpretation of clinical trials are not

---

1. National Institutes of Health Grants P01 HL46925 and RR 00059.

2. Departments of Pathology and Pediatrics, DeGowin Blood Center, University of Iowa College of Medicine, Iowa City, IO, USA.

always in agreement – often, being diametrically opposed with some trials establishing efficacy and others refuting efficacy of the therapy in question. In attempts to understand with the contrary clinical trials do not agree, they are examined critically to detect differences in characteristics of the patients enrolled, differences in how either the investigational and/or the standard therapies were administered (i.e., dose, schedule, route, duration and timing during the course of illness) and differences/flaws in experimental design and statistical analysis. This examination of reported clinical trials can take the form of review articles or commentaries/editorials in which an expert critically analyzes existing trials in the most complete and objective fashion possible and, then, offers recommendations for clinical practices, future studies, etc. The quality and completeness will depend on the knowledge, energy and zeal of the expert. Formal meta-analysis offers another form of critical analysis of multiple clinical trials that follows a more structured plan.

Meta-analysis is a statistical method/tool for the quantitative synthesis of existing primary clinical trials [1]. Meta-analysis depends on the quality and quantity of primary clinical trials available for analysis and, thus, is always observational (i.e., the meta-analyst can work only with available trials; she/he can not transform flawed studies into sound ones). A good meta-analysis is conducted according to a well-defined protocol consisting of a comprehensive literature search, blinded quality assessment, coding of results, analysis (including sensitivity analyses) and reporting [1]. The literature search is key, and attempts must be made to include all relevant articles or, at the very least, a sound representative sampling – the latter being the less desirable option, as bias is difficult to avoid. When conducted properly, meta-analysis is well suited to investigating the influence of study quality on observed/reported treatment differences, trends in trial results over time, the impact of covariance adjustments, and gaps in research that require additional data. Benefits of meta-analysis include an increase in statistical power and precision, a broadening of the scope of inference, development of information on the influence of study-level attributes, and identification of gaps in knowledge – with the potential to improve design, analysis and reporting of subsequent clinical trials [1].

Meta-analysis and Evidence-based Decisions in Neonatology

In neonatology, as in other medical disciplines, meta-analysis is performed to gain an overall view of multiple, randomized trials that address a specific topic/problem/issue. Properly-designed clinical trials in which study subjects are prospectively enrolled and randomly assigned to investigational versus control groups are difficult to perform in neonates and infants because of their small size, precarious clinical condition, difficulties in performing laboratory studies and the imprecision in defining/ recognizing/ achieving primary and secondary outcomes. Accordingly, many neonatology practices are based on logic and best of intentions, rather than sound scientific data. Despite these obstacles, randomized, controlled clinical trials have been conducted in infants, and meta-analyses performed to provide neonatal practice guidelines.

As described earlier, meta-analysis involves a formal statistical analysis of clinical trials that fulfil predetermined criteria (selected to be scientifically desirable) for inclusion. Because many reported clinical trials fail to fulfill the inclusion criteria, firm recommendations for practice are not always evident even following meta-analysis. Accordingly, practices may have to be based on both the results of formal meta-analysis plus a critical "clinical" review of all available literature (i.e., evidence-based medicine per expert commentary or editorial). As an example, the role of recombinant human erythropoietin therapy rHEPO in the treatment of the anaemia of prematurity will be discussed in the following sections to illustrate how both of these processes contribute to decision making.

Pathophysiology of Erythropoietin in the Anaemia of Prematurity

During the first weeks of life, all infants experience a decline in circulating RBCs caused both by physiological factors and, in sick premature infants, by phlebotomy blood losses. In healthy term infants, the nadir blood haemoglobin value rarely falls below 9 g/dL at an age of approximately 10–12 weeks [2]. In preterm infants, this decline occurs at an earlier age and is more pronounced in severity – the mean haemoglobin concentration falls to approximately 8 g/dL in infants of 1.0–1.5 kg birth weight and to 7 g/dL in infants < 1.0 kg [3]. Because this postnatal drop in haemoglobin level is universal and is well tolerated in term infants, it is commonly referred to as the "physiologic anaemia" of infancy. However, in preterm infants, this marked decline in haemoglobin frequently is exacerbated by phlebotomy blood losses and may be associated with symptomatic anaemia requiring RBC transfusions – making the anaemia of prematurity unacceptable as a benign "physiologic" event.

Physiological factors influencing erythropoiesis and erythropoietin (EPO) biology are critical in the pathogenesis of the anaemia of prematurity. Growth is extremely rapid during the first weeks of life, and RBC production by neonatal marrow must increase commensurately. The circulating life span of neonatal RBCs in the bloodstream is shorter than that of adult RBCs. A key clinical factor is the need for repeated blood sampling to monitor critically ill neonates. Another key reason is the relatively diminished EPO level in the plasma of preterm infants in response to anaemia. Although anaemia provokes EPO production in premature infants, the plasma levels achieved are lower than those observed in older persons with comparable degrees of anaemia and, when related quantitatively, rising EPO levels and falling blood haemoglobin concentrations correlate weakly [4]. This relatively ineffective EPO response limits compensation for anaemia in the newborn caused by rapid growth and RBC loss due to phlebotomy, clinical bleeding, haemolysis, etc.

Erythroid progenitor cells in the blood and marrow of premature infants are quite responsive to recombinant EPO. Because it is the inadequate quantity of

EPO that is the major cause of anaemia – not a subnormal response of erythroid progenitors to the EPO that is present – it is logical to assume that use of rHEPO to treat EPO deficiency and, in turn, the anaemia of prematurity would be beneficial. Unfortunately, rHEPO has not been widely applied in clinical neonatology practice – particularly, in the United States [5] – because its efficacy is debatable. Clonogenic erythroid progenitors from neonates respond well to rHEPO *in vitro* and, when given in sufficient doses to human infants, rHEPO and iron effectively stimulate erythropoiesis *in vivo* as evidenced by increased blood reticulocyte and RBC counts (i.e., efficacy demonstrated at the marrow level). However, when the primary goal of rHEPO therapy is to eliminate RBC transfusions, rHEPO often fails (i.e., efficacy at the clinical level has not been consistently or convincingly demonstrated) [5].

Meta-Analysis of Clinical Trials Studying rHEPO in the Anaemia of Prematurity

By the end of 1999, over 20 controlled clinical trials assessing the efficacy of rHEPO in attempts to eliminate RBC transfusions in the anaemia of prematurity were published, but the relevance of their findings to contemporary neonatal transfusion practice has been debated [5-8]. To investigate the extent and reasons for the variation/inconsistencies in the results of published clinical trials, a meta-analysis was conducted of the controlled clinical studies investigating the efficacy of rHEPO in the anaemia of prematurity published between 1990 and 1999 [9]. Per the protocol/experimental design of the meta-analysis, to be eligible for inclusion a reported study had to prospectively enroll a treatment group of preterm infants under four months of age treated with rHEPO and a concurrent control group not given rHEPO. Moreover, data had to be reported in such a way to permit calculation one or more of three outcome measures – namely, the odds ratio of RBC transfusions in rHEPO-treated infants versus controls, the mean difference in the volume (mL/kg) of RBCs transfused to controls minus the volume of RBCs transfused to rHEPO-treated infants, and/or the mean difference in the number of RBC transfusions per infant given to controls minus the number of RBC transfusions per infant given to rHEPO-treated infants. Studies were excluded from the meta-analysis if they failed to compare infants treated with rHEPO versus concurrent controls not given rHEPO, reported the same study population included in previous publications, enrolled infants older than 4 months of age, or did not report at least one of the aforementioned three outcome measures.

Twenty-one reports were eligible for inclusion in the meta-analysis [9]. However, because the experimental design and conduct of the studies was extremely variable, only four reports [10-13] were judged to fulfill all of the highly desired characteristics of being effectively blinded, having high quality experimental design (i.e., randomized, placebo-controlled, all dropouts well-explained, etc), using conservative RBC transfusion practices (rather than liberal) and enrolling a majority of very preterm infants with birth weight <1.0 kg.

Two major conclusions emerged from the meta-analysis [9]. First, the controlled trials of rHEPO to treat the anaemia of prematurity differed from one another in multiple ways and, consequently, produced markedly variable results that could not be adequately explained. Hence, it was judged premature to make firm recommendations regarding use of rHEPO in clinical practice to treat the anaemia of prematurity. Second, when only the four studies with highly desired characteristics were analyzed, rHEPO was found to be efficacious in significantly reducing RBC transfusion needs. However, the magnitude of the effect of rHEPO on reducing the total RBC transfusions given to infants throughout their initial hospitalization was, in fact, relatively modest and of questionable clinical importance [9]. For example, in the multicentre trial of Shannon et al. [10], significantly fewer RBC transfusions were given during the defined study period to rHEPO-treated infants than to placebo-treated controls (mean of 1.1 transfusions per infant vs 1.6), but rHEPO exerted only a modest effect on overall RBC transfusion needs during the entire hospitalization (mean of 4.4 transfusions per infant for rHEPO-treated infants vs 5.3 for placebo-treated infants).

Evidence-Based Medicine beyond Meta-Analysis for Making Medical Decisions

As described in the preceding section, meta-analysis critically and quantitatively assessed the existing controlled clinical trials, but was unable to clearly recommend how best to use rHEPO in clinical practices. Consequently, neonatologists wishing to prescribe rHEPO for treatment of anaemia in preterm infants are in a dilemma. The relatively large or stable preterm infants, shown to respond best to rHEPO plus iron at the marrow level, are given relatively few RBC transfusions with today's conservative transfusion practices and, accordingly, have little need for rHEPO when the goal is to avoid RBC transfusions. Extremely small preterm infants, who are critically ill and unstable and have the greatest need for RBC transfusions shortly after birth, have not consistently responded to rHEPO plus iron when the outcome measure is to reduce need for RBC transfusions – thus, questioning rHEPO efficacy at the clinical level. Accordingly, there is no compelling need to prescribe rHEPO as standard/routine practice to treat the anaemia of prematurity because its role in substantially altering RBC transfusion practices is unclear.

As another factor contributing to the dilemma of whether or not to prescribe rHEPO to preterm neonates and infants, is the potential for adverse effects. An occasional infant experienced sudden infant death syndrome after receiving rHEPO – a situation not reported in the vast majority of clinical trials and, likely, unrelated to rHEPO therapy – but so rare that definitive information is unavailable. Preterm infants have marginal iron stores, when born before the major transport of iron from their mothers late in gestation, and are prone to iron deficiency – unless they receive iron postpartum via multiple RBC transfusions – so that infants given fewer transfusions as a benefit/response to rHEPO exhibit lower plasma ferritin levels than infants not treated with rHEPO. Presumably, iron is committed to erythropoiesis under the stimulation of pharmacologic doses of rHEPO, and the concern is that iron may be limiting/unavailable for nonerythropoietic needs of rapidly growing infants – despite attempts to provide iron supplements. The safety of rHEPO and iron, especially when given in high doses to drive erythropoiesis, is worrisome because of the threat of oxidative injury, and increased rates of the retinopathy of prematurity have been reported in infants given rHEPO [14] – possibly as a manifestation of oxidant damage.

Finally, rHEPO may exert broad systemic effects. Multiple tissues contain the genetic and metabolic factors necessary to produce EPO and EPO receptors [15]. For example, there is evidence suggesting that neural tissues produce EPO locally, rather than rHEPO being transported across the blood-brain barrier from plasma to the cerebrospinal fluid, as a mechanism to explain the presence of EPO in intracranial fluids [16]. This is important because EPO can have profound effects on neural tissues in experimental settings – presumed to be of a beneficial "neuroprotective" nature. Nonetheless, the potential for widespread systemic effects – beyond those desired/expected of simply increasing erythropoiesis – when pharmacologic doses of rHEPO are given to preterm neonates and infants is worrisome. Although most of the possible adverse effects of rHEPO remain unproven, their avoidance is desirable – particularly, in the absence of a clear benefit from rHEPO (i.e., consistently eliminating the need for RBC transfusions).

Because meta-analysis has not given firm guidelines for the use of rHEPO in clinical practice [9], neonatologists must critically assess reports beyond those included in the meta-analysis to determine if more recent information will facilitate evidence-based decision making. Several reports published after 1999 have provided useful information. Donato et al. [17] randomized 114 neonates with birth weight <1.25 kg to receive either rHEPO or placebo during the first two weeks of life, followed by a six week treatment period during which all infants were given rHEPO. All infants were given iron and folic acid. During the first three weeks of life, rHEPO increased reticulocytes and haematocrit values, but there was no difference in RBC transfusions given early in life. However, at the end of all treatment (eight weeks), a subgroup of infants beginning rHEPO shortly after birth with birth weight <0.8 kg and phlebotomy losses >30 mL/kg were given fewer RBC transfusions throughout their entire course than infants initially given placebo (3.4 ± 1.1 vs 5.4 ± 3.7, $p<0.05$). Similarly, Yeo et al. [18] found a modest advantage for very low birth weight infants given rHEPO versus control infants given no rHEPO. In a randomized, but nonblinded controlled trial, 100 neonates <33 weeks gestation were given either rHEPO or no drug from day 5 to 40; iron was given beginning day 10. Infants given rHEPO had higher reticulocyte counts and haematocrit values, but RBC transfusions were not different than controls. However, a subgroup of infants with birth weight 0.8 to 0.99 kg were given fewer RBC transfusions with rHEPO than control infants not given rHEPO (2.1 ± 1.9 vs 3.5 ± 1.6, $p<0.04$). A third randomized, blinded trial by Meyer et al. [19] found an advantage for very low birth weight infants given rHEPO. Neonates with birth weight <1.7 kg and meeting criteria that predicted a likely need for RBC transfusions were randomized either to receive rHEPO beginning shortly after birth (exact day not reported) and continued until either 34 or 36 weeks of completed gestation or to experience a sham treatment to simulate placebo injections. Iron was given to all infants, but at a much lower dose (unfortunately) to control infants not given rHEPO than to infants given rHEPO – thus, creating two variables/differences being assessed in rHEPO treated vs control infants. Reticulocytes and blood haemoglobin values were higher in infants given rHEPO, but there was no overall difference in RBC transfusions. In a subset of infants with birth weight <1.0 kg, RBC transfusions given only after 30 days of age were reduced by rHEPO vs controls (0.5 ± 0.7 vs 1.6 ± 1.1, $p=0.01$).

Two reports assessed the highly desirable outcome of "success" defined by maintaining a haematocrit of ≥30% completely without need for any RBC transfusions. Maier et al. [20] randomized 219 neonates with birth weights 0.5 to 0.99 kg to receive either early rHEPO from the first week of life for nine weeks, late rHEPO from the fourth week of life for six weeks, or no rHEPO. All infants received iron. "Success" was modest (13% of early rHEPO infants, 11% late rHEPO infants, 4% control infants) with only early rHEPO infants being significantly superior than no rHEPO ($p=0.026$). Avent et al. [21] randomized 93 neonates with birth weight 0.9 to 1.5 kg to receive either low dose rHEPO (250 units/kg) high dose rHEPO (400 units/kg), or no rHEPO. Treatment began within 7 days of life and continued until discharge (median duration of hospitalization was approximately 32 days with a maximum of 74 days). All infants received iron. "Success" was met by 75% of low dose rHEPO infants, 71% of high dose rHEPO and 40% of control infants ($p<0.001$). However, the actual number of RBC transfusions given to all infants treated with rHEPO vs controls was not significantly different, and the authors concluded that in stable infants with birth weight 0.9 to 1.5 kg, when phlebotomy losses are small and RBC transfusions given per stringent transfusion criteria, rHEPO does not significantly decrease RBC transfusions.

The observation by Avent et al. [21] that the benefits of rHEPO in reducing the number of RBC transfusions given can be equalled by stringent/conservative transfusion criteria has been made by many – including a fairly recent report [22]. Franz and Pohlandt assessed both the number of RBC transfusions given and the RBC transfusion criteria used to guide transfusions in four reported prospective, randomized trials of rHEPO given to preterm neonates. To be selected for analysis, the clinical trials had to include ventilated infants (i.e., sick infants likely to receive RBC transfusions). The authors found that, when restrictive transfusion guidelines were followed, the number of RBC transfusions and the volume of RBCs transfused were similarly low in control infants not given rHEPO to values reported for infants receiving rHEPO treatment [22] — thus, questioning the need for rHEPO when the desired outcome is the reduction/elimination of RBC transfusions. In a very small controlled trial, Amin and Alzahrani [23] found the number of RBC transfusions to be similar, whether or not rHEPO was given to preterm infants with birth weight ≤1.0 kg, when RBC transfusions were given per strict transfusion criteria.

The potential for adverse/toxic effects of rHEPO and iron remain undefined. For the most part, significant toxicity has not been well documented. However, the occurrence and severity of possible adverse effects, likely, will be related to dose, route and schedule of administration – all of which have been extremely variable among reports, making definitive observations/conclusions difficult. Pollak et al. [24] found plasma malondialdehyde (a measure of possible oxidant injury) to be increased in infants given rHEPO plus intravenous iron compared to infants given rHEPO plus oral iron or only oral iron. Somewhat in contrast, Akisu et al. [25] found malondialdehyde levels to be reduced in infants given rHEPO plus oral iron starting day 10 of life compared to infants given neither rHEPO nor iron during the period of study.

Conclusions

Although valiant attempts have been made – including many prospective randomized trials, critical analysis commentaries by experts, and formal meta-analysis – to provide firm guidelines for the use of rHEPO in the treatment of the anaemia of prematurity, no recommendations are universally accepted by most neonatologists. Clearly, rHEPO has efficacy in stimulating increased erythropoiesis as evidenced by increased reticulocytes and more stable haematocrit values when compared to controls not given rHEPO. However, when the desired goal/success is the elimination or marked reduction in need for RBC transfusions, efficacy is questionable with either no statistically significant success proven, statistical differences of a magnitude too small to be of clinical significance, or success demonstrated in only certain subsets of infants.

The greatest hope of success in reducing need for RBC transfusions seems likely in preterm infants of birth weight <1.0 kg given rHEPO at a dose of 250 to 400 units/kg three times per week subcutaneously (e.g., Monday, Wednesday and Friday) plus iron, beginning within the first few days of life and extending for several weeks (e.g., six to eight weeks) – particularly, if phlebotomy losses can be minimized. For larger infants of birth weight >1.0 kg, RBC transfusions can be reduced by following stringent/ conservative transfusion criteria – regardless of whether or not rHEPO is given. Because the risk of transmitting donor infectious diseases can be markedly reduced by limiting donor exposures (i.e., using stored units of RBCs reserved for specific infants), many neonatologists prefer to give RBC transfusions, per "single donor" programs, only when needed, instead of dealing with the uncertainties of rHEPO and iron therapy. Each physician or institution must critically analyze the available information and then decide what is best to meet the needs of infants receiving care locally. Regardless of the approach to preterm infants, in general, many physicians prescribe rHEPO and iron for preterm infants born of Jehovah Witness parents, as a means to, hopefully, avoid RBC transfusions and religious/medical/legal conflicts.

References

1. Louis TA. Meta-analysis of clinical studies: the whole is greater than the sum of its parts. Transfusion 1993;33:698-70.
2. Strauss RG. Current issues in neonatal transfusions. Vox Sang 1986;51:1-9.
3. Stockman JA. Anemia of prematurity. Current concepts in the issue of when to transfuse. Pediatr Clin North Am 1986;33:111-28.
4. Brown MS, Phibbs RH, Garcia JF, et al. Postnatal changes in erythropoietin levels in untransfused premature infants. J Pediatr 1983;103:612-17.
5. Strauss RG. Managing the Anemia of Prematurity: RBC Transfusions vs Recombinant Erythropoietin. Transf Med Rev 2001;15:213-23.
6. Widness JA, Strauss RG. Recombinant erythropoietin in the treatment of the premature newborn. Semin Neonatal 1998;3:163-71.
7. Wilimas JA, Crist WM. Erythropoietin – not yet a standard treatment for anemia of prematurity. Pediatrics 1995;95:9-10.
8. Doyle JJ. The role of erythropoietin in the anemia of prematurity. Sem Perinatol 1997;21:20-27.
9. Vamvakas EC, Strauss RG. Meta-analysis of controlled clinical trials studying the efficacy of recombinant human erythropoietin in reducing blood transfusions in the anemia of prematurity. Transfusion 2001;41:406-15.
10. Shannon KM, Keith JF III, Mentzer WC, et al. Recombinant human erythropoietin stimulates erythropoiesis and reduces erythrocyte transfusions in very-low-birth-weight preterm infants. Pediatrics 1995;95:1-8.
11. Ohls RK, Harcum J, Schibler KR, et al. The effect of erythropoietin on the transfusion requirements of preterm infants weighing 750 grams or less: A randomized, double-blind, placebo-controlled trial. J Perinatol 1998;18:173-77.
12. Kumar P, Shankaran S, Krishnan RG. Recombinant human erythropoietin therapy for treatment of anemia of prematurity in very-low-birth-weight infants: A randomized, double-blind, placebo-controlled trial. J Perinatol 1998; 18:173-77.
13. Ohls RK, Ehrenkranz RA, Lemons JA, et al. A multicenter randomized double-masked placebo-controlled trial of early erythropoietin and iron administration to preterm infants. Pediatrics 2001;108;934-42.
14. Romagnoli C, Zecca E, Gallini F, Girlando P, Zuppa AA. Do recombinant human erythropoietin and iron supplementation increase the risk of retinopathy of prematurity? Eur J Pediatr 2000;159:627-34.
15. Juul SE, Yachnis AT, Christensen RD. Tissue distribution of erythropoietin and erythropoietin receptor in the developing human fetus. Early Human Development 1998;52:235-49.
16. Juul SE, Stallings SA, Christensen RD. Erythropoietin in the cerebrospinal fluid of neonates who sustained CNS injury. Pediatr Res 1999;46:543-47.
17. Donato H, Vain N, Rendo P, et al: Effect of early versus late administration of human recombinant erythropoietin on transfusion requirements in prema-

ture infants: Results of a randomized, placebo-controlled, multicenter trial. Pediatrics 2000;105: 1066-72.

18. Yeo CL, Choo S, Ho LY. Effect of recombinant human erythropoietin on transfusion needs in preterm infants. J Paediatr Child Health 2001;37:352-58.
19. Meyer MP Sharma E, Carsons M. Recombinant erythropoietin and blood transfusion in selected preterm infants. Arch Dis Child Fetal Neonatal Ed 2003;88:F41-F45.
20. Maier RE, Obladen M, Müller-Hansen I, et al. Early treatment with erythropoietin b ameliorates anemia and reduces transfusion requirements in infants with birth weights below 1000 g. J Pediatr 2002;141:8-15.
21. Avent M, Cory BJ, Galpin J, et al. A comparison of high versus low dose recombinant human erythropoietin versus blood transfusion in the management of anemia of prematurity in a developing country. J Trop Pediatr 2002; 48:227-33.
22. Franz AR, Pohlandt F. Red blood cell transfusions in very and extremely low birthweight infants under restrictive transfusion guidelines: is exogenous erythropoietin necessary? Arch Dis Child Fetal Neonatal Ed 2001;84:F96-F100.
23. Amin AA, Alzahrani DM. Efficacy of erythropoietin in premature infants. Saudi Med J 2002;23:287-90.
24. Pollak A, Hayde M; Hayn M, et al. Effect of intravenous iron supplementation on erythropoiesis in erythropoietin-treated premature infants. Pediatrics 2001;107:78-85.
25. Akisu M, Tuzun S, Arslanoglu S, Yalaz M, Kultursay N. Effect of recombinant human erythropoietin administration on lipid peroxidation and antioxidant enzymes(s) activities in preterm infants. Acta Med Okayama 2001; 55:357-62.

PLACENTAL BLOOD BANKING IN THE YEAR 2003[1]

L. Lecchi, S. Giovanelli, I. Ratti, S. Cimoni, F. Garcea, P. Rebulla[2]

Introduction

The blood which remains in the placenta after delivery, also known as placental or cord blood, can be easily collected by venipuncture of the cord vessels. The biological and medical interests in placental blood rose steadily in the last two decades, following the discovery that placental blood contains a number of haemopoietic progenitor cells capable of reconstituting a human myeloablated recipient [1], although the number of cells may be sub-optimal in larger adult patients [2]. Further interest was triggered by recent observations suggesting that haemopoietic progenitor cells can change their developmental programme under strict environmental control, a cell capability termed 'plasticity' or 'trans-differentiation', which is currently the object of active investigation and hot debate [3-11].

Regular public banking activities for allogeneic transplantation were started in February 1993 in New York (NY) by Dr. Pablo Rubinstein, in Milan (Italy) by Dr. Girolamo Sirchia, and in Düsseldorf (Germany) by Dr. Peter Wernet. Currently, there are approximately 150,000 cord blood donations stored in more than 30 internationally accessible banking programmes (Figure 1). Cord blood immunogenetic data can be accessed at the Bone Marrow Donors Worldwide (BMDW) web site, together with bone marrow donor registry data. Approximately 70,000 cord blood donations are stored in banks linked to an organisation named NETCORD [12] (Table 1), which developed jointly with the Foundation for the Accreditation of Cell Therapy (FACT) the NETCORD-FACT standards for cord blood banking. Furthermore, NETCORD is currently implementing a real-time compatible unit search system capable of exploring the combined inventory of the member banks, which is termed the 'Virtual Office'.

---

1. Supported in part with grants from Ricerca Finalizzata 2002 (Criobanca automatizzata di materiale biologico); Project QLRT-1999-30887 (Implementation of a cord blood allocation network); Project QLRT-2001-01918 (EUROCORD III).

2. Milano Cord Blood Bank, Centro Trasfusionale e di Immunologia dei Trapianti, IRCCS Ospedale Maggiore, Milan, Italy.

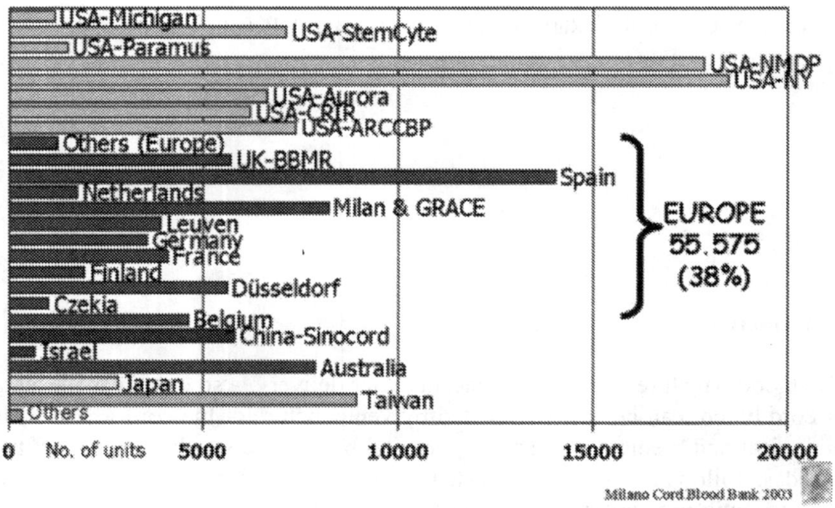

Figure 1. 148.343 Umbilical cord blood units in the BMDW, October 2003.

Table 1. The NETCORD inventory

CB Bank	Inventory	Transplanted	Children	Adults
Barcelona	5715	136	75	61
Düsseldorf	7301	193	142	51
France Cord	3980	111	82	29
Helsinki	1940	0	0	0
Jerusalem	723	12	12	0
Leiden	1764	5	5	0
Leuven	4553	22	18	4
Liège	3949	45	28	17
London	4878	57	41	16
Milan (Graco)	8269	272	167	105
New York	18390	1505	899	606
Sydney	7591	35	23	10
Tokyo	2789	199	86	113
Total	**71842**	**2592**	**1578**	**1012**

So far, more than 2,500 unrelated cord blood transplants have been performed world wide. Of them, 182 were carried out with units released by the Milano Cord Blood Bank, whose inventory of fully characterised and HLA-ABDRB1 typed donations totalled 4,763 units in September 2003.

In this article we describe the process of cord blood banking developed during 1993-2003 at the Milano Cord Blood Bank [13], which was awarded a cer-

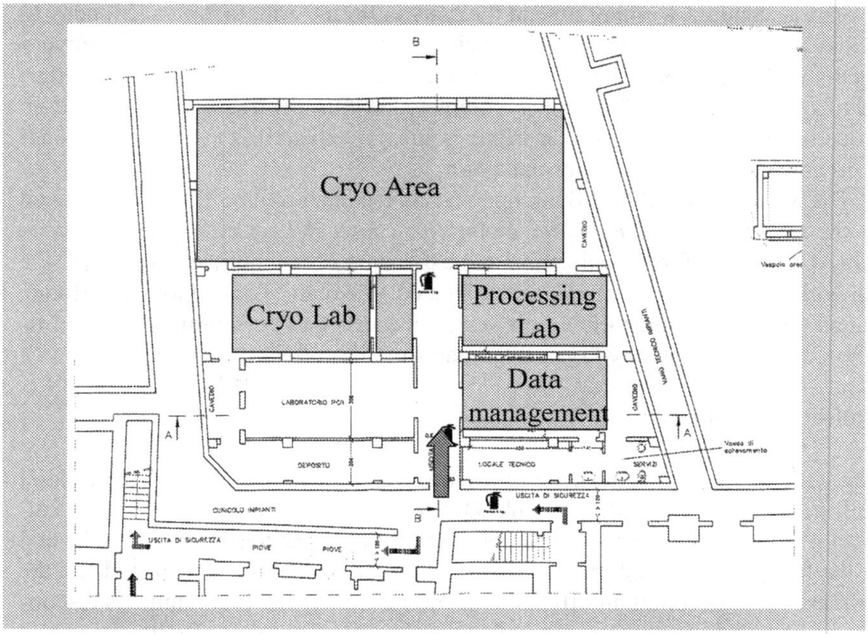

Figure 2. A map describing the location of laboratory, administrative and cryogenetic space at the Milano Cord Blood Bank.

tificate of compliance to the ISO 9002 standard in 1997 and which recently submitted a request of accreditation to the FACT.

The Milano Cord Blood Bank

The Milano Cord Blood Bank is located at the Centro Trasfusionale e di Immunologia dei Trapianti (CTIT) of the Ospedale Maggiore, Milan. The processing laboratories, administrative offices and cryogenic repository cover an area of approximately 250 sqm (Figure 2). The objectives of the Milano Cord Blood Bank are listed in Table 2.

Table 2. Objectives of the Milano Cord Blood Bank

- To ensure a service of cord blood collection and cryopreservation for allogeneic unrelated and related clinical transplantation.
- To ensure safety and efficacy of cord blood units through the adoption of a Quality System.
- To implement co-operation at the national level (Italian network GRACE, GITMO) and at the international level (NETCORD, EUROCORD, EBMT, BMDW).
- To monitor the clinical outcome of cord blood transplantation.
- To investigate cord blood biological characteristics.

As the standard working time at the bank is from 9 a.m. to 7 p.m., Monday to Friday, the time allowed for allogeneic unrelated donation at the 15 delivery rooms collecting cord blood for the Milano Cord Blood Bank is determined so as to ensure that unit freezing is completed within 36 hours from collection. Outside the limits of standard working hours, on call staff is available for donations collected for related transplantation.

The Milano Cord Blood Bank operates as the central hub of the banks linked in the *Gruppo per la Raccolta e Amplificazione delle Cellule Emopoietiche* (GRACE, Group for the collection and expansion of haemopoietic cells) [13], a network of Italian cord blood banks located in Milan, Turin, Florence, Rome, Padua and Pavia. Compatible unit search requests can be submitted to the Milano Cord Blood Bank by fax or by e-mail (micb@policlinico.mi.it).

Collection Centres

The collection centres are delivery rooms which develop a formal cord blood collection agreement with the bank. Delivery rooms applying for a formal collection agreement become provisional collection centres for one year. At the end of the first year the number and quality of the collected units is reviewed and the delivery room becomes an official collection centre or the programme is discontinued according to the outcome of the review. The number of delivery rooms collecting cord blood for the Milano Cord Blood Bank has been expanded to a maximum of 15 sites during 1993-2003. This number was not exceeded based on historical experience, so as to ensure that all the requirements of the quality system, in particular the local training and qualification and the quality audits, could be properly managed [14]. Locations up to approximately 200 miles from Milano have been accepted following a strict definition of transportation rules and times. The Milano Cord Blood Bank is responsible for the training and qualification of the personnel involved in cord blood collection and for the design of the quality system and of the operative procedures.

Donor Selection and Informed Consent

Cord blood collection centres schedule a meeting well before delivery to collect the medical family history from both the mother and the father and the mother's written informed consent to cord blood collection and its donation for allogeneic non family-related use. This is usually done at pre-delivery courses. The father's medical history should be collected through a direct interview, although this is not always possible before delivery. In addition to donor enrolment at pre-delivery courses, gynaecologists and midwives of the collection centres can select potential cord blood donors at the time of hospital admission or during clinical monitoring before delivery. In no case donors are enrolled in the program during labour. Although verbal informed consent to collection is sufficient if previous written consent is not available, written consent including both collection and banking is mandatory within 24 hours after delivery.

Exclusion Criteria

The donor exclusion criteria used at the Milano Cord Blood Bank are described below:

5. Known risk behaviour in the father and/or in the mother for transmissible diseases:
   - Use of heavy drugs
   - Sex with partners at risk
6. Positive serology of the mother and/or the father for:
   - Hepatitis: HBsAg, anti-HCV, HCV-RNA
   - AIDS: anti-HIV
   - Syphilis: TPHA or VDRL
   - Anti-HTLV I-II
7. Genetic diseases of the mother and/or the father and/or the baby.
8. Denied consent.
9. Cumulative stay for more than six months in the United Kingdom during 1980 to 1996.
10. Obstetrical exclusion criteria:
    - Delivery before 34 weeks of gestation
    - Congenital abnormalities in the newborn
    - Membranes rupture more than 12 hours before
    - Fever in the mother on the day before or after delivery
    - Foetal distress.

A detailed list of conditions excluding the collection is enclosed in the operative instructions located at the bank and at the collection centres.

The designated personnel have the responsibility to collect accurately the family medical history, providing the mother and the father with the detailed information necessary to fully understand the importance of this data collection.

Cord Blood Collection, Transportation and Receipt at the Bank

Cord blood is collected in a closed system by venesection of a cord vessel from the placenta in situ in physiological deliveries and after placental delivery in caesarean sections. A sample of venous blood is taken from the mother at the time of cord blood collection for serological screening and for HLA typing.

The cord blood units are transported to the cord blood bank under controlled temperature conditions. Temperature is monitored by a device located in the container used for transportation. Monitoring includes time of packaging, start and end of transportation and name of the operators.

The units and the maternal samples are not accepted if:

- they are mislabelled
- the bag is damaged

– the cord blood was collected more than 36 hours before
– the medical history form reports exclusion criteria.

Unit Processing, Characterisation and Quality Control

Units with net volume below 60 ml or greater than 60 ml but with post-processing number of total nucleated cells (NC) below 800×10^6 are discarded or used for research or quality control. Unit volume is reduced with a bottom-and-top procedure operated with the automated blood component device Compomat G-4 (Fresenius, Germany). This procedure consists in the removal of most plasma and red cells and the collection of the white cell fraction, which includes most CD34+ cells, in the buffy coat. The percent NC recovery from all processed units is recorded on a quality control chart.

Table 3. List of tests and laboratories involved in unit characterisation at the Milano Cord Blood Bank

Test	Laboratory
Nucleated cell count by automated haematology counter before and after volume reduction	Blood Bank Clinical Chemistry (F. Mozzi, D.Sc.)
Nucleated red cell count	Milano Cord Blood Bank
Evaluation of clonogenic potential (colonies)	Milano Cord Blood Bank
Haemoglobin screening	Blood Transfusion Centre ICP (V. Tantalo, MD)
ABO and Rh	Blood Bank Immunohaematology (AABB accredited; F. Morelati, D. Riccardi D.Sc)
Serological screening on mother's serum: HBsAg, anti-HIV 1-2, anti-HCV, HCV-RNA, HIV-RNA, TPHA, ALT, anti-HTLV I-II, anti-CMV and anti-Toxoplasma IgG and IgM, anti-HBc.	Blood Bank Clinical Chemistry
Serological screening on a sample of the unit: HBsAg, anti-HIV 1-2, anti-HCV, anti-HTLV I-II.	
CMV-DNA	Hospital Clinical Chemistry (A. Pagano, MD)
Search for aerobic and anaerobic bacteria and antibiogram if positive	Hospital Clinical Chemistry
CD34+ cell count	North Italy Transplant programme Flow Cytometry Laboratory (L. Porretti, D.Sc.)
Serological and genomic HLA-typing on unit and maternal samples tested at different times	North Italy Transplant programme Immunogenetics Laboratory (EFI accredited, F. Poli, D.Sc.)

In order to complete unit characterisation without wasting the primary precious material, tests performed to characterise the unit are carried out not only on samples removed from the collection bag, but also from the bags containing plasma and red cells to be discarded after volume reduction. Moreover, characterisation requires the access to samples from the freezing bag before freezing and to segmented samples connected to the frozen bag. Finally, the blood samples taken from the mother at cord blood collection and six months after delivery are used. The latter control is performed to reduce the chance that a unit released for transplantation was donated during a window phase for transmissible diseases [15].

Table 3 lists tests and laboratories where the tests are performed for the Milano Cord Blood Bank. Until the serological and microbiological results are available the unit is quarantined in liquid nitrogen vapours. As reported in Figure 3, unit HLA typing is carried out on different samples tested at different times, so as to increase the chance of detecting mistakes which may occur during the banking process. Mother's HLA typing is carried out to verify the Mendelian inheritance of HLA type. Based on previous studies on the variability of the clonogenic assays, the number of colonies per plate, which is recorded on a control chart, must range between 20 and 100. Corrective actions are developed when nonconformities are detected.

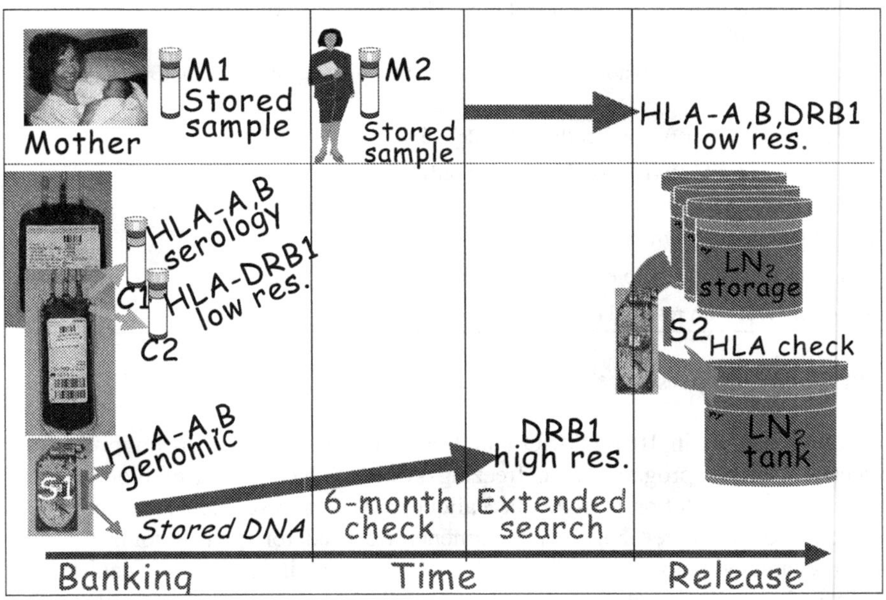

Figure 3. The HLA typing process

Table 4. Type and amount of mother and newborn biological samples stored at the Milano Cord Blood Bank

Biological sample	Amount
Maternal serum collected at delivery	
Until 1996	2-4 ml
Since 1997	4 ml
Maternal serum collected 6 months after delivery	
Until 1996	2-4 ml
Since 1997	4 ml
Cord blood plasma removed at volume reduction, available from 1/12/1997	6 ml
Residual buffy-coat from the bottom and top bag, available from 15/3/1999	about 500 μl
Segments frozen and preserved in the same conditions of the frozen bag, with vital cells.	
Units with volume reduction	0.8 ml
Units without volume reduction	2 ml
Segment of the frozen bag (only if 50 ml Baxter bag; available since 11/2000)	About 300 μl
DNA extracted from 1 ml whole cord blood or 0.6 ml buffy-coat	Mean 71 μg (36-132)
Maternal serum (or buffy-coat) collected at delivery	1.5-5 ml
Maternal serum (or buffy-coat) collected 6 months after delivery	1.5-5 ml
Whole blood (or DNA) from cord blood recipients	2-5 ml
Serum from cord blood recipients	0.5-2 ml
Thawed segment with residual cord blood	Variable

Cord Blood Cryopreservation

The unit is frozen in 10% DMSO (final concentration) within 36 hours from collection using a programmable freezing system. The mixture of blood and cryopreservation solution is frozen in 3 aliquots. At least 6 segments per unit are connected to the frozen bags. The segments are used for quality control and further characterisations. The frozen bags are stored in aluminium canisters within racks in liquid nitrogen tanks equipped with a temperature monitoring system. An alarm system covers the whole cryobiology area with acoustic and visual alarms installed inside and outside the facility. Environmental oxygen percentage is continuously monitored. The correct safety interval is maintained through an automatic ventilation system capable of recycling from 6 to 20 air volumes per hour. The temperature inside the tanks is monitored through a pre-alarm at –145°C and an alarm at –135°C. Moreover, the alarm system monitors the liquid nitrogen level in the tanks.

The location of each bag, which is recorded in the bank data management system, is easily traceable through multiple options such as unit code, date of freezing, tank and rack numbers.

The access to the bank and to the cryobiology area is regulated according to levels of authorisation based on the kind of personnel allowed to enter the area. The cryogenic area and the unit freezing laboratory have been constructed to ensure the safety of the operator (continuous control of ambient oxygen) and the protection of the product (continuous control of liquid nitrogen level and tank temperature). Personnel safety is ensured by the acoustic and visual alarms, which allows appropriate actions in emergency conditions. Tools for emergency resuscitation are available close to the entry door of the cryogenic area. A hospital emergency plan has been developed by the hospital technical department.

When unit transfer from a non-functioning tank becomes necessary, storage priority is given first to related cord blood bags, then to units of apheresis stem cells stored for autologous transplantation, and finally to cord blood donations stored for unrelated transplantation. Regular quality control of the cryopreservation procedure is ensured by testing the nucleated cell number and viability, the clonogenic potential and the sterility of one unit every two months. A parallel biorepository is in place to store the mother and newborn biological samples. The type and amount of samples are reported in Table 4.

Cord Blood Unit Validation

Supervisors from each laboratory report to the bank the results of the performed analysis. At the bank, the report is validated and registered in the data management system, and stored in paper format in the unit folder. The HLA typing laboratory staff transfer the data directly into the computer using a dedicated menu of the data management system.

Unit validation consists in the control that all the reports are present and have been checked for coherence and completeness, that the frozen unit has been fully characterised and that exclusion criteria that should have prevented the donation are not present. Validated units become selectable for a specific patient. The unit is not validated and is eventually rejected if:

- The informed consent form is not available,
- The medical history discloses exclusion criteria,
- The serological screening is positive for HBsAg, anti-HCV, anti-HIV, TPHA, anti HTLV I-II, HCV-RNA or ALT >40 U/ml (on maternal serum collected delivery),
- The sterility test is positive for pathogenic bacteria, such as Streptococcus haemolytic of A or B group,
- Alterations are disclosed during haemoglobin screening,

Table 5. Critical control points of the cord blood banking process used at the Milano Cord Blood Bank

Critical control points	**Aim**
Training of the personnel	Personnel qualification
Staff performance	Control that the activity is uniformly and regularly carried out
Collection centres audit	Control of cord blood collection, acquisition of informed consent and medical history
Monitoring of equipment	Control that equipment performance is regular during time
Cryobiology area automated management	Personnel and product safety. Continuous control of the cryopreservation conditions
Alarm system in the cryobiology area	Personnel and product safety
Daily recording of percent nucleated cell recovery	Check volume reduction procedure
Monthly and annual review of nucleated cell recovery at collection and at cryopreservation.	Cord blood inventory annual evaluation
Monthly review of the percent CD34+ cell and colony recovery, after volume reduction. Test performed on 5 banked cord blood units.	Check volume reduction procedure
Every two months, determination of nucleated cell number and viability, colonies and CD34+ cell counts on a thawed cord blood unit.	Monitoring cryopreservation procedure
Daily recording in a control chart of the number of colonies per plate (must be between 20 and 100)	Monitoring colony procedure
Identity of data reported on the original documents and printed by the computer. Two operators control the data.	Control of data entry

– Problems occur during freezing, e.g. the programmable freezing system does not work properly or the frozen bag appears to be damaged.

The data of the selectable units are recorded into the inventory of selectable units, which is periodically sent to the NETCORD central data base and to the BMDW.

Mother and Newborn Check Six Months after Delivery

Mothers and newborns are controlled six months after delivery to disclose transmissible infectious, genetic or inherited diseases not detected at the time of collection. Units that represent a unique chance for specific patients can be select-

Table 6. Indicators of the cord blood banking process used at the Milano Cord Blood Bank

Indicators	Aim
Number of units collected per month.	Monitoring of the collection activity
Number of collected and cryopreserved units by collection centre and month	Monitoring of the collection activity in each collection centre
Number of units unsuitable for freezing, unsuitable for transplantation, suitable for transplantation and released per year (global and by collection centre)	Monitoring of the bank activity
Number of deferred units by deferral reasons and collection centres	Monitoring main causes of cord blood unit deferral
Number of 6 month checks	Monitoring mother's compliance
Number of unrelated and related units released by the Milano Cord Blood Bank by year and transplant centre	Monitoring unit release
Survival analysis of the patients transplanted with cord blood units released by Milan and GRACE banks	Monitoring clinical outcome of cord blood transplantation
Time (days) of reporting unit characteristics	Monitoring efficiency
Time of reporting HLA high resolution typing	Monitoring efficiency
Time of reporting to DNA shipment request	Monitoring efficiency
Number of units reserved for >1 month	Control of the application of GRACE protocol
Number of equipment extraordinary maintenance events	Optimisation of equipment management
Number and type of mistakes in record data transfer from GRACE banks to the hub	Monitoring central hub quality
Time of transmission of further investigations requests from the hub to the banks	Monitoring central hub efficiency
Number of searches of compatible units	Monitoring hub activity
Number of released units by GRACE banks	Monitoring GRACE activity

selected and transplanted also in the absence of the 6-month control. The final choice is made by the patient's treating physician. The 6-month control program is run in cooperation with a group of trained volunteers. Two months after delivery, a cord blood bank volunteer calls the mothers who had donated cord blood units banked two months before, as a sign of appreciation for their donations and as a reminder of the retesting appointment scheduled at 6 months.

Soon before the date of the appointment at six months, the mothers are contacted again by phone to attend the bank or the collection site. During the check a fresh maternal blood sample is collected to repeat serology performed at delivery. A trained operator interviews the mother to perform an additional check of the mother's medical history form collected at donation and to collect the postnatal baby's medical history. The purpose of this action is to reduce the possibility that the baby is a carrier of evident genetic abnormalities or congenital malformations. The health conditions of the baby are recorded on the medical history form. If checks are uneventful, the unit suitability is confirmed, otherwise the unit is discarded. A detailed description of the programme and its main results have been published elsewhere [15].

Cord Blood Banking Process Monitoring

A number of critical control points and indicators are used to monitor the cord blood banking process. They are listed in Tables 5 and 6 respectively.

Conclusions

The clinical data so far collected indicate that cord blood is a useful sources of haemopoietic progenitor cells for myeloablated recipients [16-18]. Moreover recent evidence suggest that also adult patients treated with reduced – intensity conditioning regimens can benefit from cord blood transplantation [19].

In spite of its demonstrated clinical effectiveness, cord blood is an expensive resource [20]. This requires careful planning of collection and banking programs. While the former need to be expanded so as to allow the collection of large-volume units, preferentially ethics groups with HLA phenotypes poorly represented in the current inventories, consolidation of the latter is of outmost importance, to ensure that the banking programmes reach the critical mass necessary to release a number of units sufficient to recover the costs.

International efforts aimed at harmonising the national programmes have been promoted to reach the above objectives.

References

1. Gluckman E, Broxmeyer HA, Auerbach AD, et al. Hematopoietic reconstitution in a patient with Fanconi's anemia by means of umbilical-cord blood from an HLA-identical sibling. N Engl J Med 1989;321:1174-78.
2. Laughlin MJ, Barker J, Bambach B, et al. Hematopoietic engraftment and survival in adult recipients of umbilical cord blood from unrelated donors. New Engl J Med 2001;344:1815-22.
3. Bjornson CR, Rietze RL, Reynolds BA, Magli MC, Vescovi AL. Turning brain into blood: a hematopoietic fate adopted by adult neural stem cells in vivo. Science 1999;283:534-37.
4. Zubair AC, Silberstein L, Ritz J. Adult hematopoietic stem cell plasticity. Transfusion 2002;42:1096-101.
5. Orlic D, Kajstura J, Chimenti S et al. Bone marrow cells regenerate infarcted myocardium. Nature 2001;410:701-05.

6. Krause DS, Theise ND, Collector MI, et al. Multi-organ, multi-lineage engraftment by a single bone marrow-derived stem cell. Cell 2001;105:369-77.
7. Morshead CM, Benveniste P, Iscove NN, van der Kooy D. Hematopoietic competence is a rare property of neural stem cells that may depend on genetic and epigenetic alterations. Nat Med 2002;8:268-73.
8. McKinney-Freeman SL, Jackson KA, Camargo FD, Ferrari G, Mavilio F, Goodell MA. Muscle-derived hematopoietic stem cells are hematopoietic in origin. Proc Natl Acad Sci USA 2002;99:1341-46.
9. Terada N, Hamazaki T, Oka M, etal. Bone marrow cells adopt the phenotype of other cells by spontaneous cell fusion. Nature 2002;416:542-45.
10. Ying QL, Nichols J, Evans EP, Smith AG. Changing potency by spontaneous fusion. Nature 2002;416:545-48.
11. Orkin SH, Zon LI. Hematopoiesis and stem cells: plasticity versus developmental heterogeneity. Nat Immunol 2002;3:323-28.
12. Hakenberg P, Kogler G, Wernet P. NETCORD: a cord blood allocation network. Bone Marrow Transplant 1998; 22:S17-18.
13. Lazzari L, Corsini C, Curioni C, et al. The Milan Cord Blood Bank and the Italian Cord Blood Network. J Hematother 1996;5:117-22.
14. Sirchia G, Rebulla P, Lecchi L, Mozzi F, Crepaldi R, Parravicini A. Implementation of a quality system (ISO 9000 Series) for placental blood banking. J Hematotherapy 1998;1:19-35.
15. Lecchi L, Rebulla P, Ratti I, et al. Outomes of a program to evaluate mother and baby 6 month after umbilical cord blood donation. Transfusion 2001; 41:606-10.
16. Gluckman E. Current status of umbilical cord blood hematopoietic stem cell transplantation [Review]. Exp Hematol 2000;28:1197-205.
17. Rubinstein P, Carrier C, Scaradavou A, et al. Outcomes among 562 recipients of placental-blood transplants from unrelated donors. New Engl J Med 1998;339:1565-77.
18. Gluckman E, Rocha V, Boyer-Chammard A, et al. Outcome of cord blood transplantation from related and unrelated donors. New Engl J Med 1997; 337:373-81.
19. Barker JN, Davies SM, DeFor T, et al. Survival after transplantation of unrelated donor umbilical cord blood is comparable to that of human leukocyte antigen-matched unrelated donor bone marrow: results of a matched-pair analysis. Blood 2001;97: 2957-61.
20. Sirchia G, Rebulla P, Tibaldi S, Lecchi L. Cost of umbilical cord blood units released for transplantation. Transfusion 1999;39:645-50.

DISCUSSION

Moderators: N. Luban and C.Th. Smit Sibinga

N. Luban (Washington DC, USA): So for those of you who are from institutions that use Epo, please raise your hands if you are using EPO in your prematures. Interesting, one hand went up.

R.G. Strauss (Iowa City, IA, USA): How many take care of preterm infants who have elected not to use erythropoietin? I want to know the denominator.

Would any of you mention why you have decided not to use recombinant erythropoietin? Do you follow the same rationale I mentioned or are there specific reasons that we can learn from you why you don't use it? Costs too much money or what is the reason?

P.T. Pisciotto (Farmington, CT, USA): Our neonatologists went through the same analysis that you had just gone through and they really felt that, with the babies that we were taking care of we wouldn't see very much effect.

N. Luban: Let me just point out an interesting phenomenon and it maybe because of the group that has been assembled here. In the Washington area, there are a number of university hospitals and then there are at least two very large private hospitals with immense delivery services and tertiary care nurseries. They too care for very sick babies, but they are not university-based. What we find very fascinating is that at particularly one of those two institutions, they use EPO routinely on all of their prematures and believe in giving EPO to term infants who may or may not ever require a transfusion. The rationale is that they use it actually as a selling point - if you are delivered in their hospital and you go to their neonatal intensive care unit, then you can be pretty much assured that your child will not be transfused. Not with any supporting documentation, I might add. So the three university-based NIC units use no EPO and the private hospitals use it regularly. Anybody else have that kind of a phenomenon in their area?

R.G. Strauss: To me, the fallacy in that sort of thinking is that in the future perhaps that will turn-out to be true. But right now, without knowing the potential toxicities that I mentioned, deprivation of iron from other sites in the body where iron is needed, rather than red cells, may be found harmful in long term follow-up neuro-developmental studies done of the age of ten years or so in these infants. I think we are exposing babies to risks that we really don't understand, or the potential for risks that we don't understand.

J. Power (Cork, Ireland): Just to make a comment. We have one neonatologist of three who uses EPO, but they haven't come together to decide policy. I think he is just going of on his own trail. I think we need to focus again from the studies on who might be the most benefited by EPO, that has been very helpful.

C. Dame (Berlin, D): A very short comment. There are three papers published[1] during the last one and a half years, reporting that erythropoietin and erythropoietin -receptor are expressed in the retina, and ophthalmologists have the concept to use Epo as the protective agent, for example in certain degenerative ophthalmologic diseases[2]. The second point is a question. There is still a controversy about the use of erythropoietin in preventing transfusions in 'late' anaemia. In Europe, some neonatologists treat these babies with recombinant erythropoietin, some groups don't. Can you give a short overview on the situation. My impression is that half of the centres are treating with Epo.

R.G. Strauss: None of my responses are short, but I will make two comments. The first one. We were talking the other day following your talk about the fact that many tissues have the genetic material to either make a cytokine or a receptor for a cytokine. Repeatedly, in the literature pertaining to the brain, the eye and other places such as the GI-tract, investigators state that growth factors must have a protective function of some kind, neuroprotective, ophthalmologic protective, GI protective. This may be totally true, but remember we are giving these drugs in pharmacologic doses that may be a thousand times or so higher than the physiological level. We are playing God, in a way, and does God really think that those receptors are going to respond the same way to a physiologic dose as they do to tremendously high pharmacologic doses? I don't know, I just think there is the potential for harm. One of the major ways in which erythropoietin works is to prevent apoptosis. I think all of you remember from embryology how apoptosis is very important for the remodelling of organs and tissues in the developing foetus and newborn. If we block that process, are we potentially harming development? I don't know, but I am worried that just because

---

1. A. Grimm C, Wenzel A, Groszer M, et al. HIF-1-induced erythropoietin in the hypoxic retina protects against light-induced retinal degeneration. Nat Med. 2002;8:718-24. B. Bocker-Meffert S, Rosenstiel P, Rohl C, et al. Erythropoietin and VEGF promote neural outgrowth from retinal explants in postnatal rats. Invest Ophthalmol Vis Sci. 2002;43:2021-26. C. Junk AK, Mammis A, Savitz SI, et al. Erythropoietin administration protects retinal neurons from acute ischemia-reperfusion injury. Proc Natl Acad Sci U S A. 2002;99:10659-64.
2. Becerra SP, Amaral J. Erythropoietin--an endogenous retinal survival factor. N Engl J Med. 2002;347:1968-70.

there are receptors and/or the ability to make the growth factor, that giving the factor is always helpful.

In terms of the late anaemia, the papers are really mixed, and I don't really know the right answer. I think there are two clinical settings where we think about using erythropoietin. One is for later transfusions that are needed because of the anaemia of prematurity. Unless you begin erythropoietin and iron very early after birth (don't wait until the infant is four or five weeks of age, because it is too late) you will not be able prevent late transfusions. But giving it early and continuing does seem to work. So if you feel that preventing late transfusions is desirable, I would begin erythropoietin and iron early and continue it.

Another situation for erythropoietin is in alloimmunisation to K1 or Kell and alloimmunisation to D, where infants have prolonged marrow hypoplasia. Several studies have shown that if you give erythropoietin, you can "jump-start" the marrow and prevent or diminish the need for late transfusions. Others have not always found that to be true. At our institution, these infants would get a transfusion or two and, then, if their marrow did not begin to work, they probably would get started on erythropoietin and iron.

R.G. Strauss: Dr. Lecchi, on the harvesting of placental blood, are placentas delivered and taken ex utero or do you collect blood while the placenta is still in utero following a vaginal delivery?

L. Lecchi (Milan, I): In vaginal delivery we collect with the placenta in utero. After birth we clamp the cord, and when you wait for the extrusion of the placenta, you have about 5 minutes, but that is sufficient to collect cord blood. During Caesarean delivery the cord blood collection is performed after expulsion of the placenta, which is held at its edge and suspended with the foetal side and the cord down.

N. Luban: What was the rationale between the US and Eurocord in performing the six month follow-up visit for the mother and the infant. As many of you know and if you don't know I will tell you, in the US that six months visit is not performed.

L. Lecchi: I know, because we have discussed this point very often with other colleagues. We perform this check for two reasons. To collect the history of the newborn during the six months and to repeat the serological test on the maternal serum as an attempt to disclose transmissible infectious and genetic or inherited diseases not detected at the time of collection. As regard serological tests new advanced tests such as molecular test could solve the problem, but it is very important to understand if in the first time of the life of the newborn we have some sign of a specific disease. Because for example for genetic disease we haven't the possibility to screen all the possible diseases. So far, the only way to have an answer or to have a check is collect a history of the newborn. Some investigators reported difficulties in tracing mothers and that the programme is very expensive. In our experience we have a compliance of 94% of the mothers to the programme.

N. Luban: I noticed that you didn't list any screening for specific genetic diseases. You, did mention serology. Are there specific molecular tests that you do to rule out haemoglobinopathies or other commonly known genetic diseases?

L. Lecchi: For haemoglobinopathy screening, we screen in particular for thalassaemia. We carry out haemoglobin fractions to disclose alterations of the haemoglobin associated with beta-thalassaemia or alfa-thalassaemia.

P.T. Pisciotto: I noticed only about 40 to 50 percent of the cord blood you have collected was suitable, is that correct? Among the cord bloods that you collect, it appeared that only 40 percent went on to final process, 60 percent looked like they were discarded. What were the reasons for the discard?

L. Lecchi: The principle reason is low volume. Our target is 60 ml. The second reason is a low number of nucleated cells, because we want not less than 800 million. Another reason is related to the clinical history collected regarding the mother and the father. This is the most important. Other reason could be the presence of clots in the bag, so it is not a good collection. But the volume discarded is about 60 percent.

J. Power: If I understand you correctly about 5000 units that you have available in the cord blood bank at the moment. Within your own experience in the last two or three years, what has been the number of requests and what has been the number of clinical applications from your own bank?

L. Lecchi: We have about 1000 requests per year from transplant centres and we are releasing about 20-24 units per year.

C.Th. Smit Sibinga (Groningen, NL): Dr Manno, the foetal stem cell transplantation, very small volumes as you said, an advantage as you need very few cells. Have these 26 cases that you spoke about been done with cord stem cells? Given the fact that that is a small volume and you have a limited number of cells and they or very potential.

C.S. Manno (Philadelphia, PA, USA): The sources were mixed. Some of them were bone marrow harvested and some were cord blood.

C.Th. Smit Sibinga: Do you see a future for cord blood in foetal stem cell transplantation?

C.S. Manno: Sure. Particularly based on the low risk of a Graft versus Host Disease.

C.Th. Smit Sibinga: Would these cells also be more easily to manipulate?

L. Lecchi: We don't use foetal cells. Because for cord blood we can collect only if we have 34 weeks of gestation. It is not an ethical practice to collect from foetus for cord blood transplantation.

R.G. Strauss: Can I just follow up on that. In an investigation or experimental setting, cord blood cells, especially the CD 34 subsets from preterm infants, have growth advantages and characteristics that make them very amenable to gene therapy, at least in a theoretical way. Could you give us an idea of whether there is a lot of research interest in using placental blood from preterm infants, to exploit these advantages?

L. Lecchi: For research could be. Because we have more progenitor cells when we have less weeks of gestation. My interest is in a cord blood bank for transplant, so I have not such experience. I know that there is a great ethical debate if we want to use them or don't want to use. Our experience in research is only on the newborn, not on the foetus.

C.Th. Smit Sibinga: Another question which also came up at our 26th symposium.[1] Why is it that we went for anamnestic screening for inherited diseases in potential cord cell donors, why don't we do that for the regular stem cell collections, both bone marrow as well as peripheral blood if we use allogeneic? There is discrepancy. What is your idea?

L. Lecchi: I work in a cord blood bank, I don't work in a bone marrow transplantation setting or in peripheral blood collection. So I am not experienced in this. I know for example that the stem cells collected from peripheral blood in our transfusion centre is linked to the bone marrow transplant. I know that they require a questionnaire for the risk of inherited diseases. But I think that also in that situation it is necessary to define a standard, because without standard every centre makes its own policy.

C.Th. Smit Sibinga: The point is that in a number of genetically defined diseases the abnormal gene has given, as a consequence, an abnormal organ or cell complex. If you deal with a patient who has a normal organ, the target organ will not be affected by a gene that is abnormal. So that doesn't make that much sense therefore.

L. Lecchi: Yes, it is a very complicated question. Because we have no answer now to apply this in the routine. We need more studies in this way.

---

1. Transmissible Diseases and Blood Transfusion. Smit Sibinga CTh and Dodd RY, eds. Kluwer Acad. Publ. Dordrecht/Boston/London 2002:160 (discussion).

A. Suranto (Jakarta, Ind): First how long will the cord blood be stored, because there will be many blood bags stored and the freezer will be full. Second: do they have to pay for the storage?

L. Lecchi: Theoretically we can store the bag indefinitely, because they are in a liquid nitrogen. We have a bank that has stored units for more than 10 years.

For the storage we cannot ask payment, because we are a public cord blood bank. In a public health system we cannot ask money. When we release a unit of course we ask money from the requesting institution, but this is the only way for reimbursement.

C.S. Manno: With regard to the concern about dosage that the cord doesn't supply a dose that is large enough. You suggested that one strategy going forward, would be to combine donations, is that true?

L. Lecchi: This is the last way that some transplant centre follow. You remember that I showed that twelve multicord transplants were performed. It is a possible way.

C.S. Manno: What would be the concerns about that approach?

L. Lecchi: For example we released the units for 6 of these kind of transplants. The choice of the clinician was one HLA mismatch, with one difference between the two units. So you can recognise which of the infused units determine the engraftment. The intention is to infuse an higher number of cells . But in the first result it could be that only one of the two cords determines the engraftment. That means that the genes recognise only one HLA. It is yet to understand why this happens.

R.G. Strauss: When you do that then is there an advantage for using highly-purified CD 34 cells, to avoid lymphocytes?

L. Lecchi: In the cord blood we don't perform any selection, because the number of cell is too small. This practice is good if you have bone marrow or if you have peripheral blood after stimulation.

C.Th. Smit Sibinga: Dr Manno, I was intrigued by the information you provided on the activation of silence oncogenes and the insertion induced mutagenesis using retroviral vectors. What, to your opinion would be the best alternative in terms of the vector to be used if you want to induce through manipulation a healthy gene function? What would be the vector of choice?

C.S. Manno: So the vector that provides for long term expression. Using that, does require integration, but without integration in the region of an oncogene. So if you have a gene, a vector that would integrate at some site that was specific, repeatedly, and that site would be guarantee to be away from an area that would induce oncogenesis. Obviously that would be preferable.

C.Th. Smit Sibinga: Could you think of any of the existing practice that might give us that advantage?

C.S. Manno: Retroviruses really felt to be that sort of vector. The lentiviruses have long-term expression. And then some of their herpes viruses also have that advantage, but their herpes viruses are difficult to engineer. They take quite a bit more processing then adenoviruses, retrovirus. But they do result in long term expression. AAV is a very nice virus, but its coding sequence is very small, so most genes that you want to fit into the coding sequences, don't fit into the AAV. You have to truncate the coding sequences.

EPILOGUE

These symposium, organized by Prof. Dr. Cees Smit Sibinga and ongoing since 1976, have always been ahead of their time: addressing apheresis in 1976, cytokines in the 80's, molecular testing in the early 90's and cell-based therapies in the late 90's. They have stimulated young investigators to pursue laboratory efforts, trained health care professionals from around the world and provided the opportunity during tea/coffee breaks and at social functions to engage in discussions that have resulted in long term international collaborations.

While neonatology has not been the primary topic at any of the earlier symposia, neonates have not been excluded. Topics of direct relevance have included transfusion safety, immunohaematological topics and of course, hereditary bleeding and clotting disorders.

It is in many ways fitting that the last of these symposia should end with neonatal blood transfusion. The most fragile, least well studied and most at risk population requires special care and concern. We need to expand our knowledge of their unique physiology, biochemical pathways and in planning treatment and interventions, always "do no harm." In the course of this last symposium, there have been presentations on developmental immunology, the molecular basis of haematopoeisis, physiological basis of bleeding and thrombosis, transfusion risks and benefits and lastly, future therapies. Infants provide us with much to learn but in turn they will be the providers of (through cord blood) and the recipients of (through cellular engineering) the best that science can offer. Translational research, which has been the thrust of these presentations for 28 years, will benefit them in a way that no scientist could have ever predicted.

We thank Prof. Smit Sibinga for his dedication to the science of transfusion medicine, to his ability to recognize critical topics before their time and to ensure focused symposia that have benefited our field for close to three decades.

Dr. Noami Luban
Washington DC, USA

INDEX

www.ingramcontent.com/pod-product-compliance
Lightning Source LLC
Chambersburg PA
CBHW080200230226
40107CB00025B/617
* 9 7 8 0 3 8 7 2 3 5 9 9 8 *